·

Cellular Oscillatory Mechanisms

ADVANCES IN EXPERIMENTAL MEDICINE AND BIOLOGY

A Continuation Order Plan is available for this series. A continuation order will bring delivery of each new volume immediately upon publication. Volumes are billed only upon actual shipment. For further information please contact the publisher.

Cellular Oscillatory Mechanisms

Edited by
Miguel Maroto
College of Life Sciences, University of Dundee, Dundee, Scotland, UK

Nicholas A.M. Monk
School of Mathematical Sciences, University of Nottingham, Nottingham, UK

Springer Science+Business Media, LLC
Landes Bioscience / Eurekah

Springer Science+Business Media, LLC
Landes Bioscience

Printed in the USA.

Springer Science+Business Media, LLC, 233 Spring Street, New York, New York 10013, USA
http://www.springer.com

Please address all inquiries to the Publishers:
Landes Bioscience, 1002 West Avenue, Austin, Texas 78701, USA
Phone: 512/ 637 6050; FAX: 512/ 637 6079
http://www.landesbioscience.com

Cellular Oscillatory Mechanisms edited by Miguel Maroto and Nicholas A.M. Monk, Landes Bioscience /
Springer Science+Business Media, LLC dual imprint / Springer series: Advances in Experimental Medicine
and Biology

ISBN: 978-0-387-09793-0

Library of Congress Cataloging-in-Publication Data

Cellular oscillatory mechanisms / edited by Miguel Maroto, Nicholas A.M. Monk.
    p. ; cm. -- (Advances in experimental medicine and biology ; v. 641)
  Includes bibliographical references and index.
  ISBN 978-0-387-09793-0
 1. Circadian rhythms. 2. Cellular signal transduction. 3. Biological rhythms. I.
Maroto, Miguel. II. Monk, Nicholas A.M. III. Series.
  [DNLM: 1. Circadian Rhythm. 2. Oscillometry. 3. Biological Clocks. 4. Models,
Biological. 5. Signal Transduction. W1 AD559 v.641 2008 / QT 167 C393 2008]
  QP84.6.C38 2008
  612'.022--dc22
                        2008025234

PREFACE

Living systems are fundamentally dynamic and adaptive, relying on a constant throughput of energy. They are also, by definition, self-sustaining over the full range of length and time scales (from sub-cellular structures to species considered as a whole). This characteristic combination of constant adaptive flux and emergent persistence requires that the properties of all living systems must, at some level, be cyclical. Consequently, oscillatory dynamics, in which system properties rise and fall in a regular rhythmic fashion, are a central feature of a wide range of biological processes. The scale of biological oscillations covers enormous ranges, from the sub-cellular to the population level, and from milliseconds to years.

While the existence of a number of biological oscillations—such as the regular beating of the human heart or the life-cycle of a unicellular organism—is widely appreciated, there are many oscillatory phenomena that are much less obvious, albeit no less important. Since oscillations reflect periodic quantitative changes in system properties, their detection and characterisation relies on the quantitative measurement of a system over an extended period. Until recently, such measurements were difficult to obtain at cellular or sub-cellular resolution, and relatively few cellular oscillations had been described. However, recent methodological advances have revealed that oscillatory phenomena are as widespread in cells as they are at larger scales.

The chapters in this book provide an introduction to a range of both well known and less familiar cellular oscillations and serve to illustrate the striking richness of cellular dynamics. The contributions focus particularly on elucidating the basic mechanisms that underlie these oscillations. The essentially quantitative nature of oscillations has long made them an attractive area of study for theoretical biologists (see, for example, refs. 1-3), and the application of complementary modelling and experimental approaches can yield insights into oscillatory dynamics that go beyond those that can be obtained by either in isolation. The benefits of this synergy are reflected in the contributions appearing in this book.

That oscillations play central roles in phenomena at all levels of cellular organisation is illustrated by the range of examples detailed in this book. Chapters by Lloyd and by Aon and colleagues describe coherent oscillations in cellular metabolism, a process clearly common to all living cells. Similarly, the cell cycle, discussed by Csikász-Nagy and colleagues, is a fundamentally cyclical process common to all cells. Rougemont and Naef describe models for circadian rhythms, which are critical in allowing organisms to entrain their cellular activities to imposed daily changes in their environment. The chapters by Lahav and by Momiji and Monk focus on recently-discovered oscillations in cellular response systems, in which the combined requirements of sensitive response and signal termination result in unexpected oscillatory instabilities. Oscillations contribute not only to temporal organisation within cells, but can also direct spatio-temporal organisation in multicellular tissues. Thul and colleagues review the central role played by oscillatory changes in calcium concentration in processes spanning these scales. A striking and well known example of oscillatory patterning at the multi-cellular level is the aggregation of developing cells of the slime mold *Dictyostelium discoideum*. Loomis discusses the critical role played by oscillatory cAMP signalling in this phenomenon. More recently discovered illustrations of the role of oscillations in spatial patterning are provided by the chapters of Lutkenhaus and of Palmeirim and colleagues. Lutkenhaus describes the way in which many bacteria localise their cell division plane through oscillations of Min proteins. Palmeirim and colleagues review oscillatory mechanisms underlying the segmentation of vertebrate embryos.

The current resurgence in interest in interdisciplinary approaches to cell and molecular biology (often referred to as systems biology) stems in part from the increasing availability of system-wide data on the state of the components of cellular regulatory networks. A limiting factor in these approaches is often the lack of suitable ways of characterising a network state in terms of summary quantitative features. Without such features, it is typically difficult to gain new qualitative insight into the operating logic of all but the simplest networks. In this regard, oscillatory phenomena provide ideal exemplars for systems approaches, since oscillations have clear summary features (such as period, amplitude and phase) that prove invaluable in combining mathematical models with experimental data.

Miguel Maroto, PhD
Nicholas A.M. Monk, PhD

1. Goodwin, B. C. Temporal Organization in Cells: A Dynamic Theory of Cellular Control Processes. New York: Academic Press, 1963.
2. Winfree, A. T. The Geometry of Biological Time. New York: Springer, 1980.
3. Goldbeter, A. Biochemical Oscillations and Cellular Rhythms. Cambridge: Cambridge University Press, 1996.

ABOUT THE EDITORS...

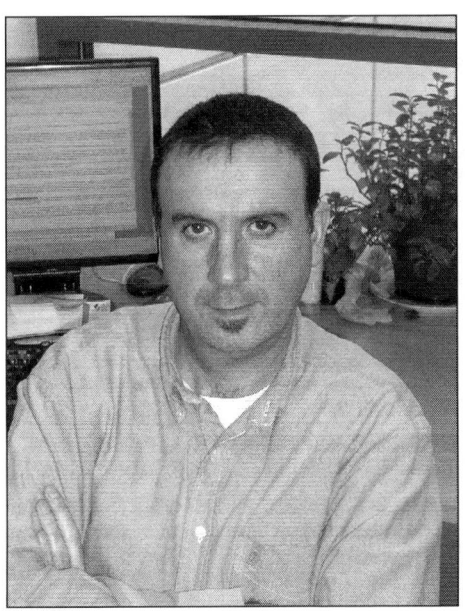

MIGUEL MAROTO, PhD, is a MRC Career Development Fellow and Lecturer at the University of Dundee, UK. He received his PhD in Biochemistry and Molecular Biology from the Department of Biochemistry of the Universidad Autonoma of Madrid, Spain. His research interests include investigating the biochemical basis of different signalling mechanisms implicated in the acquisition of specific cell fates during vertebrate development. More recently, he has been involved in the analysis of the mechanism of the molecular clock involved in the control of the process of somitogenesis.

ABOUT THE EDITORS...

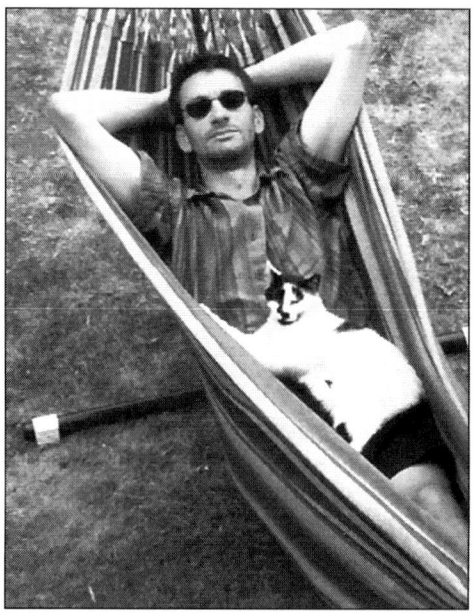

NICHOLAS A.M. MONK, PhD, is an Associate Professor and Reader in Applied Mathematics at the University of Nottingham, UK. Having received his PhD in theoretical physics from the University of London, his research changed focus to centre on the mathematical and computational modelling of biological systems. Particular areas of interest include pattern formation, developmental biology, complex network dynamics and mechanisms of intercellular signalling.

PARTICIPANTS

Miguel A. Aon
Division of Cardiology
Institute of Molecular Cardiobiology
The Johns Hopkins University
Baltimore, Maryland
USA

Tomas C. Bellamy
Laboratory of Molecular Signalling
The Babraham Institute
Babraham, Cambridge
UK

Martin D. Bootman
Laboratory of Molecular Signalling
The Babraham Institute
Babraham, Cambridge
UK

Stephen Coombes
School of Mathematical Sciences
University of Nottingham
Nottingham
UK

Sonia Cortassa
Division of Cardiology
Institute of Molecular Cardiobiology
The Johns Hopkins University
Baltimore, Maryland
USA

Attila Csikász-Nagy
Materials Structure and Modeling
  Research Group of the Hungarian
  Academy of Sciences
and
Department of Agricultural
  and Chemical Technology
Budapest University of Technology
  and Economics
Budapest
Hungary

J. Kim Dale
College of Life Sciences
University of Dundee
Dundee, Scotland
UK

Galit Lahav
Department of Systems Biology
Harvard Medical School
Boston, Massachusetts
USA

David Lloyd
Microbiology (BIOSI 1)
Cardiff School of Biosciences
Cardiff University
Cardiff, Wales
UK

William F. Loomis
Cell and Developmental Biology
University of California-San Diego
La Jolla, California
USA

Joe Lutkenhaus
Department of Microbiology, Molecular
  Genetics and Immunology
University of Kansas Medical Center
Kansas City, Kansas
USA

Miguel Maroto
College of Life Sciences
University of Dundee
Dundee, Scotland
UK

Hiroshi Momiji
Department of Computer Science
University of Sheffield
Sheffield
UK

Nicholas A.M. Monk
School of Mathematical Sciences
University of Nottingham
Nottingham
UK

Felix Naef
Swiss Institute of Experimental Cancer
  Research
Ecole Polytechnique Fédérale
  de Lausanne
Lausanne
Switzerland

Béla Novák
Department of Biochemistry
Oxford Centre for Integrative Systems
  Biology
University of Oxford
Oxford
UK

Brian O'Rourke
Division of Cardiology
Institute of Molecular Cardiobiology
The Johns Hopkins University
Baltimore, Maryland
USA

Isabel Palmeirim
Life and Health Sciences Research
  Institute
School of Health Sciences
University of Minho
Braga
Portugal

H. Llewelyn Roderick
Laboratory of Molecular Signalling
The Babraham Institute
Babraham
and
Department of Pharmacology
University of Cambridge
Cambridge
UK

Sofia Rodrigues
Life and Health Sciences Research
  Institute
School of Health Sciences
University of Minho
Braga
Portugal

Jacques Rougemont
Swiss Institute of Bioinformatics
Lausanne
Switzerland

Ruediger Thul
School of Mathematical Sciences
University of Nottingham
Nottingham
UK

John J. Tyson
Department of Biological Sciences
Virginia Polytechnic Institute
  and State University
Blacksburg, Virginia
USA

CONTENTS

8. MITOCHONDRIAL OSCILLATIONS IN PHYSIOLOGY AND PATHOPHYSIOLOGY 98

Miguel A. Aon, Sonia Cortassa and Brian O'Rourke

9. RESPIRATORY OSCILLATIONS IN YEASTS 118

David Lloyd

10. STOCHASTIC PHASE OSCILLATOR MODELS FOR CIRCADIAN CLOCKS 141

Jacques Rougemont and Felix Naef

## CHAPTER 1

Calcium Oscillations

Ruediger Thul, Tomas C. Bellamy, H. Llewelyn Roderick, Martin D. Bootman* and Stephen Coombes

Abstract

Changes in cellular Ca^{2+} concentration control a wide range of physiological processes, from the subsecond release of synaptic neurotransmitters, to the regulation of gene expression over months or years. Ca^{2+} can also trigger cell death through both apoptosis and necrosis, and so the regulation of cellular Ca^{2+} concentration must be tightly controlled through the concerted action of pumps, channels and buffers that transport Ca^{2+} into and out of the cell cytoplasm. A hallmark of cellular Ca^{2+} signalling is its spatiotemporal complexity: stimulation of cells by a hormone or neurotransmitter leads to oscillations in cytoplasmic Ca^{2+} concentration that can vary markedly in time course, amplitude, frequency, and spatial range.

In this chapter we review some of the biological roles of Ca^{2+}, the experimental characterisation of complex dynamic changes in Ca^{2+} concentration, and attempts to explain this complexity using computational models. We consider the 'toolkit' of cellular proteins which influence Ca^{2+} concentration, describe mechanistic models of key elements of the toolkit, and fit these into the framework of whole cell models of Ca^{2+} oscillations and waves. Finally, we will touch on recent efforts to use stochastic modelling to elucidate elementary Ca^{2+} signal events, and how these may evolve into global signals.

Introduction

Biological cells use calcium (Ca^{2+}) to control many of their activities.[1] Cells draw on both intracellular and extracellular Ca^{2+} sources to generate signals that transduce exogenous stimulation into physiological output.[2] It is well known that prolonged elevations of Ca^{2+} lead to cell damage or death, so cells generally limit the temporal and spatial extent of their intracellular Ca^{2+} rises. Over the past thirty years, Ca^{2+} oscillations have emerged as a ubiquitous paradigm for cellular signal transduction.[3-5] It is generally believed that by utilising brief pulses of Ca^{2+}, instead of tonic rises, cells avoid the deleterious effects of sustained cytosolic Ca^{2+} levels. Furthermore, cells also benefit from the greater fidelity inherent in frequency-modulated, as compared to amplitude-modulated, signaling.[6] A simple Medline search for 'calcium oscillations' highlights over 3260 articles since 1980.

Ca^{2+} oscillations are now routinely recorded using fluorescent probes, but were previously characterised using techniques such as bioluminescence and measurement of membrane potential fluctuations.[7,8] Indeed, it was the latter technique that provided some of the first indications that Ca^{2+} oscillations could provide specificity and longevity in cellular signalling, whereas

*Corresponding Author: Martin D. Bootman—Laboratory of Molecular Signalling, The Babraham Institute, Babraham, Cambridge, CB22 3AT, UK. Email: martin.bootman@bbsrc.ac.uk

Cellular Oscillatory Mechanisms, edited by Miguel Maroto and Nicholas A.M. Monk. ©2008 Landes Bioscience and Springer Science+Business Media.

sustained Ca^{2+} signals caused desensitization.[9] The influx of Ca^{2+} from the extracellular space[10,11] and release of Ca^{2+} from intracellular stores can both give rise to pulsatile cytosolic Ca^{2+} signals.

Ca^{2+} oscillations are initiated at the moment of fertilisation in vertebrates,[12-14] and continue through life to regulate numerous physiological processes including cell maturation and differentiation,[15] cell cycle progression,[16] mitochondrial respiration,[17] chemotaxis,[18] secretion[19] and gene transcription.[20] They occur in vertebrates,[4] plants[21,22] and invertebrates.[23] Ca^{2+} oscillations have been recorded from a vast number of different cell types. It is evident that the pattern of Ca^{2+} oscillation varies substantially between cell types,[24] and even between cells of the same type,[25] due to the expression of cell-specific Ca^{2+} signalling proteomes.[1] Thus, cells can express different combinations and concentrations of the various Ca^{2+} pumps, buffers and channels that comprise a 'toolkit' of Ca^{2+} regulatory proteins. Ca^{2+} oscillation patterns can be roughly segregated into Ca^{2+} transients with a random occurrence, those having a sinusoidal appearance[26] and periodic Ca^{2+} oscillations arising from a steady baseline cytosolic Ca^{2+} concentration.[27,28] Of these different types, the baseline Ca^{2+} oscillations have been the most widely studied, and are largely the focus of this chapter.

Baseline Ca^{2+} oscillations are thought to arise due to periodic release of Ca^{2+} from intracellular stores via intracellular Ca^{2+} channels. Although a number of novel Ca^{2+}-releasing messengers and pathways have been identified recently,[2] the generation of baseline Ca^{2+} oscillations is generally considered to be due activation of two types of intracellular Ca^{2+} channel: inositol 1,4,5-trisphosphate (IP_3) receptors and ryanodine receptors. IP_3 receptors (IP_3Rs) are large (<1200 kDa) tetrameric proteins, with an amino-terminal domain projecting into the cytoplasm, and an integral Ca^{2+} channel formed by six membrane-spanning regions in the carboxy-terminal portion of each subunit.[29] IP_3 binding within residues 226-576 of the amino terminus causes a conformational change that promotes channel opening.[30] Between the IP_3 binding site and the transmembrane regions is a large stretch of amino acids where a significant proportion of regulatory interactions occur. IP_3Rs are expressed and participate in Ca^{2+} release within almost all mammalian tissue, although their function in some cell types is unclear. Three IP_3R isoforms have been cloned and splice variants have been described, leading to the possibility of heteromultimeric channels with distinctive properties based on their subunit content. Although IP_3 is necessary for channel opening, the activation of IP_3Rs is complex and their open probability is dependent on the ambient Ca^{2+} concentration. Up to approximately 500 nM, Ca^{2+} works synergistically with IP_3 to activate IP_3Rs. At higher concentrations, cytosolic Ca^{2+} inhibits IP_3R opening.[31-34]

Ryanodine receptors are structurally and functionally homologous to IP_3 receptors, albeit that they have approximately twice their mass.[35] There are three cloned forms of the ryanodine receptor. Similar to IP_3Rs, ryanodine receptor opening displays a 'bell-shaped' dependence on cytosolic Ca^{2+} concentration, although they are generally activated and inhibited by slightly higher Ca^{2+} levels.[32] Both IP_3Rs and ryanodine receptors can therefore operate as Ca^{2+}-activated Ca^{2+} release (CICR) channels; a property that is believed to lead to the autocatalytic release of Ca^{2+} during the upstroke of a Ca^{2+} oscillation.[36-38] The inhibition of IP_3R and ryanodine receptor opening by high levels of cytosolic Ca^{2+} provides a negative feedback mechanism that will terminate Ca^{2+} release, and prevent deleterious Ca^{2+} elevations.[39] It is possible that IP_3Rs may also undergo a long-term desensitisation process that can also cause Ca^{2+} release to cease.[40]

IP_3Rs are almost ubiquitously expressed within mammals, whereas ryanodine receptors have a more limited tissue distribution.[41,42] Furthermore, whilst there appears to be considerable functional redundancy between the three IP_3R isoforms, the different types of ryanodine receptor have distinct expression patterns and gating mechanisms. Type 2 ryanodine receptors, for example, are substantially expressed in the heart, where they operate as CICR channels to generate the Ca^{2+} signal that triggers cardiac contraction during each heartbeat.[43] In contrast, type 1 ryanodine receptors are largely expressed in skeletal muscle. They also provide the Ca^{2+} signal necessary to trigger muscle contraction. However, although isolated type 1 ryanodine receptors can work as CICR channels, within the intact muscle they are actually activated through direct protein-protein interactions.[44]

The effect of Ca^{2+} on IP_3Rs and ryanodine receptors illustrates the complex regulation of these channels. However, although their modulation by Ca^{2+} is important, significant control of these channels is manifest by covalent modification and numerous allosteric interactions. In particular, their interaction with accessory proteins is uncovering new regulatory mechanisms and shedding light on novel aspects of biology in which these Ca^{2+} channels are involved.[45,46] It is emerging that IP_3Rs and ryanodine receptors simultaneously bind a multitude of accessory proteins that impact their cellular location and functionality. Some of these proteins, e.g., Bcl-2, are regulators of critical cellular events. Others are enzymes, e.g., protein kinase A, which regulate the phosphorylation status of the channels and also convey information distinct from increases in Ca^{2+}. It therefore appears that IP_3Rs and ryanodine receptors are focal points for the convergence of multiple signal transduction pathways. They can modulate cellular activities through Ca^{2+} release, but in addition they may act as a signalling nexus to bring proteins into close proximity. Both IP_3Rs and ryanodine receptors have been shown to underlie Ca^{2+} oscillations in various cell types. In some cells, either IP_3Rs or ryanodine receptors are active,[47] although there are numerous examples of both channel types working synergistically to generate Ca^{2+} oscillations.[48]

Baseline Ca^{2+} oscillations typically have a rapid upstroke from the resting Ca^{2+} concentration, and the peak cytosolic Ca^{2+} signal is generally attained within a few seconds.[49] The recovery of the Ca^{2+} signal is generally slower, and requires the Ca^{2+} to be pumped either into mitochondria, out of the cell or resequestered into the intracellular stores. The spatial correlate of a Ca^{2+} oscillation is a Ca^{2+} wave (or 'tide').[50] Due to the autocatalytic activity of IP_3Rs and ryanodine receptors, subcellular Ca^{2+} events can trigger propagating Ca^{2+} signals that can passage throughout a cell.[51] The extent of Ca^{2+} wave propagation depends on the degree of cellular stimulation,[50,52] i.e., the degree of excitability of the intracellular Ca^{2+} release channels. Ca^{2+} waves can also diffuse through gap junctions to initiate Ca^{2+} signals in neighbouring cells.[53] In this way, confluent cell layers can display synchronised Ca^{2+} signals.[54-57]

A notable characteristic of Ca^{2+} oscillations is that even within a single cell their amplitude and kinetic parameters can depend on the nature of the stimulus and its concentration.[27] For example, pancreatic acinar cells secrete digestive enzymes into the small intestine in response to cholecystokinin or acetylcholine. The secretion of enzyme-containing zymogen granules is triggered by the Ca^{2+} oscillations that occur when cholecystokinin or acetylcholine are applied. Within the same pancreatic acinar cell, cholecystokinin and acetylcholine generate Ca^{2+} oscillations with an initial sharp rising phase. However, when stimulated with cholecystokinin, the Ca^{2+} oscillations tend to show a secondary, longer-lasting, component.[58]

One of the most widely studied features of Ca^{2+} oscillations is the dependence of their frequency on the strength of external stimulation.[27,59] This concept generally applies to baseline Ca^{2+} spiking. Since, in cells that display either sinusoidal Ca^{2+} oscillations or random Ca^{2+} fluctuations the frequency of the Ca^{2+} elevations can be insensitive to stimulus strength.[26] Sinusoidal Ca^{2+} oscillations have been suggested to occur due to negative feedback regulation of either IP_3 production or IP_3R activity.[60] By controlling oscillation frequency, cells can precisely regulate their Ca^{2+}-dependent activities in a way that is graded with the level of stimulus. Cells possess a substantial number of proteins that can bind Ca^{2+}, either directly or through an intermediary such as calmodulin, and are either activated or inhibited when Ca^{2+} is bound. By 'counting' individual Ca^{2+} oscillations over time, cellular processes can be switched on or off.[61] A well-known example of an enzyme that has the ability to decode the frequency of Ca^{2+} spikes and subsequently modulate a variety of cellular activities is Ca^{2+}/ calmodulin-dependent kinase.[62]

Modelling Ca^{2+} Dynamics

The striking spatiotemporal complexity of cytoplasmic Ca^{2+} signals, as outlined in the previous section, arises from the interplay of numerous cellular sources and sinks of free Ca^{2+}; a situation that lends itself naturally to computational analysis. The approach for the majority of models to date has been to treat the cell as discrete compartments (representing the cytoplasm and intracellular organelles) that act as well-mixed reactors, isolated from a limitless extracellular space. Fluxes of Ca^{2+} occur between these compartments under the control of the various channels, transporters and buffers of the Ca^{2+} toolkit, combined with a finite leak across the membranes delimiting the compartments. Within this context, early attempts to simulate Ca^{2+} dynamics used simple empirical equations to describe the elements of the toolkit. The steady-state assumption was adopted, so that the activity of channels and pumps simply tracked IP_3 and Ca^{2+} concentration. Similarly, leak currents and buffering capacity were assumed to be linear or constant.

One of the earliest attempts to model Ca^{2+} oscillations in this way came from Meyer and Stryer.[63] These authors recognised that two of the key features of the system would be cooperative activation of Ca^{2+} release by IP_3, and positive feedback of Ca^{2+} at some stage in the pathway. The authors hypothesised that this positive feedback would arise from Ca^{2+} activating PLC, leading to enhanced IP_3 production. The model successfully generated Ca^{2+} oscillations, but also predicted that IP_3 concentration would oscillate in addition to Ca^{2+}. This behaviour was shown to be unnecessary in several experimental systems,[4] and the model lost favour. A more persistently influential model was that of Goldbeter, Dupont and Berridge,[64] which is based on the existence of two intracellular Ca^{2+} pools, one of which is sensitive to IP_3 and the other not. Consequently, receptor activation leads to release of Ca^{2+} from the Ca^{2+} sensitive pool, which triggers Ca^{2+} induced Ca^{2+} release from the IP_3-insensitive pool (supplying positive feedback). With associated pump and leak currents, this minimal model successfully generated Ca^{2+} oscillations with features similar to those observed experimentally, arising from cycles of the pool emptying into, and refilling from, the cytosol. The Goldbeter-Dupont-Berridge model therefore incorporated two variables, the Ca^{2+} concentrations in the cytosol (Z) and the IP_3-insensitive pool (Y), which varied with time:

$$\dot{Z} = v_0 + v_1\beta - v_2 + v_3 + k_f Y - kZ, \tag{1a}$$

$$\dot{Y} = v_2 - v_3 - k_f V. \tag{1b}$$

The dot indicates a derivative with respect to time, i.e., $\dot{Z} = dZ/dt$. Here v_0 is leak across plasma membrane, v_1 is efflux from IP_3-sensitive stores (multiplied by the scaling constant β, which increases with PLC activation), v_2 is uptake into the IP_3-insensitive store, v_3 is efflux from the IP_3-sensitive store, k_f is leak from the IP_3-insensitive store, and k is efflux across the plasma membrane. The channels and pumps of the IP_3-insensitive store were described by empirical equations of the Hill form, such that:

$$v_2 = V_{M_2} \frac{Z^n}{K_2^n + Z^n}, \qquad v_3 = V_{M_3} \frac{Y^m}{K_R^m + Y^m} \frac{Z^p}{K_A^p + Z^p}, \tag{2}$$

where V_{M_i} are maximal rates of Ca^{2+} transport, K_R and K_A are threshold constants, and the coefficients n, m and p determine the cooperativity of the transporter/channel. A later refinement of this model[65] reduced the system to a single Ca^{2+} pool, as experimental results did not support the segregation of pools in many cell types.

These simple models were very successful in reproducing much of the non-linear behaviour of IP_3-induced Ca^{2+} signalling, which demonstrated that the complexity of cellular signalling could arise from simple principles of cooperativity and feedback regulation. Nevertheless, discrepancies with experimental evidence remained, in particular, the requirement for stores to empty during an oscillatory cycle.[66] This approach remains in common use, but as experimental data accumulated on the biophysical properties of the components of the toolkit, more detailed models incorporating this extra complexity, were introduced.

Mechanistic Models

In the early 1990s, several groups[31-33,67] published experimental evidence that the IP$_3$ receptor is regulated by Ca^{2+} in a biphasic manner: low concentrations of Ca^{2+} rapidly activate the receptor, whilst high concentrations inactivate the receptor more slowly. The functional consequence of this activity is positive feedback of Ca^{2+} release following the initial IP$_3$ signal, followed by negative feedback after cytosolic Ca^{2+} concentration has reached hundreds of nanomolar. This behaviour is sufficient to generate Ca^{2+} oscillations, and so the IP$_3$ receptor became a focus in efforts to model cellular Ca^{2+} dynamics. It also prompted a switch in approach from the use of empirical models that described the steady-state behaviour of the receptor, to the adoption of mechanistically realistic models that postulate the existence of multiple states of the receptor, with transitions between states determined by microscopic rate constants. Such an approach has distinct advantages; principally that these models can describe both the mass action kinetics of an ensemble of receptors, and the stochastic behaviour of individual molecules. Such a strategy has been highly successful in elucidating the relationships between structure and function in plasma membrane ion channels.[68]

In the following sub-sections, we summarise a number of mechanistic models that have been proposed for key elements of the Ca^{2+} signalling toolkit.

The IP$_3$ Receptor

An early and influential model was that of De Young and Keizer.[69] We will take this as our archetype for consideration of IP$_3$R models to date, and adopt its nomenclature for later models, wherever possible.

De Young and Keizer argue that a receptor consists of three binding sites: an activating and an inhibitory Ca^{2+} binding site as well as an activating IP$_3$ binding site. Therefore, the state of a receptor can be specified by a binary triplet $ijk \in [0,1]^3$. The first index represents the IP$_3$ binding site, the second the Ca^{2+} activating binding site, and the last the Ca^{2+} inhibiting binding site. An index equals 1 when a site is occupied and 0 otherwise. Hence the state 110 refers to IP$_3$ and Ca^{2+} bound to the activating sites, respectively, and an empty inhibiting Ca^{2+} binding site. The resulting eight states are shown in Figure 1. The binding rate constants for IP$_3$ activation are given by a_1 and a_3, whereas a_2 and a_4 refer to Ca^{2+} inhibition. Ca^{2+} activation is controlled by a_5. The dissociation rates for the above processes are denoted by b_1 through b_5.

The reactions that occur at a receptor are binding and unbinding of Ca^{2+} and IP$_3$. They determine the state of one receptor. In an ensemble of receptors these processes lead to a fraction

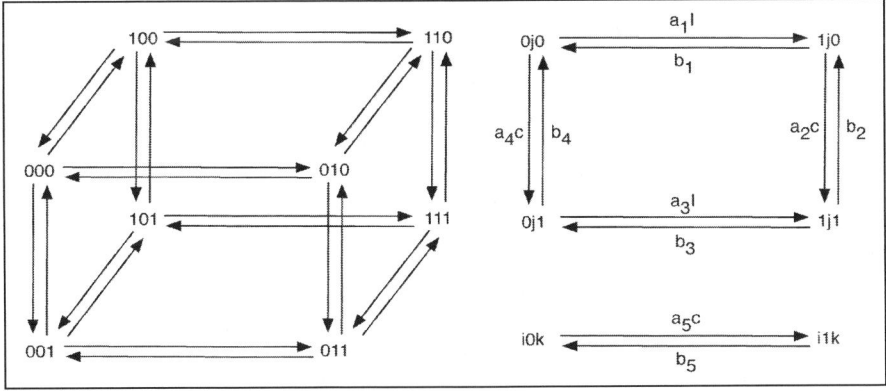

Figure 1. Transition scheme of the De Young–Keizer model. See Table 1 for parameter values.

p_{ijk} of receptors in a state *ijk*. If the ensemble is large enough and homogeneous, these fractions can be described by rate equations. For instance, the time evolution of p_{110} is governed by

$$\dot{p}_{110} = -[b_5 + a_2c + b_1]\,p_{110} + a_5cp_{100} + b_2p_{111} + a_1Ip_{010}, \tag{3}$$

with *I* being the IP$_3$ concentration and *c* the cytosolic Ca^{2+} concentration. The negative term on the right hand side represents the processes that reduce the value of p_{110}. This can result from unbinding of IP$_3$ with rate b_1, unbinding from the activating Ca^{2+} site with rate b_5 and binding to the inhibiting Ca^{2+} binding site with rate a_2c. The remaining three terms control the increase of p_{110}. This happens for example through binding with rate a_5c to the activating Ca^{2+} site of a receptor that is in the state 100. Together with the remaining seven rate equations the state of the ensemble is fully characterised. We may discard one of these equations and use instead the conservation law

$$\sum_{\{ijk\}\in[0,1]^3} p_{ijk} = 1. \tag{4}$$

This states that each receptor belongs to one of the fractions p_{ijk} and that the number of receptors is conserved. In general the Ca^{2+} concentration is not constant in time, so that a closed solution for the fractions p_{ijk} is not accessible. However, we can compute the stationary values, $\bar{p}_{ijk}$, analytically. They read

$$\bar{p}_{000} = d_1d_2d_5\gamma_1, \qquad \bar{p}_{100} = d_2d_5I\gamma_1, \tag{5a}$$

$$\bar{p}_{010} = d_1d_2\bar{c}\gamma_1, \qquad \bar{p}_{001} = d_3d_5\bar{c}\gamma_1, \tag{5b}$$

$$\bar{p}_{011} = d_3\bar{c}^2\gamma_1, \qquad \bar{p}_{101} = d_5\bar{c}I\gamma_1, \tag{5c}$$

$$\bar{p}_{110} = d_2\bar{c}I\gamma_1, \qquad \bar{p}_{111} = \bar{c}^2I\gamma_1, \tag{5d}$$

with $\gamma_1^{-1} = (\bar{c}d_3 + \bar{c} + d_5)(d_1d_2 + \bar{c}I + d_2I)$. Here $d_i = b_i/a_i$ denotes the dissociation constants for IP$_3$ activation, Ca^{2+} activation and inhibition, respectively.

Table 1 shows the binding rate constants a_i and the dissociation constants d_i that De Young and Keizer used in their original work. Note that only 4 of the 5 dissociation constants are independent due to the thermodynamic constraint of detailed balance, i.e., $d_1d_2 = d_3d_4$.[70] The constants in Table 1 were obtained by fitting steady state data by Bezprozvanny et al.[32] This has lead to some criticism during the last years, because an IP$_3$ receptor almost never reaches a steady state under physiological conditions. The kinetic response to a change in the Ca^{2+} and IP$_3$ concentration seems to be more relevant for its role in intracellular Ca^{2+} dynamics. This idea was taken up by Sneyd et al,[71] suggesting a new set of parameter values based on superfusion experiments.[72]

The IP$_3$ receptor is an integral part of the IP$_3$ receptor channel, through which Ca^{2+} is released from the endoplasmic reticulum. Biochemical experiments and electron microscopy revealed that the IP$_3$ receptor channel consists of 4 subunits and that it is conducting when at

---

Table 1. Binding rate constants a$_i$ and dissociation constants d$_i$, i = 1,...,5 of the De Young–Keizer model [34]

$a_1 = 400\ (\mu Ms)^{-1}$	$d_1 = 0.13\ \mu M$
$a_2 = 0.2\ (\mu Ms)^{-1}$	$d_2 = 1.049\ \mu M$
$a_3 = 400\ (\mu Ms)^{-1}$	$d_3 = 943.3\ \mu M$
$a_4 = 0.2\ (\mu Ms)^{-1}$	$d_4 = 144.5\ nM$
$a_5 = 20\ (\mu Ms)^{-1}$	$d_5 = 82.34\ nM$

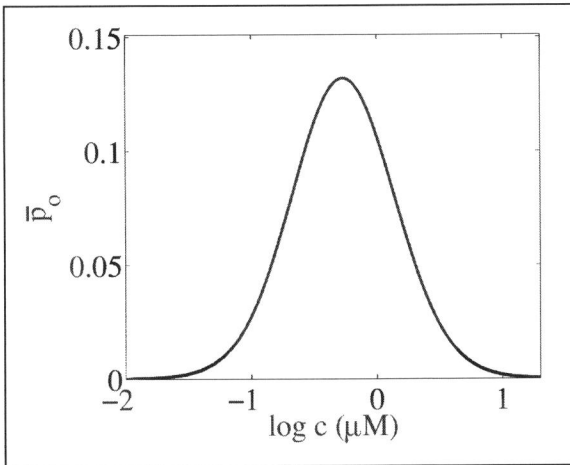

Figure 2. Stationary value of the open probability $\bar{p}_o$ of an IP$_3$ receptor channel. Parameter values as in Table 1 and $I = 0.4\ \mu M$.

least 3 of the 4 subunits are activated.[32,73,74] In the De Young-Keizer model, the configuration with IP$_3$ and Ca^{2+} bound to the activating binding sites, but with an unoccupied Ca^{2+} inhibiting binding site is the activated state of the receptor. Consequently, the open probability of an IP$_3$ receptor channel is given by

$$p_o = 4 p_{110}^3 - 3 p_{110}^4. \tag{6}$$

Figure 2 depicts the stationary value of the open probability as a function of the Ca^{2+} concentration using equation (5). At low Ca^{2+} concentrations, an increase in Ca^{2+} leads to a significant increase in the open probability. However, when the Ca^{2+} concentration becomes too high, a further increase reduces the open probability. Such a bell shaped dependence of the stationary open probability on Ca^{2+} is present in a wide range of Ca^{2+} models (see e.g., section *The Ryanodine Receptor*).

An alternative and simpler model to De Young-Keizer was proposed by Othmer and Tang,[75] in which the binding of IP$_3$ and Ca^{2+} to the channels occurred sequentially (Fig. 3). This model

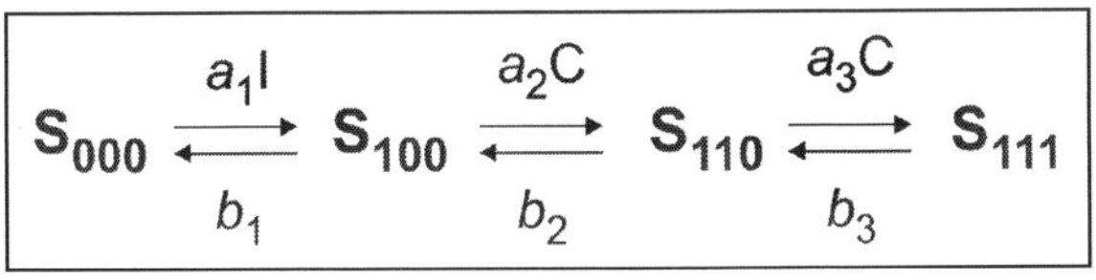

$$S_{000} \underset{b_1}{\overset{a_1 I}{\rightleftharpoons}} S_{100} \underset{b_2}{\overset{a_2 C}{\rightleftharpoons}} S_{110} \underset{b_3}{\overset{a_3 C}{\rightleftharpoons}} S_{111}$$

Figure 3. Transition scheme of the Othmer-Tang model. See Table 2 for parameter values.

Table 2. Binding rate constants a_i and unbinding rates b_i, $i = 1, 2, 3$ of the Othmer-Tang model

$a_1 = 12\ (\mu Ms)^{-1}$	$b_1 = 8\ s^{-1}$
$a_2 = 15\ (\mu Ms)^{-1}$	$b_2 = 1.65\ s^{-1}$
$a_3 = 0.8\ (\mu Ms)^{-1}$	$b_3 = 0.21\ s^{-1}$

consists of three coupled ordinary differential equations (ODEs), and was justified on the basis that experimental evidence suggested much faster binding of IP$_3$ and activating Ca^{2+} to the receptor than inactivating Ca^{2+}.[75]

Bezprozvanny[76] introduced a further step to a simple sequential model of this type: a conformational change that was essential to the activation process (Fig. 4). This additional step allows the efficacy of channel opening, and thereby the open probability, to be fixed at a defined maximum, whereas earlier models could in principle yield higher open probabilities than are observed experimentally.[32]

Despite the advantages of a mechanistic approach, the system of ODEs that describes models of this type cannot be solved analytically, and so computationally expensive numerical integrations must be carried out for non-equilibrium conditions. Accordingly, several attempts have been made to simplify the above models, based on the assumption of a quasi-steady state for those steps that are significantly faster than the rate limiting step.

The most commonly used simplification was introduced by Li and Rinzel.[77] They took advantage of the experimental findings that IP$_3$ and Ca^{2+} activation are much faster than Ca^{2+} inhibition. Consequently, they eliminated these two dynamics adiabatically, which resulted in a single equation for the fraction p_h of receptors that are not inactivated yet:

$$\dot{p}_h = -a_6 c p_h + b_6 (1 - p_h).\tag{7}$$

Here, the constants a_6 and b_6 are related to the parameters of the original De Young-Keizer model through $a_6 = a_2$ and $b_6 = b_2(I + d_1)/(I + d_3)$. With its single equation for an effective gating variable, the Li-Rinzel model represents the strongest approximation of the De Young-Keizer model. In some circumstances as e.g., the initiation stage of Ca^{2+} puffs, this might be too far a step, so that models with fewer eliminations were proposed, such as a 4-state model[78] or a 3-state model.[79]

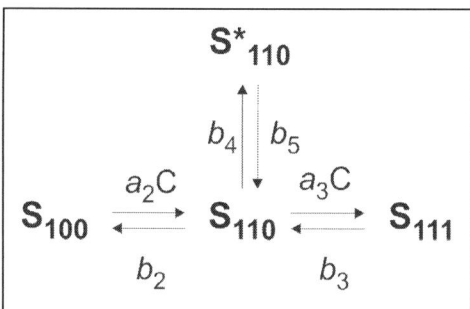

Figure 4. Transition scheme of the Bezprozvanny model when IP$_3$ is already bound. See Table 3 for parameter values.

Table 3. Binding rate constant a_3, unbinding rate b_3, and transition rates b_4 and b_5 of the Bezprozvanny model when IP$_3$ is bound. The transition rate constant a_2 remains as an open parameter, but it fixes the unbinding rate $b_2 = 0.2\mu M\ a_2$.

$a_3 = 4\ (\mu Ms)^{-1}$
$b_3 = 0.8\ s^{-1}$
$b_4 = 25.2\ (\mu Ms)^{-1}$
$b_5 = 224\ s^{-1}$

A comprehensive reduction of this type has been presented by Tang, Stephenson and Othmer.[75] These authors analysed the models discussed above and concluded that they can all be simplified to a single equation of a form that resembles that of a gating variable in the Hodgkin-Huxley formulation of action potential generation:[75]

$$\dot{y} = (y_\infty - y)/\tau , \tag{8}$$

where y is the fraction of receptors with Ca^{2+} bound to the inhibitory site. This simplification holds within certain ranges of parameters that result in quasi-steady states for binding interactions and conformational changes which are faster than receptor inactivation by Ca^{2+} binding. Strikingly, this simplified system can successfully model a range of the complex Ca^{2+} dynamics observed in cells.[75]

Valuable as this approach has been in elucidating the core behaviours underlying non-equilibrium behaviour in Ca^{2+} signalling, it fails to accommodate some of the functional properties of IP_3 receptors in an experimental setting. Two new models that have extended mechanistic models in the light of non-equilibrium experimental data obtained by rapid perfusion techniques[72,80] have been recently published.[81,82]

Sneyd and Dufour[81] have elaborated on the traditional mass action deterministic model by incorporating a rapidly equilibriating step at each transition of the receptor between states. By making the equilibration dependent on Ca^{2+} concentration, the result is a model system in which transitions exhibit Ca^{2+} dependency, but with saturable rather than simple mass action kinetics. They illustrate this principle with the Ca^{2+}-dependent transition of receptor from an active (A) to inactive (I) state, as shown in Figure 5. Here, the intermediates $\tilde{A}$ and $\bar{A}$ are in instantaneous equilibrium, such that $c\tilde{A} = L_1/l_1\bar{A}$, where $c = [Ca^{2+}]$. Therefore, as $A = \tilde{A} + \bar{A}$ the variation in the proportion of active receptors with time is described by:

$$p_A = (k_{-1} + L_2) p_I - \varphi(c)p_A, \tag{9}$$

with

$$\phi(c) = \frac{c\left(k_1 L_{-1}/l_1 + l_2\right)}{c + L_{-1}/l_1}. \tag{10}$$

In effect, by postulating the existence of rapidly interconverting intermediates at each step of receptor activation/inactivation, the resultant model has a function of Ca^{2+} ($\varphi(c)$) in place of the mass action constant of proportionality (k). This modification was introduced to accommodate the observation that the rate of receptor inactivation does not vary linearly with Ca^{2+} concentration (as would be predicted for a simple binding interaction), but its mechanistic basis is unclear.

A closer inspection of the scheme in Figure 5 reveals that upon cycling through the states $\bar{A}$, $\tilde{A}$, I and back to $\bar{A}$, a Ca^{2+} ion is picked up in the first transition and is not released before the

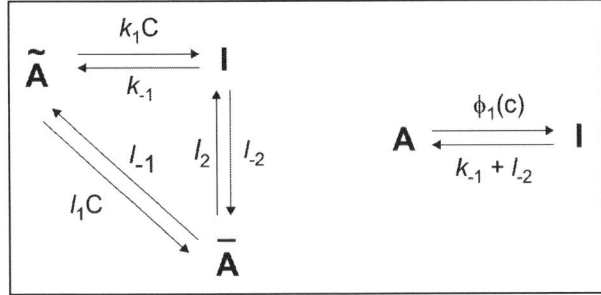

Figure 5. Transition scheme of the Sneyd-Dufour model.

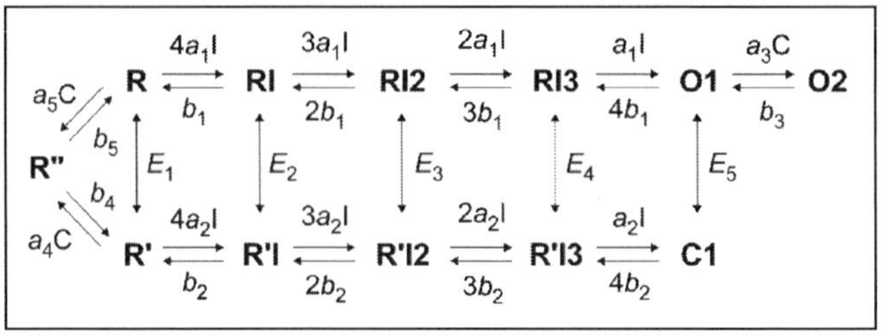

Figure 6. Transition scheme of the Dawson-Lea-Irvine model. See Table 4 for parameter values.

Table 4. Binding rate constants a_i, unbinding rates b_i and transition rates e_i and e_{-i}, $i = 1,...,5$ of the Dawson-Lea-Irvine model

$a_1 = 1000\ (\mu Ms)^{-1}$	$b_1 = 1000\ s^{-1}$	$e_1 = 1\ s^{-1}$	$e_{-1} = 100\ s^{-1}$
$a_2 = 100\ (\mu Ms)^{-1}$	$b_2 = 10\ s^{-1}$	$e_2 = 1\ s^{-1}$	$e_{-2} = 10\ s^{-1}$
$a_3 = 100\ (\mu Ms)^{-1}$	$b_3 = 10\ s^{-1}$	$e_3 = 1\ s^{-1}$	$e_{-3} = 1\ s^{-1}$
$a_4 = 10\ (\mu Ms)^{-1}$	$b_4 = 0.01\ s^{-1}$	$e_4 = 10\ s^{-1}$	$e_{-4} = 1\ s^{-1}$
$a_5 = 1\ (mMs)^{-1}$	$b_5 = 0.1\ s^{-1}$	$e_5 = 10\ s^{-1}$	$e_{-5} = 0.1\ s^{-1}$

return to Ã. This can be overcome be introducing an additional stateĨ as proposed by Falcke[83] and recently implemented by Ullah and Jung.[84]

Finally, Dawson, Lea and Irvine have introduced an 'adaptive' model for the IP$_3$R,[82] developed from a similar model for the ryanodine receptor.[85] The model postulates that the IP$_3$R exists in two gross conformational states (R and R'), in equilibrium, and that the conducting states of the channel can be reached only from one conformation (R). IP$_3$ binds to the R' state with slower kinetics, but higher affinity than the R state, and consequently, addition of IP$_3$ results in a transient opening of the channel before equilibration shifts the majority of receptors into the (closed) R' state. This scheme is summarised in Figure 6.

In the simulations (used by the authors in ref. 82), the rate constant for IP$_3$ binding to the R state (a_1) is ten times faster than the rate constant for binding to the R' state (a_2). Similarly, for the off rates, $b_1 = 100b_2$. The equilibrium constants for transition to the R' state (shown here as E_i for simplicity) increasingly favour the R' state as I increases (i.e., as more IP$_3$ molecules bind): $E_1 = e_1/e_{-1} = p_{R'}(\infty)/p_R(\infty) = 0.01$, whereas $E_5 = 100$. Therefore, if the rate at which equilibrium is reached is slower than the rate of binding to the R states, a step change in IP$_3$ concentration will result in a transient increase in the fraction of receptors reaching the open states (O1 and O2), followed by a slower progression to favour the C1 state as time passes.

The principal virtue of this model is the elegant mechanism by which quantal Ca^{2+} release is achieved. The IP$_3$R in this scenario opens in response to changes in IP$_3$ concentration, rather than giving a steady-state conductance at fixed IP$_3$ concentrations. This feature can also offer an explanation as to why unitary Ca^{2+} events are transient, and do not lead to uncontrolled positive feedback and global Ca^{2+} elevation. The authors took the model further, however, by incorporating the effect of a local domain of Ca^{2+} in the vicinity of the channel pore, by adding a second open state (O2), with higher open probability, which is reached by binding Ca^{2+}. Feedback of Ca^{2+} concentration in this way resulted in several effects: an increase in the cooperativity of IP$_3$ activation, dependence on luminal Ca^{2+} concentration (due to the pore microdomain), and a left shift in the IP$_3$ concentration response as receptor density increased. They also incorporated a Ca^{2+}-bound inactivated state (R''). These additional features can rationalise a large body of experimental work on quantal Ca^{2+} release, the existence of stores with different apparent IP$_3$ sensitivities, and the tendency for elementary Ca^{2+} events to occur in 'hotspots', simply by postulating variation in the density of adaptive IP₃Rs in different regions of the cell ER. A final, cautionary note, is that the fitting of an empirical (Hill) equation to ensemble IP₃ concentration-response curves does not, necessarily, give any information about the underlying biophysics of individual receptors, as Hill coefficients larger than one (and adaptive kinetics) can be obtained even with a single IP₃ binding site.

We have only presented here an overview of some of the more popular IP₃R models. In fact there are many others, (see for instance refs. 86-89). For a recent review of IP₃R models see reference 90.

The Ryanodine Receptor

Here we discuss ryanodine receptor modelling that relates specifically to the geometry of cardiac myocytes. This receptor resembles in many aspects the IP₃ receptor presented in the previous section. For instance it is known that it can be activated or inhibited by Ca²⁺.[91,92] However, the close proximity of ryanodine receptor channels in the SR membrane and L-type Ca²⁺ channels in the plasma membrane has led to slightly different modelling approaches. Instead of considering a single receptor, the receptor channel as a whole is mostly modeled.[93] Figure 7 shows such a gating scheme, which was proposed by Tang and Othmer.[94] Note the structural similarities to the IP₃ receptor model in Figure 1. The binary tuple in Figure 7 represents Ca²⁺ binding sites, with the first digit referring to activation and the second to inhibition. An index equals 1 when Ca²⁺ is bound and 0 otherwise. Hence, 10 refers to the state with Ca²⁺ bound only to the activating binding site.

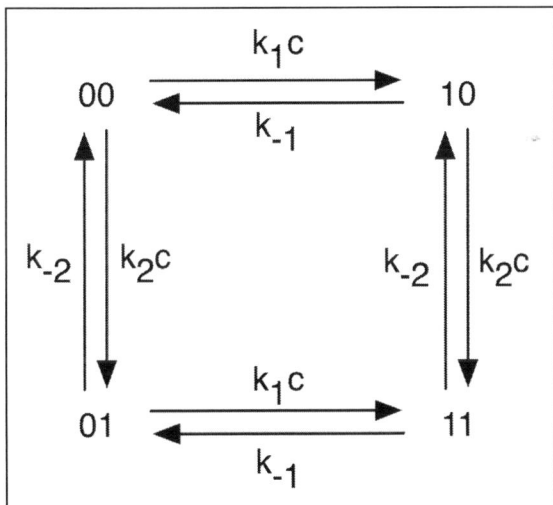

Figure 7. Transition scheme of the Tang-Othmer model. See Table 5 for parameter values.

Table 5. Binding rate constants l_i and unbinding rates l_{-i}, i = 1, 2 of the Tang-Othmer model

$k_1 = 15\ (\mu Ms)^{-1}$	$k_{-1} = 7.6\ s^{-1}$
$k_2 = 0.8\ (\mu Ms)^{-1}$	$k_{-2} = 0.84\ s^{-1}$

In case of a large number of channels, the fraction of channels in a given state is determined by an equation similar to equation (3), e.g., we find for channels in the state 10

$$\dot{p}_{10} = -(k_2 c + k_{-1})p_{10} + k_1 c p_{00} + k_{-2} p_{11}. \tag{11}$$

Since the Ca^{2+} concentration changes in time, solutions to equation (11) are not available in closed form. However, the stationary states can be readily computed, which yields

$$\bar{p}_{00} = K_1 K_2 \gamma_2, \qquad\qquad \bar{p}_{10} = K_2 \bar{c} \gamma_2, \tag{12a}$$

$$\bar{p}_{01} = K_1 \bar{c} \gamma_2, \qquad\qquad \bar{p}_{11} = \bar{c}^2 \gamma_2, \tag{12b}$$

with $\gamma_2^{-1} = K_1 K_2 + (K_1 + K_2)\bar{c} + \bar{c}^2$ and the dissociation constants $K_i = k_{-i}/k_i$. Note that $\bar{p}_{00} + \bar{p}_{01} + \bar{p}_{10} + \bar{p}_{11} = 1$ in analogy to equation (4). In a similar fashion to De Young and Keizer, Tang and Othmer consider the channel to be open when Ca^{2+} is only bound to the activating Ca^{2+} binding site, but not to the inhibiting. Hence, 10 represents the conducting state of the ryanodine receptor channel. Figure 8 depicts the stationary open probability $\bar{p}_{10}$ as a function of the Ca^{2+} concentration. We find a similar bell shaped curve as for the De Young-Keizer model.

The above analysis demonstrates that modelling IP_3 receptors and ryanodine receptors can proceed along the same lines, which greatly facilitates theoretical investigations of their dynamics. Yet, the prominent opposition of ryanodine receptor channels and L-type Ca^{2+} channels led early to the conclusion that geometry is crucial for the Ca^{2+} dynamics—an insight that is just about to make its breakthrough for IP_3 receptor channels.

When Ca^{2+} is liberated from the SR, it enters the tiny volume of the dyadic cleft, where it reaches concentrations as high as several hundred micromolar—orders of magnitude higher than bulk concentrations in a cell. Therefore, the gating mechanisms of the ryanodine receptor channel are not influenced by averaged concentrations, but by the highly elevated Ca^{2+} concentration in the dyadic cleft. Stern took up this idea and proposed *local control* models.[95] They consist of separate equations that govern the time evolution of Ca^{2+} in the dyadic cleft, the rest of the cytosol, and the lumen, respectively. Since then, various aspects of the interplay between the geometry of the dyadic cleft and its dynamics have been discussed, (see e.g., refs. 96-98).

The SERCA Pump

SERCA pumps belong to a group of enzymes known as P-type ATPases, so a natural step to model the dynamics of these pumps is to employ tools from enzyme kinetics.[99] The current

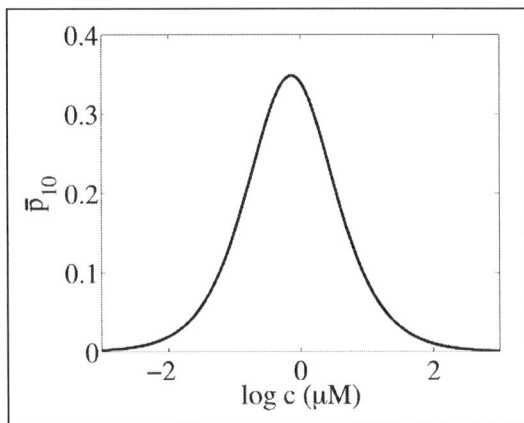

Figure 8. Stationary value of the open probability $\bar{p}_{10}$ of the Tang-Othmer model.

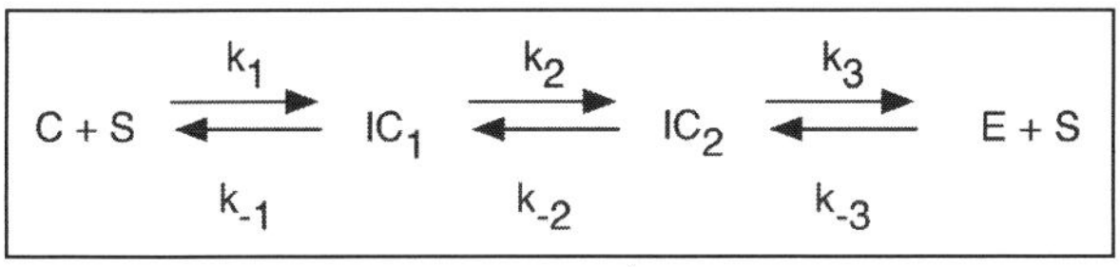

Figure 9. Reaction scheme for a SERCA pump. The SERCA pump with no Ca^{2+} bound is denoted by S, whereas IC_1 and IC_2 refer to Ca^{2+} bound transition states. C and E refer to the cytosolic and luminal calcium.

picture as obtained by pharmacological studies and electromicroscopy[100-102] indicates that once cytosolic Ca^{2+} is bound to the ATPase, the enzyme undergoes several transformations including large conformational changes to the point when it releases Ca^{2+} into the lumen. A simplified model of this transport mechanism is depicted in Figure 9. We assume that we can lump all intermediate states into two states: the state in which cytosolic Ca^{2+} is bound for the first time (IC_1), and the state from which Ca^{2+} is liberated into the lumen (IC_2). Consequently, the speed of the reaction is determined by the transitions between (IC_1) and (IC_2):

$$v = k_2[IC_1] - k_{-2}[IC_2]. \tag{13}$$

Using the steady-state approximation for binding of Ca^{2+} to the pump and for unbinding of Ca^{2+} from the pump, i.e., $[IC_1] = sc/K_1$ and $[IC_2] = se/K_2$ with $K_i = k_{-i}/k_i$ and e being the luminal Ca^{2+} concentration, we immediately arrive at

$$v = k_2 \frac{sc}{K_1} - k_{-2} \frac{se}{K_2} = \frac{v_{m,f} sc/K_1 - v_{m,r} se/K_2}{s_T} = \frac{v_{m,f} c/K_1 - v_{m,r} e/K_2}{1 + c/K_1 + e/K_2}. \tag{14}$$

Here, $v_{m,f} = k_2 s_T$ and $v_{m,r} = k_{-2} s_T$ represent the maximal forward and reverse velocity, respectively, and $s_T = s + [IC_1] + [IC_2]$ denotes the total SERCA concentration because the pump can be either unbound (S) or in one of the internal states IC_1 or IC_2. Note that since luminal Ca^{2+} can vary, the dynamics of e can have a strong impact on SERCA activity.[103] Equation (14) naturally incorporates that enzymatic reactions are reversible, and hence pays tribute to the experimental findings that SERCA pumps can operate in a reverse mode.

The reaction scheme in Figure 9 assumes that only one Ca^{2+} ion binds to the SERCA pump, which is then transported into the lumen. However, structural evidence has indicated that two ions are bound.[102] Assuming that they bind in a cooperative manner, equation (14) needs to be altered according to

$$v = \frac{v_{m,f}(c/K_1)^n - v_{m,r}(e/K_2)^n}{1 + (c/K_1)^n + (e/K_2)^n}, \tag{15}$$

where n represents the Hill index. Shannon et al[97] give a value of $n = 1.6$.

The complexity of equation (15) often leads to the implementation of approximations. One frequently used assumption is that the luminal Ca^{2+} concentration is constant and does not feed back on the dynamics, so that Ca^{2+} is only pumped from the cytosol into the lumen. This leads to

$$v = v_{m,f} \frac{c^n}{K_1^n + c^n} \tag{16}$$

The dominant feature of equations (15) and (16) is that the Ca^{2+} concentrations enter nonlinearly. In the limit of no cooperativity ($n = 1$) and low affinity ($c = K_1$ and $e = K_2$), both expressions can be linearised to yield

$$v = \frac{c}{\tau} - \frac{e}{\tau_e}, \tag{17}$$

or $v = c/\tau$, respectively, where we introduce the time scales $\tau = K_1/v_{m,f}$ and $\tau_e = K_2/v_{m,r}$. The advantage of the linearised expressions is that they allow us far reaching analytical investigations of intracellular Ca^{2+} dynamics, as we will illustrate later in the section *Threshold Models*.

Mitochondria

Calcium transport by mitochondria involves mainly two pathways: uptake by a Ca^{2+} uniporter and release through a Na^+/Ca^{2+} exchanger (NCX). Like most of the cellular transport mechanisms, a convenient way of describing them is to resort to enzymatic reactions. The number of transporters remains unchanged in the course of a reaction in the same way as the total number of enzymes does not change. Following a review by Gunter and Pfeifer,[104] the Na^+/Ca^{2+} exchanger is best represented by a product of 2 Hill functions:

$$v_{NCX} = v_m^{NCX} \frac{n^2}{K_n^2 + n^2} \frac{m}{K_m + m}, \tag{18}$$

where m and n denote the mitochondrial Ca^{2+} concentration and the cytosolic Na^+ concentration, respectively, and K_n and K_m refer to the dissociation constants for Na^+ and Ca^{2+} transport, respectively. The maximal velocity is given by v_m^{NCX}. Equation (18) reflects experimental findings that the Na^+/Ca^{2+} exchanger may work electrically neutral, in that it releases one Ca^{2+} ion for two Na^+ ions. However, other studies suggest a ratio larger than 2:1 (see e.g., ref. 105), which would lead to a higher Hill coefficient than 2 in equation (18). A similar controversy seems to exist for modelling the Ca^{2+} uniporter. Yet, the best fit is obtained for a Hill coefficient of 2,[104] giving rise to

$$v_{uni} = v_m^{uni} \frac{c^2}{K_u^2 + c^2}. \tag{19}$$

Here, v_m^{uni} is the maximal velocity of the uniporter, and K_u denotes the associated dissociation constant. Putting equations (18) and (19) together, the net Ca^{2+} flux of mitochondria is given by

$$J_m = v_{uni} - v_{NCX}. \tag{20}$$

Equation (20) represents a sensible starting point for incorporating mitochondrial dynamics into models of intracellular Ca^{2+}, because it captures essential experimental findings in a tractable expression. It has been successfully applied in references 106 and 107 to explain experiments in which energised mitochondria increase the speed of Ca^{2+} waves—a result that seems contradictory to the process of Ca^{2+} induced Ca^{2+} release (see next section). We note that patch-clamp data from the inner mitochondrial membrane is available to guide further detailed modelling of the Ca^{2+} uniporter.[108] In case more details for the Ca^{2+} flux than equation (20) are needed such as coupling to the membrane potential of mitochondria or the concentration of ADP, see e.g., references 109-111.

Homogenous Cell Models

A frequently used assumption in modelling cellular processes is that cells resemble well-stirred reactors, so that concentrations of any chemical compound are the same everywhere in the cell. Mathematically, this principle leads to a set of ODEs. When we focus just on the dynamics of cytosolic Ca^{2+} without fluxes over the plasma membrane, all these models possess the structure

$$\dot{c} = J_{release}(X, c, t) + J_{leak}(c, t) - J_{uptake}(c, t), \tag{21a}$$

$$\dot{X} = f(X, t), \tag{21b}$$

where J_{release} and J_{leak} denote Ca^{2+} liberation through receptor channels and a leak current from internal Ca^{2+} stores, respectively, and J_{uptake} represents Ca^{2+} uptake from the cytosol into these stores. The variable X refers to the states of the receptors involved, and hence the release current explicitly depends on it.

We will illustrate the dynamics of equation (21) with the De Young-Keizer model introduced earlier. As mentioned there, the open probability of an IP_3 receptor channel is given by equation (6), which reflects experimental findings that the channel is conducting when at least 3 of its 4 subunits are activated.[32,73,74] Consequently, we model the release current as

$$J_{\text{release}} = k_c \left(4 p_{110}^3 - 3 p_{110}^4 \right)(e - c),\qquad(22)$$

where k_c denotes its maximal value. The luminal Ca^{2+} concentration e is considered constant. Generally, a linear leak current $J_{\text{leak}} = -k_l c$ with a flux strength k_l is accepted, and the SERCA pumps are implemented by a Hill function as in equation (16) with a coefficient $n = 2$:

$$J_{\text{uptake}} = k_p \frac{c^2}{c^2 + K_p^2}.\qquad(23)$$

Taking it together, the time evolution of the Ca^{2+} concentration as governed by equation (21) requires us to solve 8 coupled nonlinear ODEs.

An elegant insight into such high dimensional dynamics is obtained by computing bifurcation diagrams. The left panel of Figure 10 depicts the stationary states of the Ca^{2+} concentration as a function of the IP_3 concentration. The prominent feature are two Hopf bifurcations.[112] If the IP_3 concentration is chosen in between these two bifurcation points, the Ca^{2+} concentration oscillates. A typical trace is shown in the right panel of Figure 10. At low IP_3 concentrations, the Ca^{2+} dynamics possesses a linearly stable fixed point. The same is true for high IP_3 concentrations.

The mechanism that underlies these oscillations is known as calcium induced calcium release (CICR). The open probability increases significantly with an increase of the Ca^{2+} concentration at low Ca^{2+} concentrations. Consequently, a gradual increase of Ca^{2+} at a closed IP_3 receptor channel might increase the open probability to such an extent that it opens. Then Ca^{2+} is liberated, and the high Ca^{2+} concentration inhibits the IP_3 receptor, leading to a closure of the channel. The Ca^{2+} concentration decreases and eventually reaches the same level as before the Ca^{2+} liberation started. Hence, the oscillation can start again. The features of an increase of the

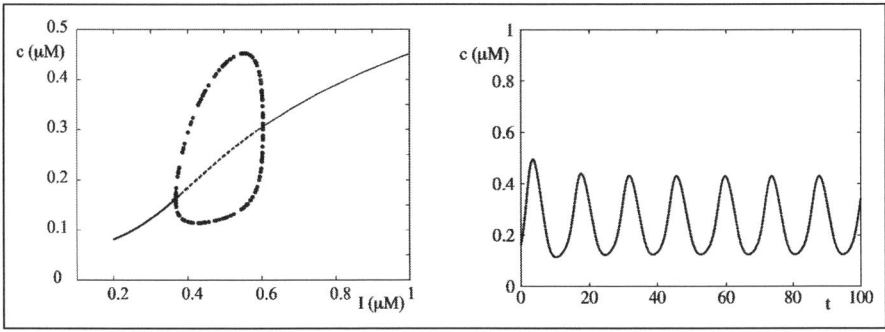

Figure 10. Left) Bifurcation diagram of the De Young-Keizer model. Solid (dashed) lines represent stable (unstable) solutions. The minimum and the maximum of the oscillations are indicated by circles. Right) Typical Ca^{2+} oscillations for $I = 0.5\ \mu M$. Parameter values as in Table 1 and $kc = 6\ s^{-1}$, $kl = 0.108\ s^{-1}$, $kp = 0.76\ (\mu Ms)^{-1}$, $Kp = 0.1\ \mu M$, and $e = 1.69\ \mu M$.

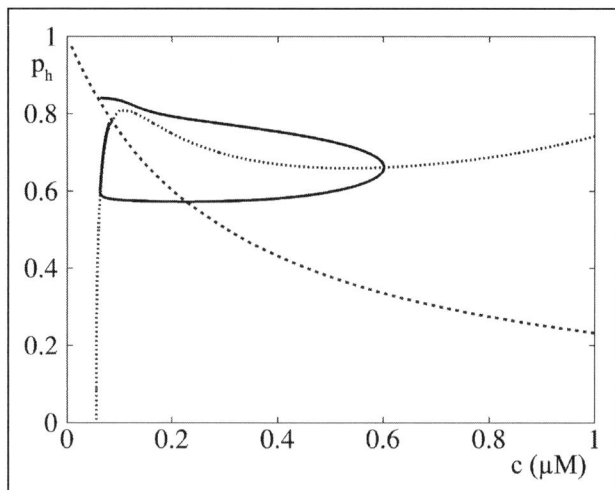

Figure 11. Nullclines of c (dotted line) and ph (dashed line) in the Li-Rinzel model. The solid line shows a trajectory with initial conditions $(c, ph) = (0.06250, 0.83959)$. Parameter values as in Figure 10 and $I = 0.2\ \mu M$, $a_5 = 10\ (\mu Ms)^{-1}$.

open probability at low Ca^{2+} concentrations and a decrease at high Ca^{2+} concentrations is also present in the stationary value of the open probability that is depicted in Figure 2.

The occurrence of a Hopf bifurcation is one possibility to generate oscillations in spatially homogeneous Ca^{2+} models. Later approaches (as e.g. in reference 86) found the same mechanism. However, it is not the only one. Another principle becomes apparent when we take X in equation (21) to be the Li-Rinzel model (equation (7)). The origin of the oscillations is best explained by investigating Figure 11. It depicts the nullclines for c and p_h, i.e., the solutions to $\dot{c} = 0$ and $\dot{p}_h = 0$. The intersection of the two curves represents a linearly stable fixed point. When c and p_h take initial values in the vicinity of the fixed point, they will always return to it. However, larger perturbations carry them away as indicated by the solid line. These excursions in phase space give rise to the observed oscillations and are known as *excitability* (see ref. 113 for a comprehensive review). A more detailed analysis reveals that the present Ca^{2+} model possesses the same structure as the seminal equations by FitzHugh and Nagumo.[114,115] Hence, the existence of excitability can be understood on general grounds.

Although Hopf bifurcations as well as excitability lead to oscillations, both mechanisms are fundamentally different. In the former case, oscillations exist intrinsically and persist forever if no perturbations are applied. On the contrast, oscillations in excitable systems can only be observed if the perturbations are strong enough. Therefore, noise can act in a destructive fashion in the presence of a Hopf bifurcation, but it is crucial in the regime of excitability. In the next section, we will explore the concept of excitability in more detail.

Threshold Models

We saw in the previous section, *Homogenous Cell Models*, that excitability is one mechanism to generate oscillations. Figure 12 illustrates that excitability is intimately related to threshold crossing. The notion of a perturbation being sufficiently strong is the same as indicating that a perturbation exceeds a threshold. If the initial perturbation is too weak, the Ca^{2+} concentration returns to its steady state. Otherwise, it crosses the threshold and evokes an oscillation.

In the case of the Li-Rinzel model, it is obvious that crossing the threshold and the exact form of the oscillation depends on both variables, the Ca^{2+} concentration c and the gating variable p_h. The latter summarises all the dynamics of the release channel, so that it essentially

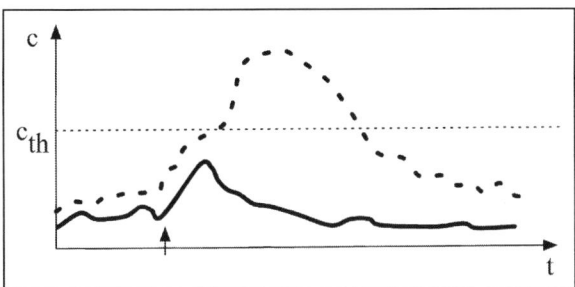

Figure 12. Concept of excitability. At the time indicated by the arrow, both Ca^{2+} trajectories are perturbed. The solid line shows a subthreshold perturbation, whereas the dashed line represents a superthreshold perturbation.

encodes for the state of the channel being either open or closed. Note that this discrete notion (on/off) is blurred by considering a population of channels and consequently fractions of open channels. This switch-like idea led to an approximation of equation (21) that is now known as a threshold model. Instead of considering the full gating mechanism as in equation (21b), this approach assumes that as long as the Ca^{2+} concentration is below a threshold, no release occurs, but as soon as it crosses threshold, Ca^{2+} is liberated from internal stores in a prescribed form. Consequently, equation (21) is replaced by a single equation with the new release term

$$J_{release} = \sum_i f\left(t - T_i\right). \tag{24}$$

The release times T_i are defined by

$$T_i = \inf \{ t \mid c \geq c_{th}, t > T_{i-1} + \tau_R \}, \tag{25}$$

where τ_R denotes an absolute refractory time-scale. Equation (25) states that release occurs when the Ca^{2+} concentration is higher than a threshold value c_{th} and that there is at least a time τ_R between consecutive release events. Given a firing time T_i, the function $f(t)$ in equation (24) governs the exact shape of the Ca^{2+} release. Assuming that liberation lasts for a time Δ with a constant flux density η, it is common to write $f(t) = \eta \Theta(t - \Delta)\Theta(t)$, where Θ is the Heaviside function with $\Theta(t) = 1$ for $t \geq 0$ and 0 otherwise. One assumption in equation (24) is that Ca^{2+} release occurs at every point in the cell. However, it is well known that release sites form either regular lattices as in cardiac myocytes or a scattered randomly as in Xenopus oocytes.[43,116] We can easily accommodate for such spatial arrangements by changing the release flux according to

$$J_{release} = \sum_{i,j} f\left(t - T_i^j\right)\delta\left(x_j - x\right), \tag{26}$$

where $\delta(x)$ is a Dirac-delta function. Release occurs now at sites labelled by the index j, so that T_i^j is the ith release event at site j.

Threshold models have greatly facilitated studies of intracellular Ca^{2+} dynamics, since they allow far reaching analytical results and cheap numerical simulations.[117-120] When using the form of release (26) such threshold models are called fire-diffuse-fire (FDF) models. Indeed they have contributed significantly to our understanding of Ca^{2+} fronts and spiral waves, which represent some of the most prominent Ca^{2+} patterns in cell biology. Note that to study wave phenomena in general, we need to append equation (21a) by a diffusive contribution, i.e.

$$\frac{\partial c}{\partial t} = D\frac{\partial^2}{\partial x^2}c + J_{release} + J_{leak}\left(c\right) - J_{uptake}\left(c\right), \tag{27}$$

where D is the diffusion coefficient of cytosolic Ca^{2+}. For a general introduction to waves see references 112 and 121.

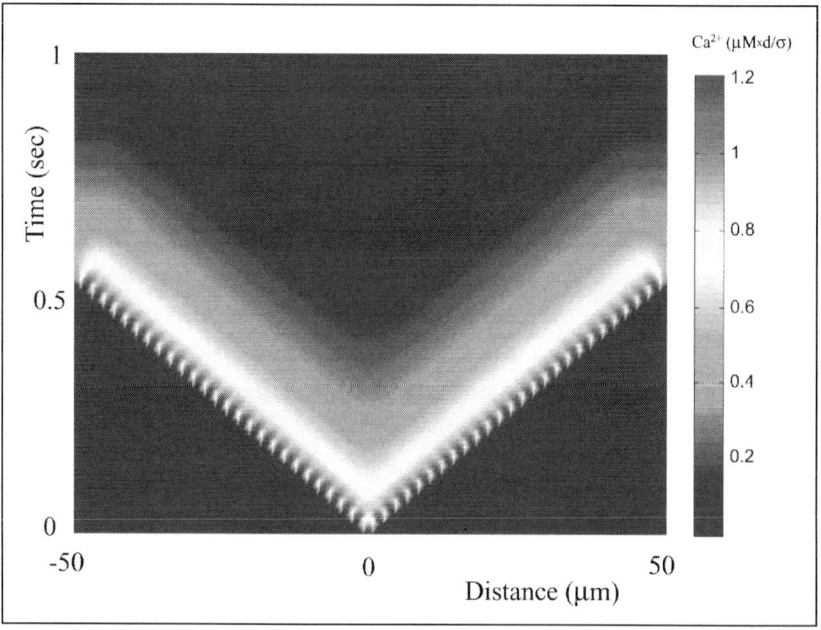

Figure 13. An example of two saltatory pulses moving out from the center of a deterministic one dimensional FDF model with 50 regularly spaced release sites and free boundary conditions. Redrawn from reference 120.

Using the release flux (26) the model is not translation invariant and one expects the emergence of saltatory waves, i.e., waves that do not propagate with a constant profile. Rather activity jumps from one release site to another, so that the speed of propagation is naturally defined in terms of the ratio of inter-release site distance to the duration of jumping. An example of such a wave is shown in Figure 13.

Despite their successes, many threshold models assume that the luminal Ca^{2+} concentration remains constant. This is only true if the lumen is infinitely large and diffusion is very fast. How quickly Ca^{2+} diffuses in the lumen is still an open question, (see refs. 122,123 for opposing views), but we can be sure about the finiteness of organelles. Consequently, a natural extension of equation (27) are the bidomain equations

$$\frac{\partial c}{\partial t} = D\frac{\partial^2 c}{\partial x^2} + J_{release}\left(c,c_{er}\right) + J_{leak}\left(c,c_{er}\right) - J_{uptake}\left(c,c_{er}\right), \tag{28a}$$

$$\frac{\partial c_{er}}{\partial t} = D_{er}\frac{\partial^2 c_{er}}{\partial x^2} - \frac{1}{\gamma}\left[J_{release}\left(c,c_{er}\right) + J_{leak}\left(c,c_{er}\right) - J_{uptake}\left(c,c_{er}\right)\right], \tag{28b}$$

$$J_{release}\left(c,c_{er}\right) = \left(c - c_{er}\right)\sum_{i,j} f\left(t - T_i^j\right)\delta\left(x_j - x\right), \tag{28c}$$

where D_{er} and γ denote the diffusion coefficient of Ca^{2+} in the lumen and the ratio of luminal to cytosolic volume, respectively. This bidomain model has recently been employed to analyse a new dynamical phenomenon of back-and-forth rocking waves (for a model with a continuous distribution of stores: $T_i^j \rightarrow T_i(x)$).[124] These types of waves have been observed in nemertean worm[125] and ascidian eggs.[126] They were first investigated in a biophysical model, with a Li-Rinzel model for the IP_3 receptor and a nonlinear SERCA pump (given by equations (7) and (16)

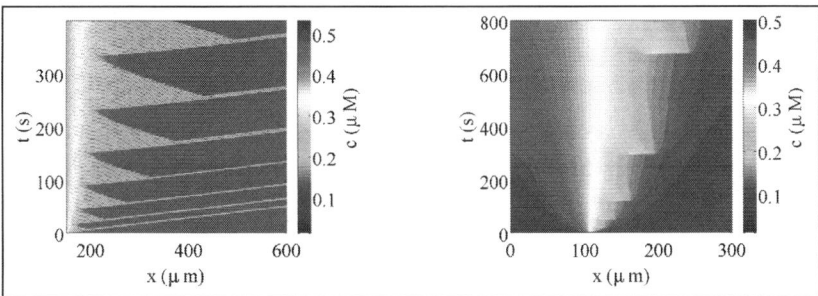

Figure 14. Different kinds of tango waves in an FDF bidomain model with $\tau R = 0.5$ s (left) and $\tau R = 0$ s (right). The pseudocolor plot shows $c(x, t)$ in μM. For further details see reference 124.

respectively). Being reminiscent of a form of classical ballroom dance they were dubbed 'tango waves'.[127] Figure 14 shows different shapes of tango waves in a threshold bidomain model. The result in the left panel was obtained for a nonzero refractory time scale, and every time the main wave reverses direction, pulses are shed off. The number of pulses varies, as there is only one pulse for the first 4 reversals, but two pulses for the subsequent ones. The right panel illustrates that the back-and-forth movement can be more compact and that isolated pulses do not necessarily exist.

Although threshold models mimic deterministic excitable systems, they can be naturally extended to describe noisy systems. For instance, the value of the threshold may be chosen to fluctuate in such a way as to approximate the stochastic gating of receptors.[128] Stochastic calcium dynamics was investigated in references 129 and 130 and can give rise to noisy waves such as those seen in Figure 15. The spark-to-wave transition in a particular stochastic threshold model is

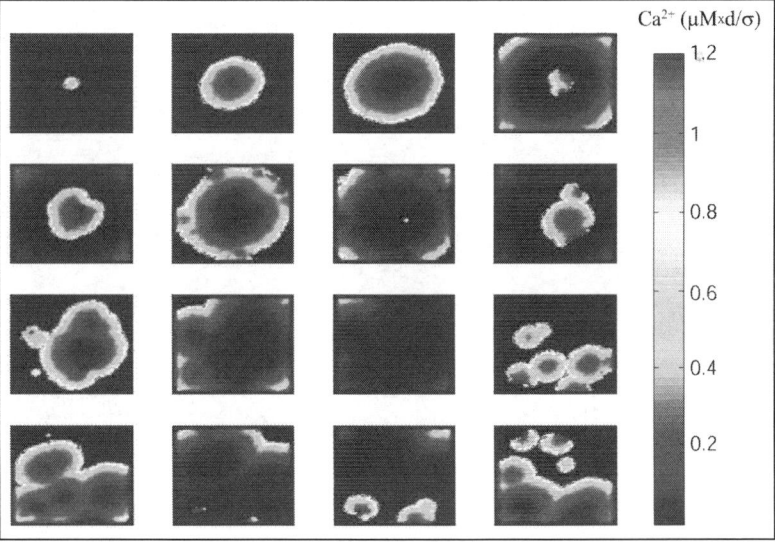

Figure 15. Temporal sequence snapshots for a two-dimensional stochastic FDF model with low noise. Frames are presented every 0.45s starting in the top left corner and moving rightward and down. An initial seed in the center of the cell model leads to the formation and propagation of a circular front. Spiral waves form in the wake of the wave by spontaneous nucleation. These can be destroyed in wave-wave collisions and created by spontaneous nucleation. Redrawn from reference 130.

analysed in reference 131. Interestingly, noise can have contrasting effects. On the one hand, it can lead to the extinction of waves that exist in the absence of noise. On the other hand, coherent oscillations can arise from a state of complete disorder, due to a form of array enhanced coherence resonance.[130] Indeed, noise can play a key role in shaping the dynamics of intracellular Ca^{2+}, and we will see some more examples of this in the next section.

Stochastic Modelling

Since the pioneering work of Hodgkin and Huxley,[132] our understanding of ion channel dynamics has greatly improved, and today there is overwhelming experimental evidence that ion channels are intrinsically noisy. Although large populations of randomly gated ion channels can generate deterministic signals,[133] detailed studies of intracellular Ca^{2+} dynamics reveal that fluctuations exist from the micro-scale of channels to the macro-scale of waves and oscillations.[83]

The reason for this persistence lies in the spatial arrangement of the Ca^{2+} release channels. They are not homogeneously distributed in the cell, but they are grouped into clusters. Indeed, in the case of IP$_3$Rs there is some evidence that they prefer to occupy positions nearer to mitochondria.[134] The exact number of channels per clusters is still unknown, but estimates range between 5-100. More specifically, Swillens et al reported cluster sizes between 5-40 for IP$_3$R channels.[135] More recent data for the number of IP$_3$Rs in a cluster can be found in reference 136. These clusters can form either regular arrays as in the case of ryanodine receptor channels,[43,137-139] or they can be less ordered as in the case of IP$_3$R channels.[116,140]

This spatial organisation has far reaching effects. The small number of channels per cluster entails that the state of a cluster in terms of the states of the channels fluctuates strongly. Consequently, Ca^{2+} release through a cluster, which is determined by the number of open channels, does not generally show regular oscillations as in the right panel of Figure 10. The interval between blips, puffs or sparks as well as the amplitude vary significantly.[116,141-144] From a modeller's perspective, this requires the replacement of the deterministic gating equations in the earlier section *The IP$_3$ Receptor* by their stochastic counterparts.

The toolbox of stochastic processes offers different methods for this goal.[145-147] We will illustrate two of them with a stochastic version of the Li-Rinzel model (equation (7)), in which a receptor is either deactivated (D) or activated (A). Hence, it obeys the transition scheme

$$A \underset{b_6}{\overset{a_6 c}{\rightleftharpoons}} D. \tag{29}$$

The most fundamental approach is to write down a master equation for a channel with N receptors, which governs the time evolution of the probability $p_n(t)$ to find n receptors in the activated state at time t:

$$\frac{dp_n(t)}{dt} = -\left[na_6c + (N-n)b_6\right]p_n(t) + (n+1)a_6cp_{n+1}(t) + (N-n-1)b_6p_{n-1}(t). \tag{30}$$

The negative term on the right hand side reflects that the probability decreases when any of the n activated receptors binds Ca^{2+} and hence deactivates, or when Ca^{2+} dissolves from any of the $(N-n)$ deactivated receptors. On the other hand, if there are $(n+1)$ activated receptors, binding of Ca^{2+} to one of them reduces this number to n activated receptors and hence increases the probability $p_n(t)$. Note that equation (30) is a system of N coupled equations, one for every n. Although being a basic equation, solving the master equation for more complicated gating schemes as e.g., the De Young-Keizer model is computationally expensive, so that approximations were suggested.

The two most frequently used approximations are either Fokker-Planck equations or Langevin equations. Instead of a set of N coupled equations, a Fokker-Planck equation is a single equation for the probability $p(x, t)$ to find a fraction $x = n/N$ receptors in the activated state. However, a master equation gives rise to several Fokker-Planck equations, which all have different properties. In the end the current question at hand decides upon a specific choice.[148] Following the ideas of Kramers and Moyal,[149,150] we find

$$\frac{\partial p(x,t)}{\partial t} = -\frac{\partial}{\partial x}\Big[b_6(1-x) - a_6cx\Big]p(x,t) + \frac{1}{2N}\frac{\partial^2}{\partial x^2}\Big[b_6(1-x) + a_6cx\Big]p(x,t). \qquad (31)$$

Both equations, (30) and (31), describe the time evolution of the *probability* to find some number or some fraction of activated subunits, respectively. Langevin took a different approach and wrote down an equation for the actually *value* of x:

$$\frac{\partial x}{\partial t} = \Big[b_6(1-x) - a_6cx\Big]x + \sqrt{\frac{b_6(1-x) + a_6cx}{N}}\,\xi(t), \qquad (32)$$

where $\xi(t)$ is zero-mean Gaussian white noise, i.e., the mean of ξ vanishes, $\langle\xi(t)\rangle = 0$, and the correlations obey $\langle\xi(t)\xi(t')\rangle = \delta(t - t')$.[151] Note that equations (30) and (31) always give the same result for identical initial conditions, respectively, whereas equation (32) yields different outcomes for every run. This is due to the the Gaussian noise. It is worth noting that equation (31) and (32) are equivalent.[145] Which to choose depends on the specific question: if the probability distribution is needed, then the Fokker-Planck equation is the first choice, whereas the Langevin equation reveals how the fraction of activated channels actually evolves in time. Both approaches have been successfully used in the past to study various aspects of intracellular Ca^{2+} dynamics.[79,84,152-155]

That fluctuations at the cluster level are necessary for a functional Ca^{2+} dynamics becomes evident when we look at the Ca^{2+} concentrations that occur at a releasing cluster. Since liberation is spatially restricted, the Ca^{2+} concentration reaches values 2-3 orders of magnitude higher than bulk concentrations.[156] Note that the IP_3 receptors experience these highly elevated Ca^{2+} concentrations, and not the bulk concentration far away from the cluster. Without any noise, such a cluster would not be able to oscillate.[157,158] The reason is that these high Ca^{2+} concentrations saturate any feedback mechanisms of the IP_3 receptor. However, they are the crucial element in driving oscillations, so that blocking them prevents the IP_3 receptors from oscillating.

We now move one structural level higher and consider a group of clusters. Taking up the idea of CICR mentioned in the section *Homogenous Cell Models*, the distance of several microns between adjacent clusters entails that they are weakly coupled by the Ca^{2+} concentration, because only little Ca^{2+} diffuses from one open cluster to the next one. Consequently, the open probability of a still closed cluster increases only slightly by the opening of one of its neighbours. Release through a single cluster is therefore insufficient to trigger a Ca^{2+} wave, which travels through the cell. This was observed experimentally and in simulations, leading to the conclusion that a minimum number of adjacent clusters needs to liberate Ca^{2+} to start a wave.[78,144,159] The time that it takes to form such a critical nucleus of conducting clusters is truly random due to fluctuations on the single cluster level and the weak coupling between clusters. Therefore, the period of Ca^{2+} oscillations is a varying quantity that demonstrates the fluctuations of intracellular Ca^{2+} dynamics on the macroscopic scale.

The insight that fluctuations occur on vastly different time scales and length scales have rendered intracellular Ca^{2+} one of today's most challenging model systems. The goal of understanding cellular behaviour needs to start at the receptor level and has to take the real geometry of cells into account. First steps in integrating processes on the receptor level into higher order dynamics have been achieved,[81,160] and it will be exciting to see how new modelling bridges between different cellular mechanisms will deepen our understanding of cellular responses.

Concluding Remarks

The models described in this chapter constitute only a few examples of the efforts made to mathematically describe the complexities of the Ca^{2+} toolkit and how they impact on Ca^{2+} oscillations. It is clear that despite significant research into the biology that controls oscillations, not all parameters that govern the 'on' and 'off' mechanisms in Ca^{2+} signalling are known. Moreover, the isoform specific differences in the biophysics of the channels, pumps and exchangers as well as how they are affected by protein-protein interactions and secondary modifications such as phosphorylation are only just beginning to emerge. Further points to consider are the spatial and Ca^{2+} buffering properties of the compartment in which Ca^{2+} signalling occurs. In the context of Ca^{2+} oscillations, the compartment can be a dyadic cleft in skeletal muscle, a neuronal spine, the entire cytosol or even a group of connected cells. Despite these caveats, modelling has already helped to identify many of the key control processes in the generation, propagation and termination of Ca^{2+} oscillations. Through a continual dialogue between experimental data and mathematical simulations we can determine which simplifications are acceptable in a given cellular context, and make quantitative predictions about the behaviour of the system, which can be tested. Furthermore, where models fail to capture the essential features of an experimental system, unrecognised signalling interactions may be suggested and sought experimentally. Ultimately, it can be hoped that new insight will be gained into how cells encode and decode the Ca^{2+} signals that drive so many aspects of physiology.

References

1. Berridge MJ, Bootman MD, Roderick HL. Calcium signalling: Dynamics, homeostasis and remodelling. Nat Rev Mol Cell Biol 2003; 4(7):517-529.
2. Bootman MD, Berridge MJ, Roderick HL. Calcium signalling: More messengers, more channels, more complexity. Curr Biol 2002; 12(16):R563-565.
3. Berridge MJ, Rapp PE. A comparative survey of the function, mechanism and control of cellular oscillators. J Exp Biol 1979; 81:217-279.
4. Berridge MJ. Calcium oscillations. J Biol Chem 1990; 265(17):9583-9586.
5. Thomas AP, Bird GS, Hajnoczky G et al. Spatial and temporal aspects of cellular calcium signaling. FASEB J 1996; 10(13):1505-1517.
6. Berridge MJ. The AM and FM of calcium signalling. Nature 1997; 386(6627):759-760.
7. Ueda S, Oiki S, Okada Y. Oscillations of cytoplasmic concentrations of Ca^{2+} and K^+ in fused L cells. J Membr Biol 1986; 91(1):65-72.
8. Yada T, Oiki S, Ueda S et al. Synchronous oscillation of the cytoplasmic Ca^{2+} concentration and membrane potential in cultured epithelial cells (intestine 407). Biochim Biophys Acta 1986; 887(1):105-112.
9. Smith PM, Gallacher DV. Acetylcholine-and caffeine-evoked repetitive transient Ca^{2+}-activated K^+ and C1-currents in mouse submandibular cells. Am J Physiol 1992; 449:109-120.
10. Schlegel W, Winiger BP, Mollard P et al. Oscillations of cytosolic Ca^{2+} in pituitary cells due to action potentials. Nature 1987; 329(6141):719-721.
11. Holl RW, Thorner MO, Mandell GL et al. Spontaneous oscillations of intracellular calcium and growth hormone secretion. J Biol Chem 1988; 263(20):9682-9685.
12. Cuthbertson KS, Cobbold PH. Phorbol ester and sperm activate mouse oocytes by inducing sustained oscillations in cell Ca^{2+}. Nature 1985; 316(6028):541-542.
13. Halet G, Marangos P, Fitzharris G et al. Ca^{2+} oscillations at fertilization in mammals. Biochem Soc Trans 2003; 31(Pt 5):907-911.
14. Miyazaki S, Ito M. Calcium signals for egg activation in mammals. J Pharmacol Sci 2006; 100(5):545-552.
15. Carroll J, Swann K, Whittingham D et al. Spatiotemporal dynamics of intracellular $[Ca^{2+}]_i$ oscillations during the growth and meiotic maturation of mouse oocytes. Development 1994; 120(12):3507-17.
16. Kapur N, Mignery GA, Banach K. Cell cycle-dependent calcium oscillations in mouse embryonic stem cells. Am J Physiol Cell Physiol 2007; 292(4):C1510-1518.
17. Hajnoczky G, Robb-Gaspers LD, Seitz MB et al. Decoding of cytosolic calcium oscillations in the mitochondria. Cell 1995; 82(3):415-424.
18. Marks PW, Maxfield FR. Transient increases in cytosolic free calcium appear to be required for the migration of adherent human neutrophils. J Cell Biol 1990; 110(1):43-52.

19. Maruyama Y, Inooka G, Li YX et al. Agonist-induced localized Ca^{2+} spikes directly triggering exocytotic secretion in exocrine pancreas. EMBO J 1993; 12(8):3017-3022.
20. Dolmetsch RE, Xu K, Lewis RS. Calcium oscillations increase the efficiency and specificity of gene expression. Nature 1998; 392(6679):933-936.
21. McAinsh MR, Webb A, Taylor JE et al. Stimulus-induced oscillations in guard cell cytosolic free calcium. Plant Cell 1995; 7(8):1207-1219.
22. Tang RH, Han S, Zheng H et al. Coupling diurnal cytosolic Ca^{2+} oscillations to the CAS- IP_3 pathway in Arabidopsis. Science 2007; 315(5817):1423-1426.
23. Espelt MV, Estevez AY, Yin X et al. Oscillatory Ca^{2+} signaling in the isolated Caenorhabditis elegans intestine: Role of the inositol-1,4,5-trisphosphate receptor and phospholipases C beta and gamma. J Gen Physiol 2005; 126(4):379-392.
24. Berridge MJ, Galione A. Cytosolic calcium oscillators. FASEB J 1988; 2(15):3074-3082.
25. Prentki M, Glennon MC, Thomas AP et al. Cell-specific patterns of oscillating free Ca^{2+} in carbamylcholinestimulated insulinoma cells. J Biol Chem 1988; 263(23):11,044-11,047.
26. Gray PT. Oscillations of free cytosolic calcium evoked by cholinergic and catecholaminergic agonists in rat parotid acinar cells. Am J Physiol 1988; 406:35-53.
27. Rooney TA, Sass EJ, Thomas AP. Characterization of cytosolic calcium oscillations induced by phenylephrine and vasopressin in single fura-2-loaded hepatocytes. J Biol Chem 1989; 264(29):17,131-17,141.
28. Bootman MD, Young KW, Young JM et al. Extracellular calcium concentration controls the frequency of intracellular calcium spiking independently of inositol 1,4,5-trisphosphate production in HeLa cells. Biochem J 1996; 314(Pt 1):347-354.
29. Taylor CW, da Fonseca PC, Morris EP. Ip(3) receptors: The search for structure. Trends Biochem Sci 2004; 29(4):210-219.
30. Bosanac I, Alattia JR, Mal TK et al. Structure of the inositol 1,4,5-trisphosphate receptor binding core in complex with its ligand. Nature 2002; 420(6916):696-700.
31. Finch EA, Turner TJ, Goldin SM. Calcium as a coagonist of inositol 1,4,5-trisphosphate-induced calcium release. Science 1991; 252(5004):443-446.
32. Bezprozvanny I, Watras J, Ehrlich B. Bell-shaped calcium-response curves of Ins(1,4,5)P3 -and calcium-gated channels from endoplasmic reticulum of cerebellum. Nature 1991; 351:751-754.
33. Iino M. Biphasic Ca^{2+} dependence of inositol 1,4,5-trisphosphate-induced Ca release in smooth muscle cells of the guinea pig taenia caeci. J Gen Physiol 1990; 95(6):1103-1122.
34. Iino M, Endo M. Calcium-dependent immediate feedback control of inositol 1,4,5-triphosphate-induced Ca^{2+} release. Nature 1992; 360(6399):76-78.
35. Berridge MJ, Cheek TR, Bennett DL et al. Ryanodine receptors and intracellular calcium signalling. In: Sorrentino V, ed. Ryanodine Receptors: A CRC Pharmacology and Toxicology Series, Basic and Clinical. CRC Press, 1995:119-154.
36. Roderick HL, Berridge MJ, Bootman MD. Calcium-induced calcium release. Curr Biol 2003; 13(R425).
37. Sneyd J, Tsaneva-Atanasova K. Modeling calcium waves. In: Falcke M, Malchow D, eds. Understanding Calcium Dynamics-Experiments and Theory, Lecture Notes in Physics. Berlin: Springer, 2003:179-199.
38. Missiaen L, Taylor CW, Berridge MJ. Spontaneous calcium release from inositol trisphosphate-sensitive calcium stores. Nature 1991; 352(6332):241-244.
39. Ehrlich BE. Functional properties of intracellular calcium-release channels. Curr Opin Neurobiol 1995; 5(3):304-309.
40. Hajnoczky G, Thomas AP. Minimal requirements for calcium oscillations driven by the IP_3 receptor. EMBO J 1997; 16(12):3533-3543.
41. Bennett DL, Cheek TR, Berridge MJ et al. Expression and function of ryanodine receptors in nonexcitable cells. J Biol Chem 1996; 271(11):6356-6362.
42. Sorrentino V, Volpe P. Ryanodine receptors: How many, where and why? Trends Pharmacol Sci 1993; 14(3):98-103.
43. Bootman MD, Higazi DR, Coombes S et al. Calcium signalling during excitation-contraction coupling in mammalian atrial myocytes. J Cell Sci 2006; 119:3915-3925.
44. Sorrentino V. Molecular determinants of the structural and functional organization of the sarcoplasmic reticulum. Biochimica at Biophysica Acta 2004; 1742(1-3):113-118.
45. Roderick HL, Bootman MD. Bi-directional signalling from the InsP3 receptor: Regulation by calcium and accessory factors. Biochem Soc Trans 2003; 31(Pt 5):950-953.
46. Hamilton SL. Ryanodine receptors. Cell Calcium 2005; 38(3-4):253-260.
47. Orchard CH, Eisner DA, Allen DG. Oscillations of intracellular Ca^{2+} in mammalian cardiac muscle. Nature 1983; 304(5928):735-738.

48. Blatter LA, Wier WG. Agonist-induced $[Ca^{2+}]_i$ waves and Ca^{2+}-induced Ca^{2+} release in mammalian vascular smooth muscle cells. Am J Physiol 1992; 263(2 Pt 2):H576-586.

49. Berridge MJ, Cobbold PH, Cuthbertson KS. Spatial and temporal aspects of cell signalling. Philos Trans R Soc Lond B Biol Sci 1988; 320(1199):325-343.

50. Bootman MD, Berridge MJ. Subcellular Ca^{2+} signals underlying waves and graded responses in HeLa cells. Curr Biol 1996; 6(7):855-865.

51. Rooney TA, Sass EJ, Thomas AP. Agonist-induced cytosolic calcium oscillations originate from a specific locus in single hepatocytes. J Biol Chem 1990; 265(18):10,792-796.

52. Parker I, Ivorra I. Localized all-or-none calcium liberation by inositol trisphosphate. Science 1990; 250(4983):977-979.

53. Boitano S, Dirksen ER, Sanderson MJ. Intercellular propagation of calcium waves mediated by inositol trisphosphate. Science 1992; 258(5080):292-295.

54. Robb-Gaspers LD, Thomas AP. Coordination of Ca^{2+} signaling by intercellular propagation of Ca^{2+} waves in the intact liver. J Biol Chem 1995; 270(14):8102-8107.

55. Jensen AM, Chiu SY. Fluorescence measurement of changes in intracellular calcium induced by excitatory amino acids in cultured cortical astrocytes. J Neurosci 1990; 10(4):1165-1175.

56. Sage SO, Adams DJ, van Breemen C. Synchronized oscillations in cytoplasmic free calcium concentration in confluent bradykinin-stimulated bovine pulmonary artery endothelial cell monolayers. J Biol Chem 1989; 264(1):6-9.

57. Neylon CB, Irvine RF. Synchronized repetitive spikes in cytoplasmic calcium in confluent monolayers of human umbilical vein endothelial cells. FEBS Lett 1990; 275(1-2):173-176.

58. Petersen CC, Toescu EC, Petersen OH. Different patterns of receptor-activated cytoplasmic Ca^{2+} oscillations in single pancreatic acinar cells: Dependence on receptor type, agonist concentration and intracellular Ca^{2+} buffering. EMBO J 1991; 10(3):527-533.

59. Hajjar RJ, Bonventre JV. Oscillations of intracellular calcium induced by vasopressin in individual fura-2-loaded mesangial cells: Frequency dependence on basal calcium concentration, agonist concentration, and temperature. J Biol Chem 1991; 266(32):21,589-21,594.

60. Bird GS, Rossier MF, Obie JF et al. Sinusoidal oscillations in intracellular calcium requiring negative feedback by protein kinase C. J Biol Chem 1993; 268(12):8425-848.

61. De Koninck P, Schulman H. Sensitivity of CaM kinase II to the frequency of Ca^{2+} oscillations. Science 1998; 279(5348):227-230.

62. Schulman H, Hanson PI, Meyer T. Decoding calcium signals by multifunctional CaM kinase. Cell Calcium 1992; 13(6-7):401-411.

63. Meyer T, Stryer L. Molecular model for receptor-stimulated calcium spiking. Proc Natl Acad Sci USA 1988; 85(14):5051-5055.

64. Goldbetter A, Dupont G, Berridge M. Minimal model for signal-induced Ca^{2+} oscillations and for their frequency encoding through protein phosphorylation. Proc Natl Acad Sci USA 1990; 87(4):1461-1465.

65. Dupont G, Goldbeter A. One-pool model for Ca^{2+} oscillations involving Ca^{2+} and inositol 1,4,5-trisphosphate as coagonists for Ca^{2+} release. Cell Calcium 1993; 14(4):311-322.

66. Bootman MD. Quantal Ca^{2+} release from InsP3-sensitive intracellular Ca^{2+} stores. Mol Cell Endocrinol 1994; 98(2):157-166.

67. Parker I, Ivorra I. Inhibition by Ca^{2+} of inositol trisphosphate-mediated Ca^{2+} liberation: A possible mechanism for oscillatory release of Ca^{2+}. Proc Natl Acad Sci USA 1990; 87(1):260-264.

68. Colquhoun D, Hawkes AG. The principle of the stochastic interpretation of ion-channel mechanics. In: Sakmann B, Neher E, eds. Single Channel Recording. Plenum Press, 1995:397-482.

69. De Young G, Keizer J. A single inositol 1,4,5-triphosphate-receptor-based model for agonist-stimulated oscillations in Ca^{2+} concentration. Proc Natl Acad Sci USA 1992; 89:9895-9899.

70. Hill TL. Free Energy Transduction in Biology. New York: Academic Press, 1977.

71. Sneyd J, Falcke M, Dufour JF et al. A comparison of three models of the inositol trisphosphate receptor. Prog Biophys Mol Biol 2004; 85(2-3):121-140.

72. Dufour JF, Arias IM, Turner TJ. Inositol 1,4,5-trisphosphate and calcium regulate the calcium channel function of the hepatic inositol 1,4,5-trisphosphate receptor. J Biol Chem 1997; 272(5):2675-2681.

73. Watras J, Bezprozvanny I, Ehrlich B. Inositol 1,4,5-trisphosphate-gated channels in cerebellum: Presence of multiple conductance states. J Neurosci 1991; 11:3239-3245.

74. Jiang QX, Thrower EC, Chester DW et al. Three-dimensional structure of the type 1 inositol 1,4,5-trisphosphate receptor at 24° a resolution. EMBO J 2002; 21:3575-3581.

75. Tang Y, Stephenson JL, Othmer HG. Simplification and analysis of models of calcium dynamics based on IP3-sensitive calcium channel kinetics. Biophys J 1996; 70(1):246-263.

76. Bezprozvanny I. Theoretical analysis of calcium wave propagation based on inositol (1,4,5)-trisphosphate (InsP3) receptor functional properties. Cell Calcium 1994; 16(3):151-166.

77. Li Y, Rinzel J. Equations for InsP3 receptor-mediated $[Ca^{2+}]_i$ oscillations derived from a detailed kinetic model: A Hodgkin-Huxley like formalism. J Theor Biol 1994; 166:461-473.

78. Falcke M. On the role of stochastic channel behavior in intracellular Ca^{2+} dynamics. Biophys J 2003; 84:42-56.

79. Thul R, Falcke M. Frequency of elemental events of intracellular calcium. Phys Rev E 2006; 73(6):61,923-61,924.

80. Marchant JS, Taylor CW. Rapid activation and partial inactivation of inositol trisphosphate receptors by inositol trisphosphate. Biochemistry 1998; 37(33):11,524-11,533.

81. Sneyd J, Dufour JF. A dynamic model of the type-2 inositol trisphosphate receptor. Proc Natl Acad Sci USA 2002; 99(4):2398-2403.

82. Dawson AP, Lea EJ, Irvine RF. Kinetic model of the inositol trisphosphate receptor that shows both steady-state and quantal patterns of Ca^{2+} release from intracellular stores. Biochem J 2003; 370:621-629.

83. Falcke M. Reading the pattern in living cells -the physics of Ca^{2+} signaling. Adv Phys 2004; 53:255-440.

84. Ullah G, Jung P. Modeling the statistics of elementary calcium release events. Biophys J 2006; 90(10):3485-3495.

85. Sachs F, Qin F, Palade P. Models of Ca^{2+} release channel adaptation. Science 1995; 267:2010-2011.

86. Atri A, Amundson J, Clapham D et al. A single pool model for intracellular calcium oscillations and waves in the Xenopus laevis oocyte. Biophys J 1993; 65:1727-1739.

87. Sneyd J, LeBeau A, Yule D. Traveling waves of calcium in pancreatic acinar cells: Model construction and bifurcation analysis. Physica D 2000; 145(1-2):158-179.

88. Mak DD, McBride SMJ, Foskett JK. Spontaneous channel activity of the inositol 1,4,5-trisphosphate (InsP3) receptor (InsP3R): Application of allosteric modeling to calcium and InsP3 regulation of InsP3R single-channel gating. J Gen Physiol 2003; 122(5):583-603.

89. Baran I. Gating mechanisms of the type-1 inositol trisphosphate receptor. Biophys J 2005; 89(2):979-998.

90. Sneyd J, Falcke M. Models of the inositol trisphosphate receptor. Prog Biophys Mol Biol 2005; 89(3):207-245.

91. Fabiato A. Two kinds of calcium-induced release of calcium from the sarcoplasmic reticulum of skinned cardiac cells. In: Frank GB, Bianchi CP, Keurs H, eds. Excitation-Contraction Coupling in Skeletal, Cardiac and Smooth Muscle, Advances in Experimental Medicine and Biology. New York: Springer, 1992:311:245-262.

92. Gyorke S, Fill M. Ryanodine receptor adaptation: Control mechanism of Ca^{2+}-induced Ca^{2+} release in heart. Science 1993; 260(5109):807-809.

93. Stern MD, Song LS, Cheng H et al. Local control models of cardiac excitation-contraction coupling: A possible role for allosteric interactions between ryanodine receptors. J Gen Physiol 1999; 113(3):469-489.

94. Tang Y, Othmer HG. A model of calcium dynamics in cardiac myocytes based on the kinetics of ryanodine-sensitive calcium channels. Biophys J 1994; 67(6):2223-2235.

95. Stern MD. Theory of excitation-contraction coupling in cardiac muscle. Biophys J 1992; 63(2):497-517.

96. Peskoff A, Langer G. Calcium concentration and movement in the ventricular cardiac cell during an excitation-contraction cycle. Biophys J 1998; 74(1):153-174.

97. Shannon TR, Wang F, Puglisi J et al. A mathematical treatment of integrated Ca dynamics within the ventricular myocyte. Biophys J 2004; 87(5):3351-3371.

98. Tanskanen AJ, Greenstein JL, Chen A et al. Protein geometry and placement in the cardiac dyad influence macroscopic properties of calcium-induced calcium release. Biophys J 2007; 92(10):3379-3396.

99. Segel IH. Biochemical Calculations. New York: John Wiley, 1976.

100. MacLennan DH, Rice WJ, Green NM. The mechanism of Ca^{2+} transport by sarco(endo)plasmic reticulum Ca^{2+}-ATPases. J Biol Chem 1997; 272(46):28,815-28,818.

101. Toyoshima C, Nakasako M, Nomura H et al. Crystal structure of the calcium pump of sarcoplasmic reticulum at 2.6° a resolution. Nature 2000; 405(6787):647-655.

102. Toyoshima C, Nomura H. Structural changes in the calcium pump accompanying the dissociation of calcium. Nature 2002; 418(6898):605-611.

103. Yano K, Petersen O, Tepikin AV. Dual sensitivity of sarcoplas-mic/endoplasmic Ca^{2+}-ATPase to cytosolic and endoplasmic reticulum Ca^{2+} as a mechanism of modulating cytosolic Ca^{2+} oscillations. Biochem J 2004; 15(383(Pt 2)):353-360.

104. Gunter TE, Pfeiffer DR. Mechanisms by which mitochondria transport calcium. Am J Physiol Cell Physiol 1990; 258(5):C755-786.
105. Jung DW, Baysal K, Brierley GP. The Sodium-Calcium antiport of heart mitochondria is not electroneutral. J Biol Chem 1995; 270(2):672-678.
106. Falcke M, Hudson JL, Camacho P et al. Impact of mitochondrial Ca^{2+} cycling on pattern formation and stability. Biophys J 1999; 77(1):37-44.
107. Falcke M, Li Y, Lechleiter JD et al. Modeling the dependence of the period of intracellular Ca^{2+} waves on SERCA expression. Biophys J 2003; 85(3):1474-1481.
108. Kirichok Y, Krapivinsky G, Clapham DE. The mitochondrial calcium uniporter is a highly selective ion channel. Nature 2004; 427:360.
109. Magnus G, Keizer J. Model of beta-cell mitochondrial calcium handling and electrical activity. II. Mitochondrial variables. Am J Physiol Cell Physiol 1998; 274(4):C1174-1184.
110. Magnus G, Keizer J. Model of beta-cell mitochondrial calcium handling and electrical activity. I. Cytoplasmic variables. American Am J Physiol Cell Physiol 1998; 274(4):C1158-1173.
111. Magnus G, Keizer J. Minimal model of beta-cell mitochondrial Ca^{2+} handling. American Am J Physiol Cell Physiol 1997; 273(2):C717-733.
112. Keener J, Sneyd J. Mathematical Physiology. New York: Springer, 1998.
113. Lindner B, García-Ojalvo J, Neiman A et al. Effects of noise in excitable systems. Phys Rep 2004; 392:321-424.
114. FitzHugh R. Impulses and physiological states in theoretical models of nerve membrane. Biophys J 1961; 1(6):445-466.
115. Nagumo J, Arimoto S, Yoshizawa S. An active pulse transmission line simulating nerve axon. Proc IRE Inst Rad Eng 1962; 50(10):2061-2070.
116. Marchant J, Parker I. Role of elementary Ca^{2+} puffs in generating repetitive Ca^{2+} oscillations. EMBO J 2001; 20:65-76.
117. Keizer J, Smith GD, Ponce-Dawson S et al. Saltatory propagation of Ca^{2+} waves by Ca^{2+} sparks. Biophys J 1998; 75(2):595-600.
118. Pearson JE, Ponce-Dawson S. Crisis on skid row. Physica A 1998; 257(1-4):141-148.
119. Dawson SP, Keizer J, Pearson JE. Fire-diffuse-fire model of dynamics of intracellular calcium waves. Proc Natl Acad Sci USA 1999; 96(11):6060-6063.
120. Coombes S. The effect of ion pumps on the speed of travelling waves in the fire-diffuse-fire model of Ca^{2+} release. Bull Math Biol 2001; 63(1):1-20.
121. Murray JD. Mathematical Biology. Berlin: Springer, 2004.
122. Olveczky BP, Verkman AS. Monte Carlo analysis of obstructed diffusion in three dimensions: Application to molecular diffusion in organelles. Biophys J 1998; 74(5):2722-2730.
123. Keller M, Kao JPY, Egger M et al. Calcium waves driven by "sensitization" wave-fronts. Cardiovas Res 2007; 74(1):39-45
124. Thul R, Smith GD, Coombes S. A bidomain threshold model of intracellular calcium release and propagating calcium waves. J Math Biol 2007, 56(4):435-63.
125. Stricker SA. Repetitive calcium waves induced by fertilization in the nemertean worm Cerebratulus lacteus. Dev Biol 1996; 176(2):243-263.
126. Yoshida M, Sensui N, Inoue T et al. Role of two series of Ca^{2+} oscillations in activation of ascidian eggs. Dev Biol 1998; 203(1):122-133.
127. Li YX. Tango waves in a bidomain model of fertilization calcium waves. Physica D 2004; 186:27-49.
128. Hille B. Ion Channels of Excitable Membranes. 3rd ed. Sunderland: Sinauer Assoicates, 2001.
129. Coombes S, Hinch R, Timofeeva Y. Receptors, sparks and waves in a fire-diffuse-fire framework for calcium release. Prog Biophys Mol Biol 2004; 85:197-219.
130. Coombes S, Timofeeva Y. Sparks and waves in a stochastic fire-diffuse-fire model of Ca^{2+} release. Phys Rev 2003; E68:021,915-1-8.
131. Keener J. Stochastic calcium oscillations. Math Med Biol 2006; 23:1-25.
132. Hodgkin AL, Huxley AF. A quantitative description of membrane current and its application to conduction and excitation in nerve. Am J Physiol 1952; 177(4):500-544.
133. Fox RF, Lu YN. Emergent collective behavior in large numbers of globally coupled independently stochastic ion channels. Phys Rev E 1994; 49(4):3421-3431.
134. Marchant JS, Ramos V, Parker I. Structural and functional relationships between Ca^{2+} puffs and mitochondria in Xenopus oocytes. American Am J Physiol Cell Physiol 2002; 282:C1374-1386.
135. Swillens S, Dupont G, Combettes L et al. From calcium blips to calcium puffs: Theoretical analysis of the requirements for interchannel communication. Proc Natl Acad Sci USA 1999; 96:13,750-13,755.
136. Shuai J, Rose HJ, Parker I. The number and spatial distribution of IP_3 receptors underlying calcium puffs in Xenopus oocytes. Biophys J 2006; 91(11):4033-4044, (DOI 10.1529/biophysj.106.088880).

137. Franzini-Armstrong C. The sarcoplasmic reticulum and the control of muscle contraction. FASEB J 1999; 13(9002):266S-270.
138. Yin CC, Lai FA. Intrinsic lattice formation by the ryanodine receptor calcium-release channel. Nat Cell Biol 2000; 2(9):669-671.
139. Hu XF, Liang X, Chen KY et al. Modulation of the oligomerization of isolated ryanodine receptors by their functional states. Biophys J 2005; 89(3):1692-1699.
140. Machaca K. Increased sensitivity and clustering of elementary Ca^{2+} release events during oocyte maturation. Dev Biol 2004; 275(1):170-182.
141. Bootman M, Niggli E, Berridge M et al. Imaging the hierarchical Ca^{2+} signalling system in HeLa cells. Am J Physiol 1997; 499(Pt 2):307-314.
142. Sun X, Callamaras N, Marchant J et al. A continuum of InsP3 mediated elementary Ca^{2+} signalling events in Xenopus oocytes. Am J Physiol 1998; 509:67-80.
143. Callamaras N, Marchant JS, Sun XP et al. Activation and coordination of InsP3-mediated elementary Ca^{2+} events during global Ca^{2+} signals in Xenopus oocytes. Am J Physiol 1998; 509(1):81-91.
144. Marchant J, Callamaras N, Parker I. Initiation of IP$_3$-mediated Ca^{2+} waves in Xenopus oocytes. EMBO J 1999; 18:5285-5299.
145. Gardiner C. Handbook of Stochastic Methods. 3rd ed. Berlin: Springer, 2004.
146. van Kampen N. Stochastic Processes in Physics and Chemistry. Amsterdam: North-Holland, 2001.
147. Risken H. The Fokker-Planck Equation. Berlin: Springer, 1984.
148. Gitterman M, Weiss G. Some comments on approximations to the master equation. Physica A 1991; 170:503-510.
149. Kramers H. Brownian motion in a field of force and the diffusion model of chemical reactions. Physica 1940; 7:284-304.
150. Moyal J. Stochastic processes and statistical physics. J R Stat Soc [Ser B] 1949; 11:150-210.
151. Schimansky-Geier L, Talkner P. Tools of stochastic dynamics. In: Ebeling W, Schimansky-Geier L, Romanovsky YM, eds. Stochastic Dynamics of Reacting Biomolecules. Hackensack: World Scientific, 2003.
152. Shuai JW, Jung P. Stochastic properties of Ca^{2+} release of inositol 1,4,5-trisphosphate receptor clusters. Biophys J 2002; 83(1):87-97.
153. Jung P, Shuai J. Optimal sizes of ion channel clusters. Europhys Lett 2001; 56(1):29-35.
154. Shuai JW, Jung P. Optimal intracellular calcium signalling. Phys Rev Lett 2002; 88(6):068,102-1-4.
155. Meinhold L, Schimansky-Geier L. Analytic description of stochastic calcium-signaling periodicity. Phys Rev E 2002; 66(5):050,901.
156. Thul R, Falcke M. Release currents of IP$_3$ receptor channel clusters and concentration profiles. Biophys J 2004; 86:2660-2673.
157. Thul R, Falcke M. Stability of membrane bound reactions. Phys Rev Lett 2004; 93:188,103-1-4.
158. Thul R, Falcke M. Reactive clusters on a membrane. Phys Biol 2005; 2:51-59.
159. Bär M, Falcke M, Levine H et al. Discrete stochastic modeling of calcium channel dynamics. Phys Rev Lett 2000; 84:5664-5667.
160. Thul R, Falcke M. Waiting time distributions for clusters of complex molecules. Europhys Lett 2007; 79:38,003.

## CHAPTER 2

Oscillations by the p53-Mdm2 Feedback Loop

Galit Lahav*

Abstract

The p53 network is perhaps the most important pathway involved in preventing the initiation of cancer. p53 levels and activity are upregulated in response to various stresses including DNA damage, hypoxia, and oncogene activation. Active p53 initiates different transcriptional programs that result in cell cycle arrest, cellular senescence or apoptosis. p53 also activates the transcription of Mdm2, which in turns target p53 for degradation, therefore creating a negative feedback loop on p53. Previous studies showed that the level of p53 increased dramatically after exposure to damaging radiation, then declined in a series of damped oscillations. Recent quantitative studies examined p53 responses in individual living cells, using time-lapse fluorescent microscopy and showed that—on an individual cell level—the oscillations are not damped. Instead, one cell may have only one pulse of p53, while its neighbor may show several repeated pulses. As the amount of irradiation increased, the percentage of cells showing a high number of p53 pulses also increased. The mean height and width of the pulses was constant and did not depend on the damage level. These observations opened new questions regarding the mechanism and function of p53 oscillatory dynamics. In this chapter I will review the different models that have been suggested for p53 oscillations, including proposed reasons for variation between cells, and will discuss potential functions for oscillatory dynamics in the p53 signaling pathway and in stress responses in general.

Introduction

The tumor suppressor protein p53 is the protein most frequently inactivated in human cancer.[1] More than half of all human cancers contain mutations in the p53 gene, and in almost all cancers the p53 regulatory circuit is functionally inactivated.[2] The protein is known as the "guardian of the genome" because it is activated when cells are under stress. For example, when cells suffer DNA damage (as skin cells do when they are exposed to excessive radiation), both the level of p53 and its transcriptional activity are increased. This may cause the cell to delay DNA replication to give extra time to repair the DNA. Sometimes, however, p53 triggers a cell death pathway instead, preventing the chance that the damaged cell may later become cancerous. If p53 is not functional, the cell cycle might continue unrestrained, leading to uncontrolled cell proliferation and cancer.

Under normal, unstressed conditions p53 is kept at low levels, primarily through a mechanism in which the negative regulator Mdm2 targets p53 to degradation. Mdm2 is one of p53's target genes and thus any increase of p53 normally leads to an increase in Mdm2 levels, which

---

*Galit Lahav—Department of Systems Biology, Harvard Medical School, Boston, MA 02115, USA. Email: galit@hms.harvard.edu

Cellular Oscillatory Mechanisms, edited by Miguel Maroto and Nicholas A.M. Monk. ©2008 Landes Bioscience and Springer Science+Business Media.

then pushes p53 back down to a low steady state level. But in various stress conditions, upstream mediators are activated and induce post-translational modification on p53 and Mdm2. For example, DNA damage activates the protein kinases ATM, ATR, Chk1 and Chk2, which phosphorylate p53 and Mdm2. These modifications disrupt the p53-Mdm2 interaction, leading to stabilization of p53 and an increase in p53 transcriptional activity. p53 then activates several stress response programs including cell cycle arrest (both reversible and irreversible, such as senescence), DNA repair and programmed cell death (apoptosis)[2-4] (Fig. 1).

Double-strand breaks (DSBs) are an important type of DNA damage, which lead to stabilization and activation of p53. They are mainly caused by ionizing radiation and radio-mimetic chemicals, and can also occur by mechanical stress on chromosomes and during DNA replication. DSBs are repaired by two main mechanisms, homologous recombination and nonhomologous end-joining. In both cases, phosphorylation of histone H2AX is an early

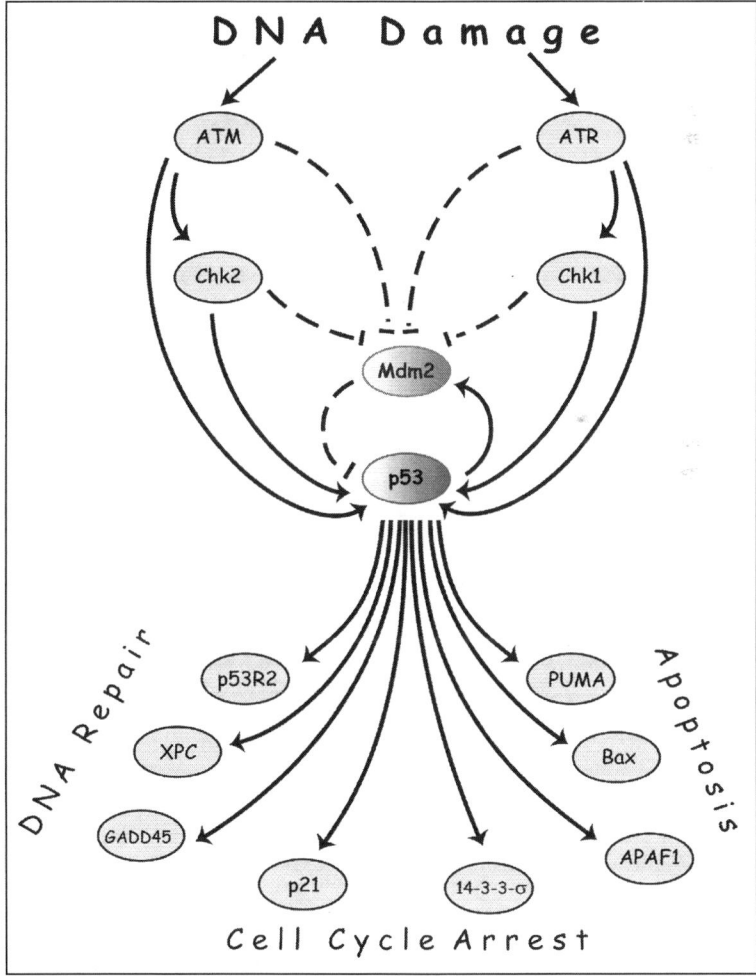

Figure 1. The p53 network. In response to DNA damage, ATM and ATR transfer the damage signal directly, and through Chk2/Chk1, to p53. p53 level and transcriptional activity increase, leading to activation of several programs including: cell cycle arrest, DNA repair and apoptosis.

event that leads to recruitment of the ATM (ataxia-telangiectasia mutated) protein, as well as other components of a sensor/repair pathway. DSBs induce rapid autophosphorylation of ATM, and increase ATM kinase activity.[5] Active ATM-P phosphorylates several substrates, including p53 and Mdm2, leading to disassociation of the p53-Mdm2 complex, and hence the stabilization of p53 and an increase in p53 protein levels. ATM also phosphorylates the checkpoint kinase Chk2, which directly phosphorylates p53 and Mdm2, further contributing to p53 stabilization.

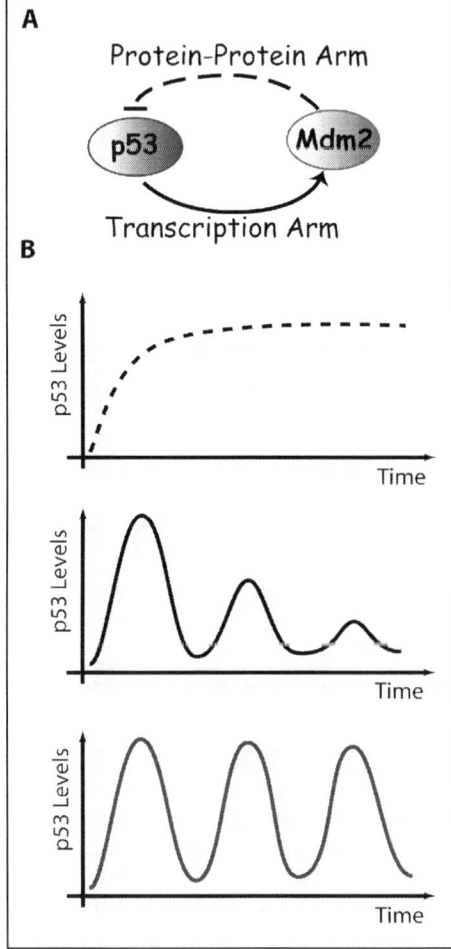

Figure 2. Negative feedback loops: structure and dynamics. A) p53-Mdm2 Negative feedback. p53 is a transcription factor that increases Mdm2 expression. Mdm2 is a E3 ligase protein that binds to p53, ubiquitinates it and targets it for degradation. B) Negative feedback loop dynamics. Negative feedback loops can give rise to a number of different behaviors depending on the relative values of feedback parameters; monotonic increase (top), damped oscillations (middle) or undamped/sustained (bottom) oscillations.

The p53-Mdm2 Negative Feedback Loop

The core regulatory circuit of p53 consists of p53 and the E3 ligase protein, Mdm2. p53 and Mdm2 form a negative feedback loop, in which p53 positively regulates Mdm2 by activating Mdm2 transcription,[6,7] and Mdm2 negatively regulates p53 by promoting its ubiquitination and degradation[8,9] (Fig. 2A). The main mechanism for p53 stabilization in response to stress signals is a reduction in its interaction with Mdm2, causing an increase in p53 levels.[10] This core negative feedback loop is embedded inside a network of additional interactions, many of which are well characterized.[11] For example, there are at least two additional target genes that create a negative feedback loop with p53: Cop1 and Pirh2.[12,13] Both are ubiquitin ligases that promote p53 ubiquitination and proteasomal degradation.

Negative feedback loops, such as that between p53 and Mdm2, are motifs found far more often than predicted by chance in biological networks.[14] The p53/Mdm2 loop is a hybrid, composed of interactions on two different timescales: a slow positive transcriptional arm and a fast negative protein-interaction arm (Fig. 2A). This type of loop can give rise to a number of different behaviors depending on the relative values of feedback parameters such as the rate at which the gene encoding the inhibitor is expressed, or the rate at which the inhibitor and the transcription factor form an inactive complex. A loop with the same logical structure can give rise to a monotonic increase in p53 levels in response to DNA damage, damped oscillations or undamped (sustained) oscillations. If the time delay between the increase in p53 and the increase in Mdm2 transcription is long, oscillatory behavior is expected.[15-18] If, on the other hand, the basal degradation rates of the proteins are high, this would tend to damp out the oscillations (Fig. 2B).

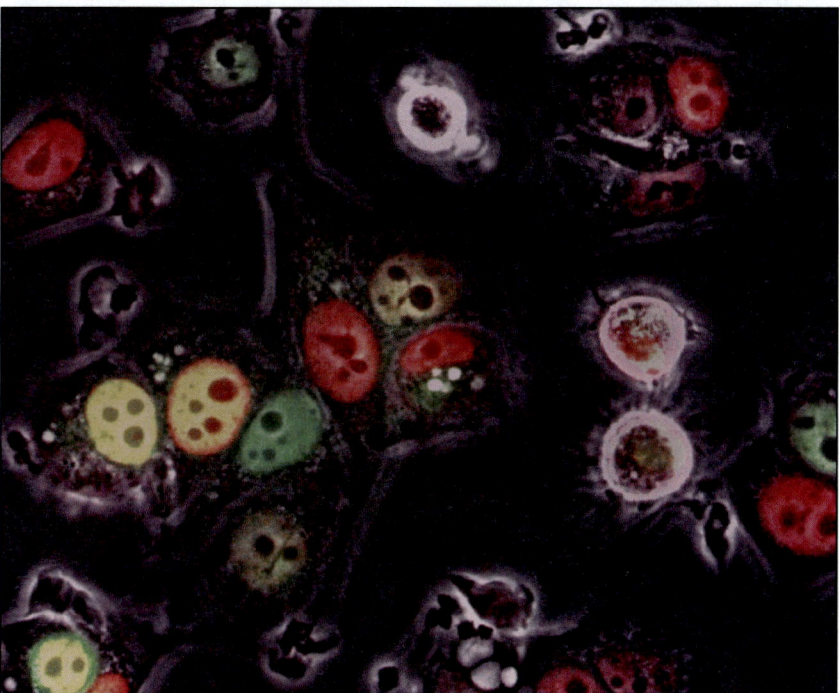

Figure 3. Variation between single cells. MCF7 breast cancer cells expressing p53-CFP (shown in green) and Mdm2-YFP (shown in red) 16h following 5Gy of γ-irradiation. Yellow represents coexpression of p53 and Mdm2.

Oscillations of p53 and Mdm2

Experimental studies in populations of cultured cells have shown that p53 and Mdm2 undergo oscillatory behavior following DNA damage caused by gamma irradiation. These oscillations appeared to be damped in assays that measure population averages.[19] The model proposed to explain these damped oscillations invoked a time delay between p53 activation and p53-dependent induction of Mdm2.[19] Later, a system for following p53 and Mdm2 dynamics in individual living cells was developed, using the MCF7 breast cancer cell line stably transfected with p53 fused to cyan fluorescent protein (p53-CFP), and Mdm2 fused to yellow fluorescent protein (Mdm2-YFP) (Fig. 3A). The p53-CFP fusion protein was active in causing apoptosis and trans-activating p53 downstream targets. The concentrations and dynamics of both fluorescently-tagged proteins were found in Western blots to reliably reproduce the dynamics of endogenous p53 and Mdm2 expressed by these cells.[20] Using time-lapse fluorescence microscopy to measure p53 levels in individual cells, it was found that p53 levels produce a series of pulses following DNA damage. Identical cells exposed to the same amount of damage show varying numbers of p53 pulses.[20] As the amount of irradiation increased, the percentage of cells showing a high number of p53 pulses also increased (Fig. 4A). The mean height and width of the pulses was constant, however, and did not depend on the damage level. In the population studies, the pulses in different cells were averaged together, giving an appearance of damped oscillations (Fig. 4B).

These findings suggest that the behavior of the p53 feedback loop can be thought as 'digital' as opposed to 'analog'. In analog circuits stronger input leads to higher and wider output. In contrast, in the p53-Mdm2 negative feedback, it is the number of p53 pulses, and not their amplitude and duration that depends on the level of input.

One remaining question is how relevant is this phenomenon to normal cells?[21] Recent in vivo studies have shown that the temporal dynamics of p53 activity following ionizing irradiation have a distinct oscillatory pattern, which confirm the oscillations seen in population and single cultured cells.[22]

The Mechanism of p53-Mdm2 Oscillations

Several mathematical models have been developed in an attempt to explain p53 oscillations. Because the behavior of even simple networks can be quite counter-intuitive, mathematical models can be useful in identifying areas where our understanding is incomplete. Undamped oscillations, like the ones seen in the p53-Mdm2 circuit, pose a challenge to modelers since the simplest models of this negative feedback loop show damped oscillations.[19] Most of the mathematical models that have been suggested to explain the dynamics of p53 in response to DNA damage aim to find a minimal way that could capture the characteristics of p53 undamped oscillations. Essentially, they all begin by examining a few core components of the process, including the basic feedback loop in which p53 transcriptionally activates Mdm2, and active Mdm2 increases the degradation rate of p53. Any of the suggested models can generate dynamics similar to the experimental data. However, they differ in mathematical details and require different ranges of parameters to fit the experimental data.

One type of model is the delay oscillator, which hypothesizes a time delay between up-regulation of p53 and the expression/maturation of Mdm2.[23-25] An expansion of this model was suggested recently by Ma et al (2005)[26] and Wagner et al (2005).[27] They suggest a model with three subsystems: a DNA damage repair module, a switch involving ATM, and the p53-Mdm2 oscillator. The oscillator subsystem also includes transcription and translational/translocation time delays to model the nuclear concentrations of Mdm2. In this model, ATM shows switch-like behavior in response to DNA damage and active ATM remains at maximal levels as long as the number of double strand breaks is above a certain threshold. Active ATM levels decay to zero once the number of breaks decreases below this threshold. The ATM module thus produces an on-off switching signal to the down stream oscillator. This model suggests

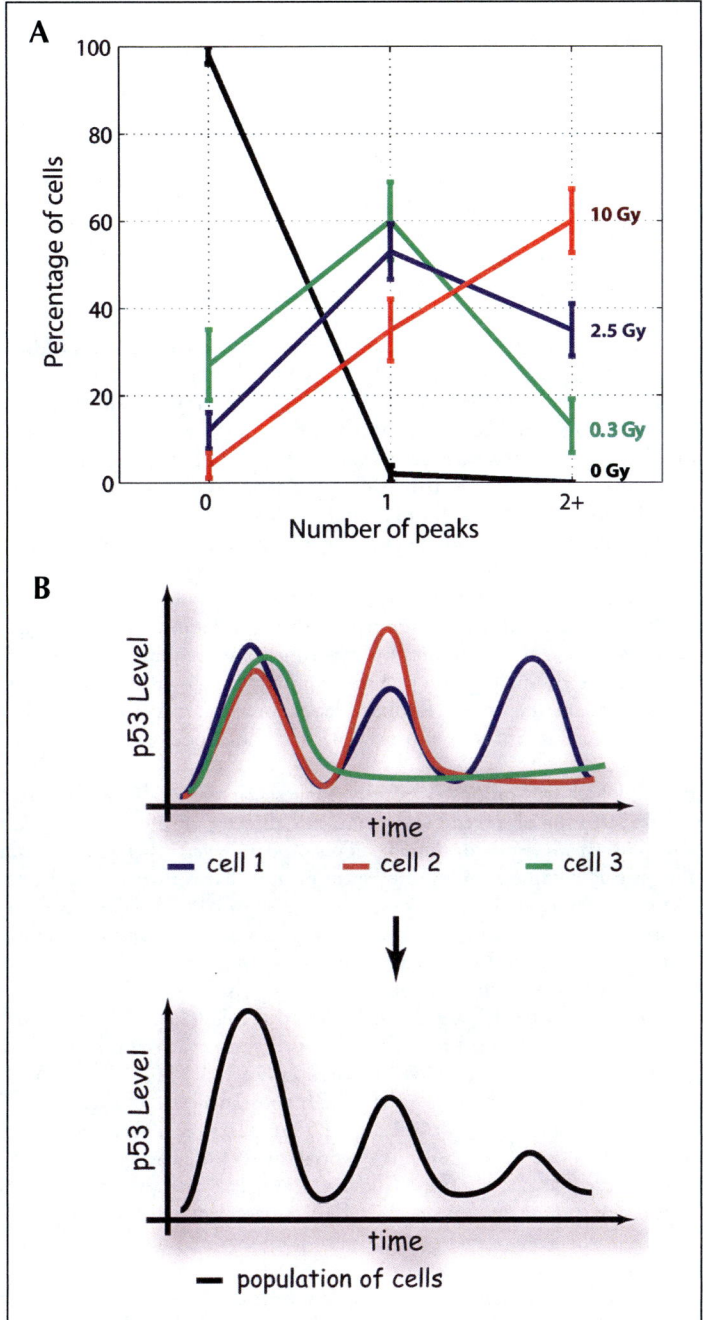

Figure 4. Single cell analysis of p53 oscillations. A) Fraction of cells with zero, one two or more pulses as a function of γ-irradiation dose. Taken from Lahav et al (2004).[20] B) Schematic diagram showing the differential p53 oscillations in individual cells. When studying populations of cells, the amplitude of the pulses is averaged, and damped oscillations are observed.

that the levels of active ATM-P should be high throughout the period when DNA damage is present, then actively switched off when the DNA is completely repaired.[26]

An alternative network structure that could explain the undamped oscillations invokes additional intermediate components for p53 and Mdm2, and an additional positive feedback loop on p53.[28] Combinations of negative and positive feedback loops are found in other biological systems that are known to produce oscillations, such as circadian clocks and the cell cycle oscillator. In the case of the cell cycle it was shown experimentally that positive feedback on Cdc2 activity is required to properly activate the negative feedback loop and that eliminating or shortening the positive feedback damped the oscillations of Cdc2 activity in Xenopus eggs extracts.[29] It is possible therefore that positive feedback loop(s) on p53, as was suggested in Ciliberto et al (2005)[28] are also essential for its oscillatory behavior.

There are several known positive feedbacks on p53 that might be crucial for its oscillatory behavior: one is via activation of PTEN, a target of p53 that down-regulates Mdm2 and thus prevents Mdm2 negative regulation of p53.[11,28,30] PTEN is not induced in MCF7 cells after gamma irradiation as was shown by us and others, implying that the positive feedback on p53 through PTEN is not active in MCF7 cells and therefore is not required for p53 oscillations. It is still possible, however, that feedback regulation through PTEN may operate via posttranslational modifications that do not require PTEN upregulation. Other known positive feedbacks on p53—through dapk1,[31] c-Ha-Ras[32] and DDR1[33]—involve the activation of p19ARF, which inhibits Mdm2. Since MCF7 cells do not have the ARF gene, it is unlikely that these loops are essential for the p53 oscillatory behavior that was observed in these cells. An additional potential positive feedback on p53 is through p21. p21 is a transcriptional target of p53 that inhibits the complex cyclinE-cdk2. This inhibition increases the formation of an Rb-Mdm2 complex that enhances activation of p53.[11] Additional experiments are required to determine whether this or other positive feedback loops on p53 are required for its oscillatory behavior; it is possible that one or more of the known feedback loops, or a so-far-unknown feedback loop is important in this behavior, but it is also possible that these loops are not connected to the oscillatory behavior.

A new model, which was proposed recently, suggests that a combination of two negative feedback loops explain the observed oscillations, one directly on p53 through Mdm2 and a longer one on an upstream regulator of p53.[34] This model suggests that a protein downstream of p53 inhibits the activity of a protein upstream of p53 that is involved in detecting DNA damage, and that the apparent oscillations are in fact repeated p53 pulses resulting from repeated examinations of the damaged DNA. This model explicitly considers the dynamics of elements upstream to p53 in the DNA damage signal response, and predicts that such elements (e.g., ATM-P or Chk2-P)[5,35-37] may also show repeated pulses.

There are at least two potential target genes of p53 that might be involved in the postulated feedback loop inhibiting up-regulators of p53. One is the protein cyclin G, which was shown to recruit protein phosphatase 2A (PP2A)[38] to dephosphorylate Mdm2 and ATM.[39,40] Breast cancer cells such as MCF7 are known to have high constant levels of cyclin G mRNA and protein in unstressed conditions,[41] yet still show p53 oscillations. This implies that the feedback involving cyclin G upregulation is not essential for p53 oscillations in MCF7 cells. The second candidate is the phosphatase Wip1 (PPM1D). Wip1 levels show a pulse during the first 6 hours in response to gamma irradiation,[42] a behavior that is predicted for the putative inhibitor. Wip1 is also a downstream target of p53. It is not known whether Wip1 directly interacts with ATM, but there is evidence that Wip1 can reverse the phosphorylation status of both p53[43] and Chk2.[44] In addition, the Ser1981 phosphorylation site in ATM-P is a strong candidate for a Wip1 target sequence, based on sequence homology.[44] These data are consistent with the notion that Wip1 may feed back on either or both of ATM and Chk2.

Additional experiments together with repeated iterative simulation and model-building are required to test the validity of any of these models, in order to have a clear comprehensive picture that robustly explains p53 oscillations.

Variability in the Response of Individual Cells

Two types of variability in the p53 pulses in individual cells can be observed: one is in the number of pulses, the other in the shape of each pulse (both amplitude and duration). A plausible hypothesis for variation in the number of p53 pulses is that it may be determined by the variable number of double-strand breaks (DSBs) in the DNA of each cell. Cells with many DSBs might oscillate for longer, as they try again and again to repair their DNA. If this is the case, the number of p53 pulses would correlate with the amount of DNA damage an individual cell has suffered, and the variable number of pulses would offer a potential mechanism for "counting" the number of attempts a cell has made to repair damage.

The canonical marker for double strand breaks is phosphorylated H2AX (γ-H2AX) which binds to the sites of damage. Clear foci of γ-H2AX, which are thought to represent individual DNA breaks, can be detected with antibody staining. The variation in the number of foci seen after damage[45] is consistent with the hypothesis that the difference in the number of p53 pulses seen in single cells may reflect a difference in the amount of DNA damage.

The variability in the shape of the oscillations appears to be mainly in the amplitude, while the duration is relatively constant. Detailed analysis revealed that these variations appear to stem from fluctuations in the protein production rates.[34] Although the cell populations studied are clonal, some of this variation may be due to cell-to-cell differences that are caused by the known genomic instability of cancer cells in culture.

The Potential Function of p53 Oscillations

Oscillations are found in diverse systems in biology such as the segmentation clock, cell cycle regulation and circadian rhythms. Since these cellular systems need to change in a cyclical pattern over time, it seems useful for them to have feedback parameters that give rise to oscillatory behavior. In the case of cellular stress, however, the need for oscillations is much less obvious. The first question to answer is whether the apparent oscillations are indeed oscillations, or repeated pulses that are individually and repetitively triggered.

If the p53 system does indeed oscillate, it is possible that the downstream effect of p53 activation is determined by the frequency of the oscillations. This is known to be the case for intracellular Ca^{2+} oscillations and for the pulsatile release of cyclic adenosine monophosphate (cAMP) signals in *Dictyostelium* amoebae. In addition, most hormones are secreted in a pulsatile rather than continuous manner, and the temporal pattern in which a hormone appears is often more important than its concentration. Changing the frequency of p53 oscillations and testing the effect of such changes on the expression of its target genes will help reveal whether this is also the case for the p53 system. An alternative explanation is that the oscillations may simply exist to allow DNA repair without the risk of irreversible consequences of continued excessive p53 levels.

If the apparent oscillations are instead repeatedly triggered individual pulses, their purpose might be more clear: in each p53 pulse the DNA repair machinery is launched and the interval between pulses is used to reevaluate the cell state by checking whether damage remains.[46]

In either case, it is possible that the number of pulses (or oscillations) may convey information. For example, the post-translational modifications on p53 may change over time as repeated pulses occur. Although gaps still exist in our knowledge regarding the role of many p53 posttranslational modifications, recent evidence showed that p53 carrying different modifications may selectively activate certain p53 target genes. For example, phosphorylation on Ser46 was found to be essential for activating transcription of genes in the apoptotic pathway, such as p53AIP1.[47-49] We do not know precisely what causes p53 to be modified in one way rather than another, but it is possible that the modifications integrate a variety of upstream signals. The importance of the pattern of modifications might offer a different explanation for the need for oscillations. After each pulse, if a decision to grow or die has not been made, the post-translational modifications may need to be erased. The modified p53 produced in the previous pulse is degraded, and new protein is synthesized from scratch in the next pulse.[46] A similar hypothesis may also explain the oscillatory dynamics observed in the NFκB-IκB feedback loop. Nelson et al showed recently that NF-κB protein trapped in the nucleus could no longer activate its target genes[50] probably because of dephosphorylation of NF-κB in the nucleus by protein phosphatase A2, or deacetylation by histone deacetylase 3. Thus, it appears that the export of NF-κB induced by IκBα is not in fact essential for turning off the transcriptional response, but instead is required to bring NF-κB back to the cytoplasm, where it can receive new signals.

Highly regulated oscillations with variable amplitude and precise timing were also recently found in the SOS DNA damage response in *E. coli.*[51] The presence of oscillations in this and the NFκB system suggest that oscillations (or repeated pulses) may play a general role in stress or damage responses. Further work is required to determine whether the unusual temporal dynamics of p53 after DNA damage have an important role and whether oscillations in general serve as a mechanism for integrating multiple signals over time.

One potential clue for the importance of oscillations comes from cells in which p53 oscillations are naturally modified. Recent studies showed that a single nucleotide polymorphism in the Mdm2 promoter (SNP309) leads to an increase in binding of the transcriptional activator Sp1, resulting in higher levels of Mdm2 RNA and protein.[52,53] SNP309 has been shown to be associated with accelerated tumor formation in humans and to cause defects in the activation of p53-dependent transcriptional programs.[52] Cell lines carrying SNP309 allow p53 up-regulation but do not show oscillations,[26] providing correlative evidence that the oscillations might be functionally important and possibly implying a role for p53 oscillations in preventing cancer.

Conclusion and Key Questions in the Field

The tumor suppressor p53 is perhaps one of the most intensely investigated proteins. Since its discovery in 1979, almost 40,000 papers have been published on this topic, and yet it can still surprise us. It is only recently that new technological developments have allowed detailed analysis of p53 kinetics in individual cells. The discovery that single cells vary in the number of p53 pulses show the limitations of population data in studying the dynamics of this system, and emphasize the importance of single cell studies to reveal protein behavior and connecting behavior to molecular mechanism.

The series of oscillations in the p53 system open several new questions in the field. For example, it is still unclear how p53 oscillations arise. Although several mathematical models have been suggested to explain p53's oscillatory behavior we are still far from having a comprehensive predictive picture of the mechanisms that generate these unusual dynamics. We also do not yet know how general this phenomenon may be—is it a consequence of changes that cell culture cells undergo, or do normal human cells, or uncultured cancer cells, also show periodic p53 pulses in response to DNA damage? Perhaps most importantly, it is still unknown what, if any, is the function of p53 oscillations and whether they play a role in elucidating the right cellular behavior in response to DNA damage. Even after a quarter century of study, p53 still has much to teach us.

Acknowledgements

I thank A. Loewer for help with illustration of figures and all the members of our laboratory for useful discussions. I acknowledge support from the Smith Family New Investigator Award Program—the Medical Foundation.

References

1. Levine AJ. p53, the cellular gatekeeper for growth and division. Cell 1997; 88(3):323-331.
2. Jin S, Levine AJ. The p53 functional circuit. J Cell Sci 2001; 114(Pt 23):4139-4140.
3. Vogelstein B, Lane D, Levine AJ. Surfing the p53 network. Nature 2000; 408(6810):307-310.
4. Hofseth LJ, Hussain SP, Harris CC. p53: 25 years after its discovery. Trends Pharmacol Sci 2004; 25(4):177-181.

5. Bakkenist CJ, Kastan MB. DNA damage activates ATM through intermolecular autophosphorylation and dimer dissociation. Nature 2003; 421(6922):499-506.
6. Barak Y, Juven T, Haffner R et al. Mdm2 expression is induced by wild type p53 activity. EMBO J 1993; 12(2):461-468.
7. Wu X, Bayle JH, Olson D et al. The p53-mdm-2 autoregulatory feedback loop. Genes Dev 1993; 7(7A):1126-1132.
8. Haupt Y, Maya R, Kazaz A et al. Mdm2 promotes the rapid degradation of p53. Nature 1997; 387(6630):296-299.
9. Kubbutat MH, Jones SN, Vousden KH. Regulation of p53 stability by Mdm2. Nature 1997; 387(6630):299-303.
10. Michael D, Oren M. The p53-Mdm2 module and the ubiquitin system. Semin Cancer Biol 2003; 13(1):49-58.
11. Harris SL, Levine AJ. The p53 pathway: Positive and negative feedback loops. Oncogene 2005; 24(17):2899-2908.
12. Dornan D, Wertz I, Shimizu H et al. The ubiquitin ligase COP1 is a critical negative regulator of p53. Nature 2004; 429(6987):86-92.
13. Leng RP, Lin Y, Ma W et al. Pirh2, a p53-induced ubiquitin-protein ligase, promotes p53 degradation. Cell 2003; 112(6):779-791.
14. Yeger-Lotem E, Sattath S, Kashtan N et al. Network motifs in integrated cellular networks of transcription-regulation and protein-protein interaction. Proc Natl Acad Sci USA 2004; 101(16):5934-5939.
15. Tyson JJ. Monitoring p53's pulse. Nat Genet 2004; 36(2):113-114.
16. Tyson JJ, Chen KC, Novak B. Sniffers, buzzers, toggles and blinkers: Dynamics of regulatory and signaling pathways in the cell. Curr Opin Cell Biol 2003; 15(2):221-231.
17. Nelson DE, Ihekwaba AEC, Elliott M et al. Oscillations in NF-{kappa}B signaling control the dynamics of gene expression. Science 2004; 306(5696):704-708.
18. Hoffmann A, Levchenko A, Scott ML et al. The IkB-NF-kB signaling module: Temporal control and selective gene activation. Science 2002; 298:1241-1245.
19. Lev Bar-Or R, Maya R, Segel LA et al. Generation of oscillations by the p53-Mdm2 feedback loop: A theoretical and experimental study. Proc Natl Acad Sci USA 2000; 97(21):11250-11255.
20. Lahav G, Rosenfeld N, Sigal A et al. Dynamics of the p53-Mdm2 feedback loop in individual cells. Nat Genet 2004; 36(2):147-150.
21. Tyson JJ. Another turn for p53. Mol Syst Biol 2006; 2:0032.
22. Hamstra DA, Bhojani MS, Griffin LB et al. Real-time evaluation of p53 oscillatory behavior in vivo using bioluminescent imaging. Cancer Res 2006; 66(15):7482-7489.
23. Mihalas GI, Simon Z, Balea G et al. Possible oscillatory behavior in p53-Mdm2 interaction computer simulation. Journal of Biological Systems 2000; 8:21-29.
24. Monk NAM. Oscillatory expression of Hes1, p53, and NF-κB driven by transcriptional time delays. Curr Biol 2003; 13(16):1409-1413.
25. Tiana G, Jensen MH, Sneppen K. Time delay is a key to apoptosis induction in the p53 network. European Physical Journal B 2002; 29:135-140.
26. Ma L, Wagner J, Rice JJ et al. A plausible model for the digital response of p53 to DNA damage. Proc Natl Acad Sci USA 2005; 102(40):14266-14271.
27. Wagner J, Ma L, Rice JJ et al. p53-Mdm2 loop controlled by a balance of its feedback strength and effective dampening using ATM and delayed feedback. IEEE Proc.-Syst Biol 2005; 152(3):109-118.
28. Ciliberto A, Novak B, Tyson JJ. Steady states and oscillations in the p53/Mdm2 network. Cell Cycle 2005; 4(3):488-493.
29. Pomerening JR, Kim SY, Ferrell Jr JE. Systems-level dissection of the cell-cycle oscillator: Bypassing positive feedback produces damped oscillations. Cell 2005; 122(4):565-578.
30. Mayo LD, Dixon JE, Durden DL et al. PTEN protects p53 from Mdm2 and sensitizes cancer cells to chemotherapy. J Biol Chem 2002; 277(7):5484-5489.
31. Martoriati A, Doumont G, Alcalay M et al. dapk1, encoding an activator of a p19ARF-p53-mediated apoptotic checkpoint, is a transcription target of p53. Oncogene 2005; 24(8):1461-1466.
32. Deguin-Chambon V, Vacher M, Jullien M et al. Direct transactivation of c-Ha-Ras gene by p53: Evidence for its involvement in p53 transactivation activity and p53-mediated apoptosis. Oncogene 2000; 19(51):5831-5841.
33. Ongusaha PP, Kim JI, Fang L et al. p53 induction and activation of DDR1 kinase counteract p53-mediated apoptosis and influence p53 regulation through a positive feedback loop. EMBO J 2003; 22(6):1289-1301.

34. Geva-Zatorsky N, Rosenfeld N, Itzkovitz S et al. Oscillations and variability in the p53 system. Molecular Systems Biology 2006; 2:E1-E13.
35. Canman CE, Lim DS, Cimprich KA et al. Activation of the ATM kinase by ionizing radiation and phosphorylation of p53. Science 1998; 281(5383):1677-1679.
36. Canman CE, Lim DS. The role of ATM in DNA damage responses and cancer. Oncogene 1998; 17(25):3301-3308.
37. Khosravi R, Maya R, Gottlieb T et al. Rapid ATM-dependent phosphorylation of MDM2 precedes p53 accumulation in response to DNA damage. Proc Natl Acad Sci USA 1999; 96(26):14973-14977.
38. Okamoto K, Kamibayashi C, Serrano M et al. p53-dependent association between cyclin G and the B' subunit of protein phosphatase 2A. Mol Cell Biol 1996; 16(11):6593-6602.
39. Ohtsuka T, Jensen MR, Kim HG et al. The negative role of cyclin G in ATM-dependent p53 activation. Oncogene 2004; 23(31):5405-5408.
40. Goodarzi AA, Jonnalagadda JC, Douglas P et al. Autophosphorylation of ataxia-telangiectasia mutated is regulated by protein phosphatase 2A. EMBO J 2004; 23(22):4451-4461.
41. Reimer CL, Borras AM, Kurdistani SK et al. Altered regulation of cyclin G in human breast cancer and its specific localization at replication foci in response to DNA damage in p53+/+ cells. J Biol Chem 1999; 274(16):11022-11029.
42. Fiscella M, Zhang H, Fan S et al. Wip1, a novel human protein phosphatase that is induced in response to ionizing radiation in a p53-dependent manner. Proc Natl Acad Sci USA 1997; 94(12):6048-6053.
43. Lu X, Nannenga B, Donehower LA. PPM1D dephosphorylates Chk1 and p53 and abrogates cell cycle checkpoints. Genes Dev 2005; 19(10):1162-1174.
44. Fujimoto H, Onishi N, Kato N et al. Regulation of the antioncogenic Chk2 kinase by the oncogenic Wip1 phosphatase. Cell Death Differ 2005.
45. Rothkamm K, Lobrich M. Evidence for a lack of DNA double-strand break repair in human cells exposed to very low X-ray doses. Proc Natl Acad Sci USA 2003; 100(9):5057-5062.
46. Lahav G. The strength of indecisiveness: Oscillatory behavior for better cell fate determination. Sci STKE 2004; 2004(264):pe55.
47. Komiyama S, Taniguchi S, Matsumoto Y et al. Potentiality of DNA-dependent protein kinase to phosphorylate Ser46 of human p53. Biochem Biophys Res Commun 2004; 323(3):816-822.
48. Oda K, Arakawa H, Tanaka T et al. p53AIP1, a potential mediator of p53-dependent apoptosis, and its regulation by Ser-46-phosphorylated p53. Cell 2000; 102(6):849-862.
49. Mayo LD, Seo YR, Jackson MW et al. Phosphorylation of human p53 at serine 46 determines promoter selection and whether apoptosis is attenuated or amplified. J Biol Chem 2005; 280(28):25953-25959.
50. Nelson DE, See V, Nelson G et al. Oscillations in transcription factor dynamics: A new way to control gene expression. Biochem Soc Trans 2004; 32(Pt 6):1090-1092.
51. Friedman N, Vardi S, Ronen M et al. Precise temporal modulation in the response of the SOS DNA repair network in individual bacteria. PLoS Biol 2005; 3(7):e238.
52. Bond GL, Hu W, Bond EE et al. A single nucleotide polymorphism in the MDM2 promoter attenuates the p53 tumor suppressor pathway and accelerates tumor formation in humans. Cell 2004; 119(5):591-602.
53. Bond GL, Hu W, Levine A. A single nucleotide polymorphism in the MDM2 gene: From a molecular and cellular explanation to clinical effect. Cancer Res 2005; 65(13):5481-5484.

cAMP Oscillations during Aggregation of *Dictyostelium*

William F. Loomis*

Abstract

For many years it has been known that developing cells of *Dictyostelium discoideum* show periodic surges as they aggregate. When it was discovered that the cells were responding chemotactically to cAMP gradients produced within the populations, experiments were carried out that demonstrated similar periodic changes in the concentration of extracellular cAMP. Moreover, homogenous populations of developed cells held in suspension could be shown to respond to cAMP by changes in cell shape. Such suspensions showed spontaneous oscillations in light scattering as well as cAMP levels as the result of entrainment of the cells. The molecular components necessary for the pulsatile release of cAMP were uncovered by analyzing the behavior of a large number of strains with defined mutations isolated from saturation mutagenic screens. Subsequent genetic and biochemical studies established the connections between a dozen proteins essential for spontaneous oscillations. Computer simulations of a molecular circuit based on these results showed that it is able to account for the temporal and quantitative aspects of the oscillatory system. The circuit also appears to be coupled to the construction and dismantling of the actin/myosin cortical layer that ensures that pseudopods are restricted to the anterior of cells during chemotaxis and that the cells do not back-track when the natural wave is behind them. Since the same molecular clock controls both signal production and signal response, these behaviors are always kept strictly in phase.

Introduction

Oscillations have been observed with a wide range of frequencies in different cell types. Neurons show periodicities in the millisecond range while circadian clocks show periodicities of about a day. Various mammalian cell types show periodicities in the range of a few minutes for the secretion of hormones.[1-3] The mechanisms underlying these oscillations depend on the time scale and the cell type, however, there are similarities to the molecular circuits that generate oscillations with similar periodicities. Many oscillations that occur every few minutes appear to be mediated in part by cAMP.[1,2,4]

cAMP is a ubiquitous second message in cells of bacteria, plants, yeast and animals. It is synthesized from ATP by adenylyl cyclase and hydrolyzed to 5'AMP by phosphodiesterases. In bacteria, cAMP activates the DNA binding protein CRP which regulates transcription of a large number of genes. In animal cells, cAMP activates the protein kinase, PKA, which phosphorylates a large number of proteins. In the social amoeba *Dictyostelium*, cAMP is not only a second message that activates PKA but also an extracellular chemoattractant that directs cellular

*William F. Loomis—Cell and Developmental Biology, University of California-San Diego, La Jolla, California 92093, USA. Email: wloomis@ucsd.edu

Cellular Oscillatory Mechanisms, edited by Miguel Maroto and Nicholas A.M. Monk.
©2008 Landes Bioscience and Springer Science+Business Media.

motility.[5,6] The high resolution genetic and biochemical techniques that can be applied to *Dictyostelium* have uncovered the molecular circuits that can account for the production and cellular responses to pulses of cAMP.[7-10] During the aggregation stage of development cAMP is produced in pulses and released into the environment where it can diffuse to neighboring cells. When cAMP binds to the the high affinity surface receptor CAR1, it triggers several signal transduction pathways one of which stimulates the adenylyl cyclase ACA while another inhibits the internal phosphodiesterase RegA.[7] cAMP accumulates rapidly and is released to relay the chemoattractant signal. The activity of adenylyl cyclase peaks about 3 minutes after ligand binding to CAR1 and then decreases resulting in oscillations in cAMP production that show a 7 minute periodicity.

Dictyostelium is a eukaryotic microorganism that diverged from the evolutionary line leading to mammals shortly after the divergence of plants.[11,12] It grows in the soil by ingesting bacteria and divides by binary fission. In the laboratory it can be grown in simple defined media with a generation time of about 8 hours generating gram quantities of homogenous cells for biochemical analyses. The fact that these cells can grow and develop equally well as haploids or diploids facilitates microbial genetic techniques to rapidly isolate rare recessive mutations from populations of millions of cells. When cells are collected from nutrient environments, washed and deposited on buffer-saturated surfaces, they initiate a developmental program that results in the formation of aggregates of about 10^5 cells in 10 hours, migrating slugs by 14 hours, and finished fruiting bodies by 24 hours. The fruiting bodies have stalks that are about 2 mm high topped by a ball of spores (Fig. 1).

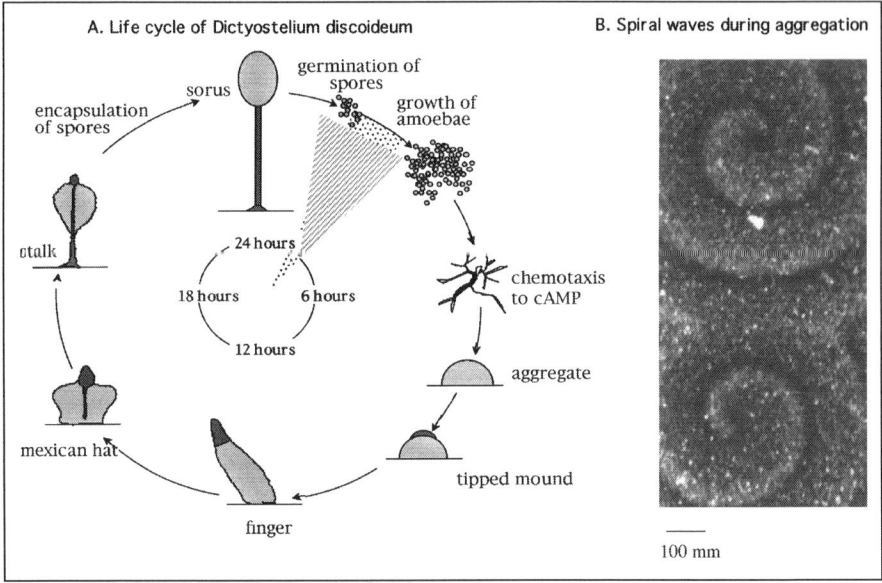

Figure 1. A) Schematic representation of the life cycle of *Dictyostelium discoideum*. Cells can grow for an indefinite period as long a there is a source of food. Upon starvation they initiate a developmental program that leads to the formation of fruiting bodies up to 2 mm high. B) Spiral waves in a chemoattractant field. About 6 hours after the initiation of development the cells become aggregation competent and signal each other with the chemoattractant molecule cAMP. Changes in cell shape in response to cAMP can be observed by dark field microscopy. There are approximately 10^6 cells in the field that are entrained by the pulses of cAMP emanating from the center and spreading as nondissipating spiral waves that mutually annihilate when they meet. Spirals rotate with a period of approximately 7 minutes.

During the first few hours following the initiation of development the cells express a dozen or so developmental genes that encode the components for extracellular signaling by cAMP. These include the receptor, CAR1, the adenylyl cyclase, ACA, the extracellular cAMP phosphodiesterase, PdsA, the Gα2 subunit of the trimeric G protein that mediates signaling from CAR1, and the MAP kinase ERK2.[13-15] Null mutations that knock out any of these genes result in strains that are unable to aggregate.[10] After about 4 hours the cells start to spontaneously release pulses of cAMP which rapidly entrain surrounding cells to release their own cAMP in phase. cAMP diffuses outward as nondissipating waves that become spirals when they encounter obstacles or nonresponding cells.[16] When cells are exposed to a wave of cAMP they not only relay the signal but also respond by modifying their cytoskeleton such that they round up and change their light scattering properties (Fig. 1). These spirals rotate with a period of about 7 minutes. A few hours after these waves first appear the cells start to move directionally towards high cAMP. They aggregate into streams that lead to mounds containing tens of thousands of cells. Pulses of cAMP continue to be released for a few hours but are then replaced by steady production of cAMP.

Proposed cAMP Oscillatory Circuit

Genes recovered from aggregateless strains that came out of saturation mutagenesis screens were cataloged as genes necessary for aggregation. As the list filled up it became apparent that simulations of the interactions of their products might account for the observed oscillations in cAMP accumulation. A successful model would generate spontaneous oscillations in cAMP with a periodicity of 7 minutes and a quantitative change in the range of 5 fold. It should also be able to account for the developmental stage at which spontaneous oscillations are observed. Critical variables could then be computationally explored.

We focused on those activities known to be controlled by cAMP or to interact with each other. It was clear that both ACA and ERK2 were activated when cAMP bound to CAR1.[10,17] ERK2 was found to inhibit the internal phosphodiesterase RegA leading to rapid accumulation of cAMP.[8,18] Most of the cAMP was secreted and slowly hydrolyzed on the outside by the secreted phosphodiesterase PdsA. The cAMP that was not secreted activated PKA which then indirectly led to the inactivation of both ACA and ERK2.[17] The connections in this circuit (Fig. 2) are all supported by biochemical studies in wild type cells as well as a wide range of mutant strains in which individual components were either missing or over-expressed. The kinetics of activation and inactivation of each component were calculated using a set of nonlinear interacting differential equations.[7,8] Parameters were set to account for the measured rate of activation of ACA, ERK2 and PKA. The remaining parameters were optimized to give rise to stable oscillations. A robust periodicity of 6 to 7 minutes was observed that did not change significantly even when individual parameters were varied 2 fold. The amplitude was affected but not the periodicity as has been observed in mutants with reduced ERK2 or RegA activities.[8,19] Only when several parameters were simultaneous changed was the periodicity affected.

Over 25 years ago Gunther Gerisch observed spontaneous oscillations in light scattering of populations of cells developing while suspended in buffer.[20,21] Since there were millions of cells in suspension that were synchronously changing their shape, it was clear that they had become entrained. When multiple cells are exposed to the external cAMP levels generated in the simulated circuit, they were found to rapidly become entrained such that they all produced cAMP at the same time.[7] Winfree[22] had predicted that cells with such oscillatory circuits will innately become synchronized if the cells interact in a common environment due to phase advancement and retardation. Gerisch found that cells in suspension had to develop for at least 3 hours before they would exhibit spontaneous oscillations and that the oscillations stopped after 7 hours of development. When the known changes in ACA and ERK2 during early development are incorporated into the circuit, the simulations captured this developmental pattern (Fig. 3). ACA activity increases at least 6 fold during the first 4 hours of development and does not produce sufficient cAMP to initiate the oscillations until 3 hours. The internal phosphodiesterase,

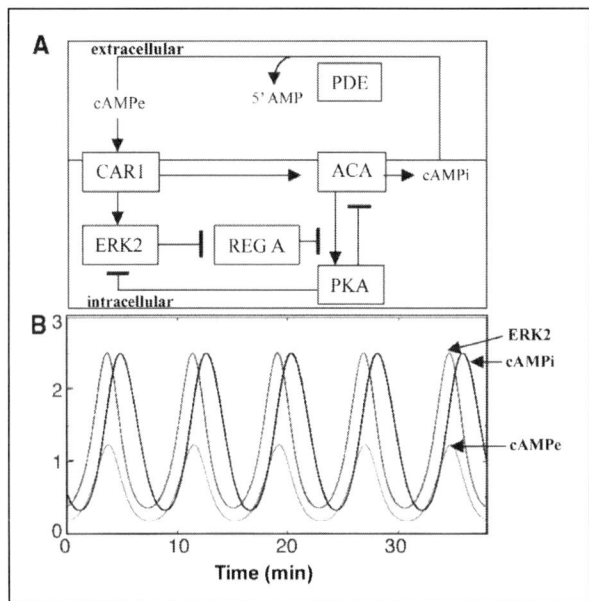

Figure 2. Proposed circuit and its output. A) cAMP accumulates as the result of activation of adenylyl cyclase (ACA) following ligand binding to the cAMP receptor CAR1 and the inhibition of the internal cAMP phosphodiesterase RegA by the MAP kinase ERK2 which is also activated following ligand binding to CAR1. Most of the cAMP is released into the extracellular space where it can stimulate adjacent cells before being broken down by the extracellular phosphodiesterase PDE. About 10% of the cAMP is retained in the cells where it can activate the cAMP dependent protein kinase PKA which indirectly inhibits both ERK2 and the stimulation of ACA activity. Phosphatases activate RegA which reduces the internal concentration of cAMP to reset the circuit. B) Using parameters that capture the kinetics at 4 hours of development, the circuit generates periodic changes in ERK2 activity and cAMP that closely mimic those observed in developing cells. (From Maeda et al, ref. 8.)

RegA, is subject to regulated turnover between 4 and 12 hours of development.[23] The circuit predicts that oscillations will stop when RegA activity decreases to 20% of peak activity.[8] Both the temporal and quantitative aspects of the measured oscillations were accurately predicted by the circuit giving considerable confidence that it includes the critical components and that the architecture is basically correct.

Intermediate steps that do not appear to be connected to the nodes were not included in the model because they just pass the signal along without modifying it. For instance, we know that ligand binding to CAR1 stimulates GTP exchange for GDP of the trimeric G protein containing $G\alpha2$ and the release of $G\beta\gamma$ which carries the signal to activation of ACA in a process dependent on CRAC, a PH-domain protein that binds to phosphatidyl (3,4,5) phosphate [PIP3] on the inner face of the cell membrane. Furthermore, it is likely that ligand binding to CAR1 activates an upstream component of a MAP kinase cascade rather than directly activating ERK2. However, it was not necessary to include these intermediate steps into the circuit for successful simulations. All of the activation steps in the circuit were considered to be zero-order in the component activated while all inactivating steps were considered first order in the component affect. Such first order inactivation would be expected when the substrate is limiting. This structure to the differential equations is essential to give the time lags necesssary to generate cAMP pulses.

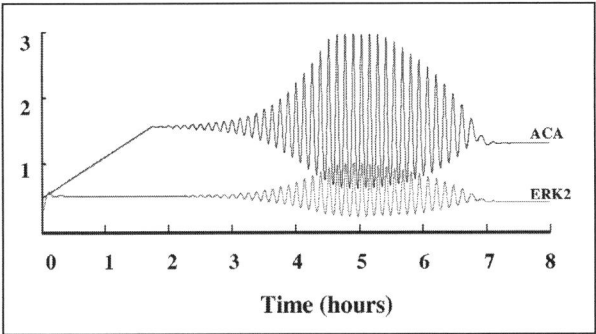

Figure 3. Developmental regulation. Spontaneous oscillations of ACA and activated ERK2 have been shown to occur only between 3 aned 7 hours of development (Gerisch et al, 1979; Maeda et al, 2004). ACA increases 6 fold during the first 4 hours of development while RegA activity decreases as the result of protein degradation. When these developmental parameters are entered into the circuit, spontaneous oscillations are limited to the developmental stage between 3 and 7 hours. (From Maeda et al, ref. 8.)

The fact that the model successfully captures the essential aspects of the observed spontaneous oscillations in cAMP and other components and can account for the transient occurance of oscillations during development suggests that most of the essential components are included and that the connections are physiologically relevant. The model has recently been used to successfully interpret the effects of the antipsychotic drugs, valproic acid and lithium, on early development of *Dictyostelium*.[24]

The model as presently implemented cannot account for the transient activation of adenylyl cyclase and ERK activity observed in cells exposed to constant saturating levels of cAMP. It is not written in kinetic terms and so cannot evaluate possible changes in the affinity of CAR1 for cAMP following activation as proposed in the model of Martiel and Goldbeter.[9] Moreover, adaptation may involve components not included in the present model such as a delayed pathway involving Gα9 or the activity of PI3 kinase that generates PIP3.[25,26] In any case, adaptation is not essential to account for the oscillations during natural waves.

Periodic Motility

Many eukaryotic cells move on a substratum by a crawling process that consists of a succession of events: cells extend an F-actin rich leading pseudopod, attach it to the substratum, and then retract the posterior in a process dependent on filamentous myosin in the cortex.[10,27] Lateral pseudopods are restricted by the cortical layer of actin/myosin that underlies the basolateral surfaces. *Dictyostelium* cells can translocate rapidly, moving about one cell length every minute, which permits high resolution analyses to be carried out using computer assisted motion analysis.[28-30] In response to periodic waves, aggregation competent cells move forward during the rising phase of the cAMP signal. At the peak of the cAMP signal, when the concentration is no longer increasing, the cells aburptly slow down. As the wave moves outward and decreases, the gradient is reversed. There is no net movement during the decreasing phase of the wave and the cells only form small pseudopods in random directions (Figs. 4, 5). As a result, the instantaneous rate of motility in natural waves shows a periodicity of 7 minutes coupled to the periodicity of cAMP release.

Somewhat surprisingly, loss of any of the components of the oscillatory circuit not only preclude the periodic production of cAMP pulses but also result in the inability of the cells to respond to natural waves produced by a surrounding population of wild type cells.[30-32] Cells lacking either RegA or ACA do not produce a leading pseudopod and dither around

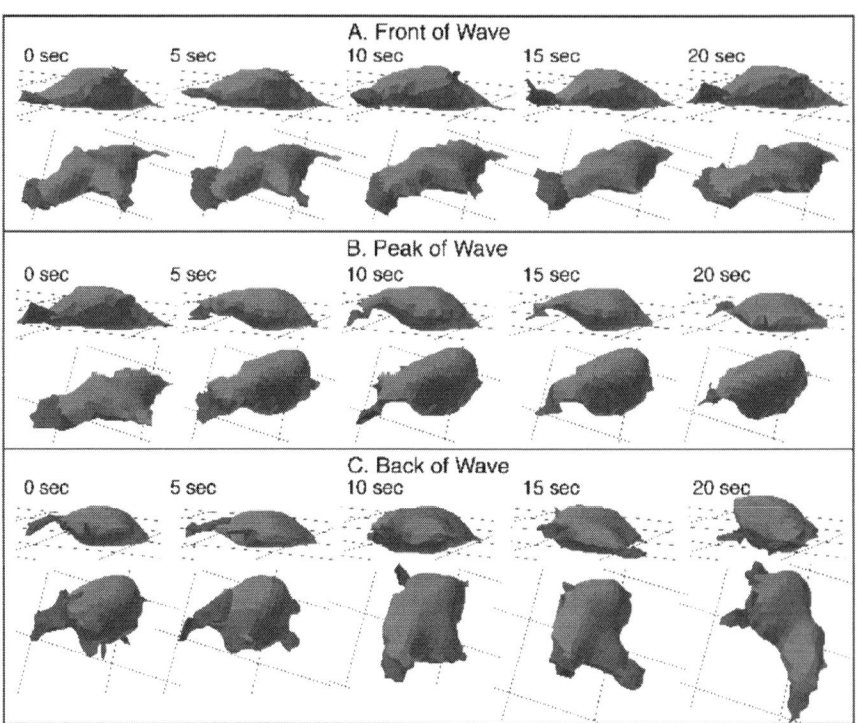

Figure 4. Responses to a wave of cAMP. Developing AX4 cells were given with a wave of cAMP that increased and decrease over a period of 7 minutes. As the cells migrated to the left, they were photographed through a confocal microscope and their shapes later reconstructed by 3D-DIAS.[32] The cell is shown at 15° and 60° from the surface as the cAMP started to increase, at the peak of cAMP at 3.5 minutes, and as the cAMP was decreasing. Nonparticulate pseudopods are darkened. (From Zhang et al,[32] with permission from the American Society for Microbiology.)

putting out small pseudopods in random directions. It is surprising that these mutant strains have almost exactly the same defects in chemotactic motility as each other since internal cAMP is high in one (*regA*⁻) and low in the other (*acaA*⁻). However, if the construction and dismantling of the cortical layer requires oscillations in internal cAMP, then the common phenotype could be explained.[31] Support for such a mechanism is based on the consequences to phosphorylation of myosin heavy chain II (MHCII). Unphosphorylated MHCII forms filaments in the cortex which dissociate when they are phosphorylated by myosin heavy chain kinases.[33] The myosin filaments associate with F-actin to form the rigid layer that precludes pseudopod formation along the sides and back of chemotaxing cells. The cortical layer is constructed during the rising phase of a natural wave and dismantled in the back of the wave. This periodic change in the cytoskeleton appears to be mediated by the oscillations in the internal concentration of cAMP.

Heid et al[34] were able to show that oscillations in phosphorylation of MHCII were critical to chemotactic movement. They studied *mhcA*⁻ cells lacking endogenous myosin heavy chain that were transformed with constructs such that the cells express modified MHC II in which the threonine moities that are phosphorylated (1823, 1833 and 2029) are replaced with either alanine or aspartate. The 3XALA protein cannot be phosphorylated while the 3XASP protein mimics the phosphorylated form of MHC II. Cells expressing either the

3XALA or the 3XASP replacement of MHC II could not stream to form aggregates even when developed in mixed populations with wild type cells. F-actin normally increases in the cortex of wild type cells during the first phase of a temporal wave when the cAMP is increasing and then returns to the cytoplasm. However, in both 3XALA and 3XASP cells there is little or no increase in F-actin in the cortex.[34] It appears that MHC II must cycle between phosphorylated and unphosphorylated forms to bring F-actin to the cortex. Unphosphorylated myosin may bind F-actin in the cytoplasm and form a cortical layer by polymerizing with other myosin chains. When MHC II is phosphorylated it dissociates from the cortex and returns to the cytoplasm where it is dephosphorylated. In the 3XALA cells the myosin cannot be phosphorylated and remains in the cortex where it may interfere with F-actin localization. However, the fact that F-actin does not become membrane associated in the front of a wave in 3XASP cells where the MHC II does not form a cortex, argues against a simple physical barrier to actin assembly. Periodic recruitment of F-actin to the cortex appears to depend upon the dephosphorylation of MHC rather than just unphosphorylated MHC. Therefore, to generate a cortex that can limit the formation of lateral pseudopodia, it is necessary to have oscillation in MHC II phosphorylation and dephosphorylation.

One of the components of the oscillatory signaling circuit is PKA, which is activated when internal cAMP rises. PKA activity may lead to activation of other kinases or phosphatases that affect the phosphorylation state of MHC II. We determined the chemotactic properties of cells with constitutive PKA activity as the result of a null mutation in the regulatory subunit.[32] *pkaR* mutant cells were found to be defective in chemotaxis and failed to respond to natural waves when incubated in a predominantly wild type aggregation field. Moreover, when the mutant cells made up the great majority of the population, wild type cells failed to show any organized chemotactic response indicating that the *pkaR* cells also failed to generate pulses of cAMP.

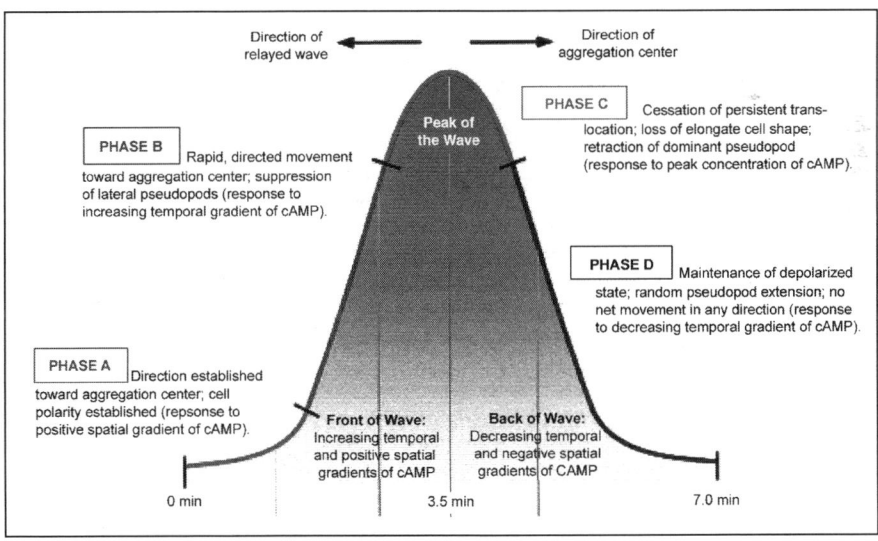

Figure 5. Phases of a natural wave. The direction of the gradient of cAMP is determined in the first minute when cAMP begins to increase. The cells orient their anterior pseudopod and move towards the high point for several minutes. When the concentration of cAMP no longer continues to increase, cells round up and cease moving. In the back of the wave, the cells extend multiple small pseudopods in random directions and show no net movement. The cortical layer is dismantled and the cells are ready to respond to the next wave. (From Zhang et al,[32] with permission from the American Society for Microbiology.)

In spatial gradients, constitutive PKA mutant cells put out twice as many lateral pseudo-pods as wild type cells and turn more frequently. Three dimensional computer asssisted reconstructions of cells in the front of a temporal wave showed that the dominant pseudo-pods were often off the substratum, waving in the buffer, accounting for the failure of the PKA mutant cells to show periodic changes in instantaneous velocity in phase with the changes in cAMP concentration.[32] Moreover, the cells are ovoid as are cells completely lacking MHC II as the result of deletion of the structural gene *mhcA*. Usually PKA reaches highest activity just after adenylyl cyclase reaches its highest activity near the peak of the wave.[7,35] In the *pkaR* mutant cells PKA activity is essentially constant. Maximum PKA activation may be necessary to dismantle polarity at the peak of the wave and allow the cells to round up.[32] The PKA mutants are always round.

Discussion

Oscillations in the time scale of minutes are often mediated by reversible enzymatic modi fications of critical components. The circuit that underlies the periodic release of cAMP pulses in *Dictyostelium* relies heavily on phosphorylation and dephosphorylation although periodic activation of PKA by changes in the internal cAMP is a central step.[7,8] PKA appears to be responsible for inhibition of the activity of ERK2 as well as attenuating the activation of adenylyl cyclase. The effects on ACA may result from PKA activity acting on any of the steps leading from CAR1 to ACA although it is unlikely to affect the subunits of the trimeric G protein.[36] Alternatively, PKA could indirectly affect ACA itself to reduce its activity.

Oscillation in PKA activity may also be indirectly coupled to the construction and disman-tling of the actin/myosin cortical layer that is essential for efficient chemotaxis. Coupling the response to the same oscillatory circuit that controls periodic release of cAMP ensures that the two processes are always in phase. If cAMP production and motility were out of phase, cells might back-track when the wave of cAMP had passed over them and the cAMP signal was being produced by cells further out from the aggregation center. PKA activity might directly or indirectly activate MHC kinases leading to the dismantling of the cortical layer in the back of the wave such that cells cannot translocate when the gradient is reversed but put out lateral pseudopods in all directions. MHCII is dephosphorylated in the cytoplasm and can then form filaments in the cortex when the next wave arrives. Recruitment of F-actin from the cytoplasm to the cortex appears to depend on the formation of new myosin filaments thereby insuring the coordinate construction of an actin/myosin layer that can direct pseudopods to the anterior.

While oscillatory signaling and responses have been far better characterized in *Dictyostelium* than other cells, there is compeling evidence that polymorphonuclear leukocytes respond in an almost identical manner to waves of chemoattractant.[37] These white blood cells move over long distances to sites of inflammation and infection. In a spatial gradient of the peptide fMLP, they move at the same rate as *Dictyostelium* cells and show excellent chemotactic directionality by suppressing lateral pseudopods. In a series of temporal waves in which the concentration of fMLP oscillated between 10^{-9}M and 10^{-7}M with a 7 minute periodicity the leukocytes showed oscillations in the instantaneous velocity similar to those of *Dictyostelium* cells exposed to tem-poral waves of cAMP. During the rising phase of each wave, they translocated more rapidly because of the suppression of lateral pseudopods. At the peak of each wave, motility decreased as the anterior psuedopod was retracted. And during the back of the wave, motility returned to basal levels as the result of extending many small lateral pseudopods.[37] These cells appear to have all the machinery to read a temporal gradient. While it is unlikely that leukocytes them-selves generate waves of chemoattractant as *Dictyostelium* cells do, there is preliminary evidence for production of nondissipating periodic waves of chemoattractant in surrounding cells (David Soll, personal communication).

Oscillatory processes have an innate resiliance to perturbation as the result of their susceptability to phase advancement and phase retardation by signals emanating from other cells in the network. The advantage for *Dictyostelium* appears to be coordinated production of cAMP as well as integrated relay of the signal over long distances. This mechanism increases the local concentration of cAMP by summing the output of multiple cells such that it is likely to be above threshold in populations over a wide range of cell densities.[38] Similar advantages may accrue from pulsatile production of hormones in metazoa.

Acknowledgements

I thank Drs. Adam Kuspa, Michael Laub, Gad Shaulsky and David Soll for many discussions of oscillations over the years. This review benefited from discussions during a symposium supported by the NSF at the Aspen Center for Physics. Recent work in my laboratory has been supported by NIH (GM60447 and GM62350).

References

1. Dyachok O, Isakov Y, Sagetorp J et al. Oscillations of cyclic AMP in hormone-stimulated insulin-secreting beta-cells. Nature 2006; 439:349-352.
2. Navarro C, Saeed S, Murdock C et al. Regulation of cyclic adenosine 3',5'-monophosphate signaling and pulsatile neurosecretion by Gi-coupled plasma membrane estrogen receptors in immortalized gonadotrophin-releasing hormone neurons. Mol Endocrinol 2003; 17:1792-1804.
3. Wetsel W, Valenca M, Merchenthaler I et al. Intrinsic pulsatile secretory activity of immortalized luteinizing hormone-releasing hormone-secreting neurons. Proc Natl Acad Sci 1992; 89:4149-4153.
4. Baillie G, MacKenzie S, Houslay M. Phorbol 12-myristate 13-acetate triggers the protein kinase A-mediated phosphorylation and activation of the PDE4D5 cAMP phosphodiesterase in human aortic smooth muscle cells through a route involving extracellular signal regulated kinase (ERK). Mol Pharmacol 2001; 60:1100-1111.
5. Konijn TM, van de Meene JGC, Bonner JT et al. The acrasin activity of adenosine-3',5'-cyclic phosphate. Proc Natl Acad Sci USA 1967; 58:1152-1154.
6. Loomis WF. Role of PKA in the timing of developmental events in Dictyostelium cells. Microbiol Mol Biol Rev 1998; 62:684.
7. Laub MT, Loomis WF. A molecular network that produces spontaneous oscillations in excitable cells of Dictyostelium. Mol Biol Cell 1998; 9:3521-3532.
8. Maeda M, Lu SJ, Shaulsky G et al. Periodic signaling controlled by an oscillatory circuit that includes protein kinases ERK2 and PKA. Science 2004; 304:875-878.
9. Martiel JL, Goldbeter A. A model based on receptor desensitization for cyclic AMP signaling in Dictyostelium cells. Biophys J 1987; 52:807-828.
10. Parent CA, Devreotes PN. Molecular genetics of signal transduction in Dictyostelium. Annu Rev Biochem 1996; 65:411-440.
11. Loomis WF, Smith DW. Molecular phylogeny of Dictyostelium dscoideum by protein sequence comparison. Proc Natl Acad Sci USA 1990; 87:9093-9097.
12. Song J, Olsen R, Loomis WF et al. Comparing the Dictyostelium and Entamoeba genomes reveals an ancient split in the Conosa lineage. PLoS Comput Biol 2005; 1:579-584.
13. Iranfar N, Fuller D, Loomis WF. Genome-wide expression analyses of gene regulation during early development of Dictyostelium discoideum. Euk Cell 2003; 2:664-670.
14. Kumagai A, Hadwiger JA, Pupillo M et al. Molecular genetic analysis of two Galpha protein subunits in Dictyostelium. J Biol Chem 1991; 266:1220-1228.
15. Segall JE, Kuspa A, Shaulsky G et al. A MAP kinase necessary for receptor-mediated activation of adenylyl cyclase in Dictyostelium. J Cell Biol 1995; 128:405-413.
16. Levine H, Aranson I, Tsimring L et al. Positive genetic feedback governs cAMP spiral wave formation in Dictyostelium. Proc Natl Acad Sci USA 1996; 93:6382-6386.
17. Aubry L, Maeda M, Insall R et al. The Dictyostelium mitogen-activated protein kinase ERK2 is regulated by ras and cAMP-dependent protein kinase (PKA) and mediates PKA function. J Biol Chem 1997; 272:3883-3886.
18. Shaulsky G, Fuller D, Loomis WF. A cAMP-phosphodiesterase controls PKA-dependent differentiation. Development 1998; 125:691-699.
19. Sawai S, Thomason PA, Cox EC. An autoregulatory circuit for long-range self-organization in Dictyostelium cell populations. Nature 2005; 433:323-326.
20. Gerisch G, Hess B. Cyclic-AMP-controlled oscillations in suspended Dictyostelium cells: Their relation to morphogenetic cell interactions. Proc Natl Acad Sci USA 1974; 71:2118-2122.
21. Gerisch G, Malchow D, Roos W et al. Oscillations of cyclic nucleotide concentrations in relation to the excitability of Dictyostelium cells. J Exp Biol 1979; 81:33-47.
22. Winfree A. Phase control of neural pacemakers. Science 1977; 197:761-763.

23. Mohanty S, Lee S, Yadava N et al. Regulated protein degradation controls PKA function and cell-type differentiation in Dictyostelium. Genes Devel 2001; 15:1435-1448.
24. Boeckeler K, Adley K, Xu X et al. The neuroprotective agent, valproic acid, regulates the mitogen-activated protein kinase pathway through modulation of protein kinase A signalling in Dictyostelium discoideum. Eur J Cell Biol 2006; 85:1097-1057.
25. Brzostowski JA, Parent CA, Kimmel AR. A Galpha-dependent pathway that antagonizes multiple chemoattractant responses that regulate directional cell movement. Genes Devel 2004; 18:805-815.
26. Comer F, Parent CA. Phosphoinositide 3-kinase activity controls the chemoattractant-mediated activation and adaptation of adenylyl cyclase. Mol Biol Cell 2006; 17:357-366.
27. Devreotes PN, Zigmond SH. Chemotaxis in eukaryotic cells: A focus on leukocytes and Dictyostelium. Annu Rev Cell Biol 1988; 4:649-686.
28. Soll DR, Wessels D, Heid PJ et al. A contextual framework for characterizing motility and chemotaxis mutants in Dictyostelium discoideum. J Muscle Res Cell Motil 2002; 23:659-672.
29. Wessels D, Voss E, Von Bergen N et al. A computer-assisted system for reconstructing and interpreting the dynamic three-dimensional relationships of the outer surface, nucleus and pseudopods of crawling cells. Cell Motil Cytoskel 1998; 41:225-246.
30. Wessels DJ, Zhang H, Reynolds J et al. The internal phosphodiesterase RegA is essential for the suppression of lateral pseudopods during Dictyostelium chemotaxis. Mol Biol Cell 2000; 11:2803-2820.
31. Stepanovic V, Wessels D, Daniels K et al. Intracellular role of adenylyl cyclase in regulation of lateral pseudopod formation during Dictyostelium chemotaxis. Euk Cell 2005; 4:775-786.
32. Zhang H, Heid PJ, Wessels D et al. Constitutively active protein kinase A disrupts motility and chemotaxis in Dictyostelium discoideum. Euk Cell 2003; 2:62-75.
33. Yumura S, Yoshida M, Betapudi V et al. Multiple myosinII heavy chain kinases: Roles in filament assembly control and proper cytokinesis in Dictyostelium. Mol Biol Cell 2005; 16:4256-4266.
34. Heid PJ, Wessels D, Daniels KJ et al. The role of myosin heavy chain phosphorylation in Dictyostelium motility, chemotaxis and F-actin localization. J Cell Sci 2004; 117:4819-4835.
35. Behrens MM, Juliani MH, Maia JCC. Periodic changes in the cAMP-dependent protein kinase activity ratio in Dictyostelium discoideum. Biochem Internat 1986; 13:221-226.
36. Janetopoulos C, Jin T, Devreotes P. Receptor-mediated activation of heterotrimeric G-proteins in living cells. Science 2001; 291:2408-2411.
37. Geiger J, Wessels D, Soll DR. Human polymorphonuclear leukocytes respond to waves of chemoattractant, like Dictyostelium. Cell Motil Cytoskel 2003; 56:27-44.
38. Song L, Nadkarni S, Bodeker H et al. Dictyostelium discoideum chemotaxis: Threshold for directed motion. Eur J Cell Biol 2006; 85:981-989.

## CHAPTER 4

Min Oscillation in Bacteria

Joe Lutkenhaus*

Abstract

Oscillation of the Min proteins is a key regulator of the division plane in many bacteria including the model organism *E. coli*. The coupled oscillation of these proteins between the ends of the cell restricts the formation of the Z ring, an essential cytoskeletal element that serves as a scaffold for the cytokinesis machinery, to a narrow region at midcell. The oscillation was discovered following the fusion of the Min proteins to green fluorescent protein. Importantly, the Min system is readily manipulated allowing rapid advances in understanding key aspects of the oscillation. In addition, details of the biochemistry of the Min proteins have emerged that provide the basis for their dynamic interaction with the membrane. Furthermore, the in vivo description of the oscillations along with the biochemical details of the Min proteins have provided the fuel for mathematical approaches to try and understand the critical features that underlie this oscillatory system. The simplicity and ease of manipulating the Min system make it a tractable model to obtain a complete understanding of a self-organizing system.

Introduction

One of the key events in the life of a cell is cytokinesis, a process which splits one cell into two daughter cells. In all cells this event involves spatial and temporal regulation of the assembly of a cytoskeletal element that determines the division plane.[1] In bacteria this cytoskeletal element is the Z ring (Fig. 1) which functions as a scaffold to recruit the other essential division proteins, of which there are about a dozen in *E. coli*. Once assembled this ensemble of proteins constitutes a fully competent cytokinetic ring. This cytokinetic ring is able to carry out the necessary steps, invagination of the cytoplasmic membrane and synthesis of new cell wall, which divides the bacterial cell.

The key event in bacterial cytokinesis is the assembly of the Z ring, since its position dictates the division site.[2] It is clear that this step is highly regulated, and under normal growth conditions the Z ring forms precisely at the center of the long axis of the rodshaped cell.[3] Information about this regulation has come from the study of various mutants and inhibitors of DNA metabolism. These studies revealed that the nucleoid (term used for the bacterial chromosome) exerts a negative effect on Z ring assembly such that a Z ring does not form over the nucleoid.[4] This inhibitory mechanism is referred to as nucleoid occlusion (Noc). Genes have been identified that mediate this effect, although the mechanism is not clear.[5,6] Another inhibitory mechanism was revealed following the isolation of a mutant designated *min*. In this mutant spatial regulation of Z ring assembly is compromised and cytokinesis occurs near the ends of the cell to produce small anucleate minicells.[7] Analysis of this mutant revealed an inhibitory system in wild type cells that prevents assembly of a Z ring near the ends of the cell while allowing it to form at midcell.[8] These two

*Joe Lutkenhaus—Department of Microbiology, Molecular Genetics and Immunology, University of Kansas Medical Center, Kansas City, KS, USA. Email: jlutkenh@kumc.edu

Cellular Oscillatory Mechanisms, edited by Miguel Maroto and Nicholas A.M. Monk.
©2008 Landes Bioscience and Springer Science+Business Media.

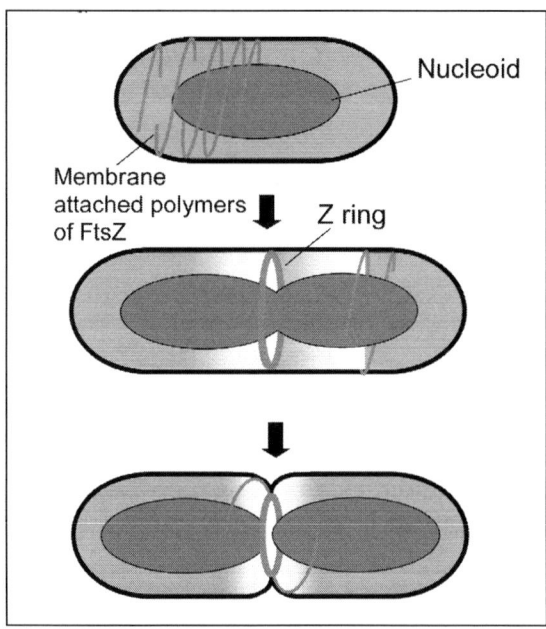

Figure 1. Spatial regulation of the Z ring formation. Dynamic polymers of FtsZ are attached to the membrane through linker proteins. These polymers coalesce at midcell to form the Z ring. The influence of negative regulators (Min and Noc) of Z ring assembly is lowest at midcell as the nucleoids segregate (indicated by the shading). Reprinted with permission from the Annual Review of Biochemistry, Volume 76 ©2007 by Annual Reviews www.annualreviews.org.

inhibitory systems (Noc and Min) cooperate to precisely position the Z ring[3] and have been recently reviewed (refs. 9,10). This chapter is about the Min system, whose components undergo a rapid oscillation between the ends of the cell to spatially regulate Z ring assembly. This oscillation generates a gradient on the membrane of an antagonist of Z ring assembly (MinC) that over time has the lowest concentration at midcell.

Z Ring

The Z ring is composed of protofilaments (a head to tail linear array of subunits) of FtsZ that are attached to the membrane through linker proteins such as FtsA.[11] The names of these proteins are derived from the filamenting phenotype resulting from a temperature sensitive mutation in the corresponding gene. The protofilaments are formed through the polymerization of FtsZ, a bacterial homologue of eukaryotic tubulin, the building block of microtubules that are the basis of the mitotic machinery in eukaryotes.[12,13] FtsZ protofilaments are extremely dynamic due to a GTPase activity that is coupled to their assembly.[14] In vivo measurements using FRAP (fluorescence recovery after photobleaching) reveals that the Z ring is also very dynamic as FtsZ subunits turn over with a half life of less than 10 seconds.[15,16] This rapid turnover in vivo is similar to the dynamics of the protofilaments observed in vitro suggesting that the turnover is dictated by the intrinsic GTPase rate. A key unanswered question is the length and arrangement of protofilaments within the Z ring.

In eukaryotes the assembly of the cytoskeleton is regulated at the nucleation step.[17] This type of regulation allows for temporal and spatial control of the positioning of these cytoskeletal structures. It appears, however, that FtsZ polymerization is not regulated at this step. The intracellular concentration of FtsZ is >5 μM which is well above the critical concentration of about 1 μM^{14} and there do not appear to be any proteins that sequester FtsZ under normal growth conditions. Thus, most of the FtsZ in the cell is likely to be in polymers. In addition, the properties of FtsZ polymerization appear similar to that of the bacterial actin homologue ParM which lacks a kinetic barrier to assembly and is continually turning over.[18] Recent observations indicate that FtsZ polymers are attached to the membrane throughout a nondividing cell.[19] The Z ring forms through the coalescence of these membrane-attached FtsZ polymers. It occurs at midcell since the influence of negative regulators of Z ring assembly, including the Min proteins, is the lowest there[11] (Fig. 1). Thus, the function of Min is to prevent the coalescence of FtsZ polymers away from midcell.

The Min System

Inactivation of the *min* locus in the rod-shaped organism *E. coli* results a loss in the spatial regulation of cytokinesis.[7] In the *min* mutant the assembly of Z rings occurs at the poles of the cell in addition to the space between the replicated nucleoids[20,21] (Noc regulation is still present). This mislocalization of the Z ring to the poles in the *min* mutant leads to polar cytokinesis and the formation of anucleate minicells, an easy to assay phenotype indicating loss of spatial regulation of Z ring assembly. Since the polar cytokinetic events occur in addition to cytokinesis between nucleoids the *min* mutant survives. This viability of the *min* mutant allows the Min system to be relatively easily manipulated. Also, the phenotype of this mutant reveals that the function of the *min* locus in wild type cells is to prevent Z ring assembly at the poles.[8] This inhibitory function of the Min system at the poles implies that the Min system has topological specificity since in wild type cells it prevents Z ring assembly at the poles of the cell while allowing it to occur at midcell.

The Min system encodes three proteins MinC, MinD and MinE, whose functions are well established (Fig. 2). MinC is an antagonist of FtsZ assembly, MinD activates MinC by recruiting it to the membrane and MinE spatially regulates the bipartite MinCD inhibitor through its interaction with MinD.[22-24] In the absence of MinE the MinCD inhibitor is distributed throughout the cell membrane and Z rings are prevented from forming anywhere in the cell. Thus, loss of the entire locus only causes minicells and is not lethal, although the loss of just MinE would be lethal as it would remove the spatial constraints on MinCD activity.

A complete understanding of the Min system requires knowledge about the proteins themselves and how they interact. Importantly, structural information about each of the proteins from diverse bacteria has been obtained. MinD is a member of a large ATPase family (ParA) that includes proteins involved in chromosomal and plasmid partitioning as well as more distant members involved in activities as diverse as detoxification of arsenic compounds and transfer of electrons by nitrogenase.[25,26] The signature feature of this family of ATPases is a variation of the Walker A motif involved in ATP hydrolysis. An additional and critical lysine present in this motif can only participate in hydrolysis following dimerization.[26,27]

NifH from the nitrogenase complex is the most studied representative of the ParA family.[28] An emerging theme of this family of proteins is ATP-dependent dimerization. The structures of all MinDs determined so far are monomers,[29-31] however, MinD has been observed to undergo ATP-dependent dimerization.[32] Recently, determination of the structure of a hydrolytic mutant of another ParA member (called Soj) revealed that it was a dimer similar to NifH.[33] This second example solidifies the dimerization theme for this large family of proteins. A second theme of this family is that dimerization increases the affinity of the protein for other biological molecules.[26] In the case of MinD the list of biological molecules includes the membrane, MinC and MinE, as well as other MinD dimers. Importantly, the ATP dependence of the dimerization makes the process reversible as ATP hydrolysis reverses the dimerization and the affinity for all partners.[32,34,35]

MinC and MinE are also dimers (Fig. 2). MinC forms a stable dimer, however, the MinE dimer has a dissociation constant estimated at 0.6 μM.[36] Since the level of MinE in the cell has been estimated at 1400 molecules per cell (~1.4 μM) the dimer-monomer equilibrium is likely

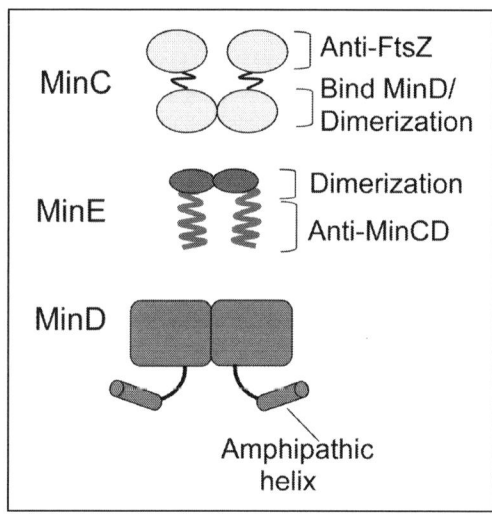

Figure 2. Min proteins are dimers. The dimerization of MinD is ATP-dependent. The MinC and MinE dimers consist of monomers with distinct functional and structural domains. The N-terminal domain of MinC anatagonizes FtsZ assembly and the C-terminal domain is responsible for dimerization and interaction with MinD. MinE consists of a C-terminal globular domain responsible for dimerization and an N-terminal domain that is thought to form a helix and interact with MinD.

to be important factor during the oscillation.[37] Both MinC and MinE are composed of monomers with two separable and functional domains. MinE is a small protein of only 88 amino acids; however, it has several important activities. The N-terminal domain comprised of the first 31 amino acids is capable of suppressing the division inhibition caused by MinCD complex.[38,39] Although it can suppress the inhibitory activity of the MinCD complex it does this throughout the cell without preference for midcell. The C-terminal domain consists of amino acids 32-88 and is required for dimerization and for the N-terminal domain to suppress MinCD in a topologically specific manner.

The MinC monomer is composed of two equal-sized domains connected by a linker of variable length in MinCs from different bacteria[40,41] (Fig. 2). The C-terminal domain is required for dimerization and binding to MinD. The N-terminal domain is primarily responsible for the antagonism of FtsZ assembly although recent evidence indicates the C-terminal domain also makes a contribution.[42] Although purified MinC can antagonize FtsZ assembly in vitro,[43] MinD is required in vivo as it enhances MinC activity by recruiting it to the membrane and concentrating it at its site of action.[8,44] The precise mechanism by which MinC antagonizes FtsZ assembly is unclear. It does not prevent FtsZ's GTPase indicating it acts after assembly of a protofilament.[22] Possibilities include the prevention of lateral interactions between protofilaments, which are thought to be important in Z ring formation, and stimulated disassembly of a protofilament.

The Oscillation

The oscillatory behavior of the Min system was discovered by observing the behavior of functional fusions of the Min proteins to GFP (green fluorescent protein).[43,45,46] These studies revealed that MinE and MinD are the essential components of the oscillator and that MinC, an antagonist of FtsZ assembly, is just a passenger. The Min proteins oscillate between the poles of the cell with a period of ~50 seconds at room temperature. More recent studies demonstrate that the period can be as short as 10 seconds at the optimum growth temperature of 37°C.[47]

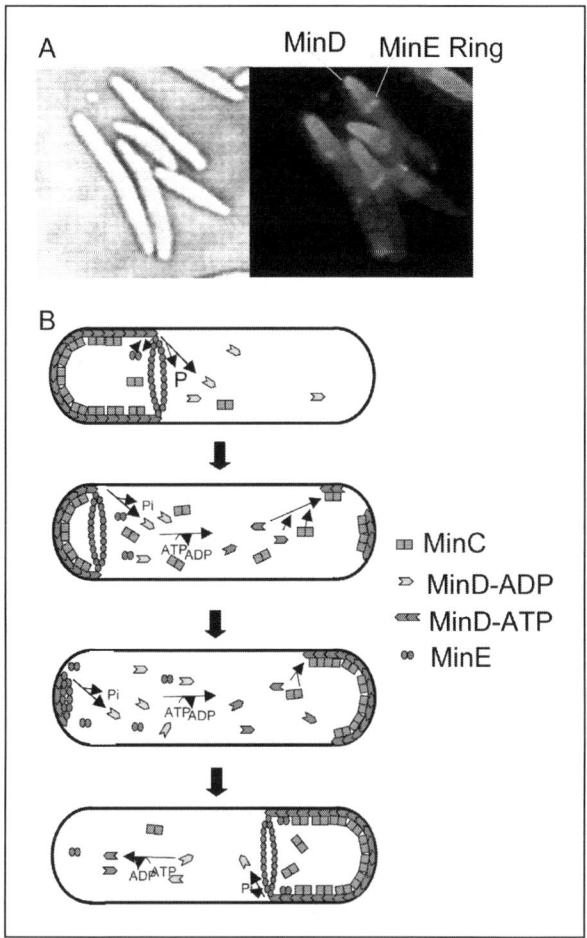

Figure 3. Min oscillation. A) Snapshot of the Min oscillation. MinD and MinE are fused to different color variants of GFP. MinD is in red and the MinE ring is blue. This figure is adapted from reference 79. Used with permission from Nature Publishing group ©2007. B) Diagram of the Min oscillation. MinD assembles into a polar zone at one end of the cell. A MinE ring assembles on the edge of the MinD zone near midcell. MinE stimulates the MinD ATPase causing the MinD zone to disassemble towards the pole. The released MinD undergoes nucle-otide exchange and a new polar zone assembles in the other half of the cell. A new MinE ring is formed and the cycle is repeated. MinC binds to MinD on the membrane. Deconvolution microscopy reveals that MinD attached to the membrane is in a spiral pattern suggesting it forms a polymer. Reprinted with permission from the Annual Review of Biochemistry, Volume 76 ©2007 by Annual Reviews www.annualreviews.org.

The fluorescence has a distinct pattern with MinD present in a test tube pattern with the open end near midcell (Fig. 3A,B). MinE is primarily present at the open end of the MinD tube, referred to as the MinE ring, although some is spread throughout the MinD zone. As the oscillation ensues the MinD tube recedes towards the pole, chased by the MinE ring.[48,49] MinD released by the MinE ring starts to establish a new polar zone at the opposite pole. When the MinE ring reaches the pole, it disassembles and forms a new ring at the edge of the nascent MinD polar zone near midcell and the process is repeated toward the opposite pole.

Several important features of the oscillation were determined in the initial study: (1) the period varies inversely with the ratio of MinD to MinE, (2) in artificially elongated cells (in which cell division is prevented from occurring) MinD and MinE switch from a pole to pole oscillation to a striped pattern with a distance between maxima of ~7.5 microns, and (3) the oscillation continues indefinitely in the absence of protein synthesis and cell growth.[45] Subsequent examination of the oscillation using deconvolution microscopy indicates that MinD is present in spirals raising the possibility that MinD assembles into a polymer during the oscillation.[37] MinC and MinE also appeared as spirals but this is entirely dependent upon MinD.

The first important feature of the oscillation identified was that the ratio of MinD to MinE determined the length of the period. This was found by holding MinE constant and increasing the level of MinD 5-10 fold. This change in the ratio slowed the oscillation sufficiently so that minicells started to form; the retention of the Min proteins at one pole allowed time for a Z ring to form at the free pole. Also, holding MinD constant and increasing MinE resulted in a shorter period. The second feature identified was revealed by blocking cell division through depletion of FtsZ. This leads to the formation of long filamentous cells that eventually die, however, as they elongate the oscillation continues but switches from a pole to pole oscillation to a striped pattern with the number of nodes increasing with cell length (Fig. 4). The third feature was revealed by adding an inhibitor of protein synthesis and demonstrated that the Min proteins were stable.

One of the possibilities raised by these observations of the Min oscillation is that the only requirements for the oscillation are MinD, MinE, a container and a source of energy. This possibility was indicated in particular by the striped pattern in elongated cells which suggested that the pole does not play a nucleating role for MinD assembly.[46] Further support for this possibility comes from the observation that the oscillation occurs in round cells.[50,51] Various mutants of *E. coli* (*rodA*, *pbpB* or *mreB*) have lost the ability to maintain a rod-shape and are more spherical. In such mutants, especially *mreB*, which has a more regular size distribution,

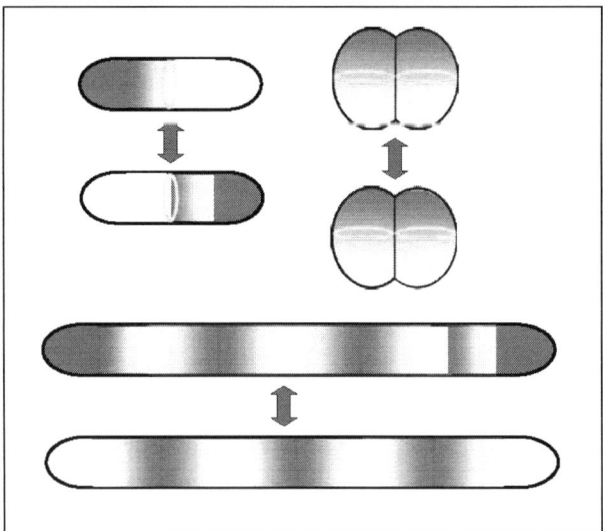

Figure 4. Oscillation in cells with altered morphology. In normal sized cells the Min proteins are observed to oscillate between the poles. If cell division is blocked the Min oscillation takes on a striped appearance with the number of nodes increasing with cell length. In mutants that grow with a spherical shape cytokinesis deforms the cells such that a long axis is generated in the nascent daughter cells. Min proteins oscillate along the long axis leading to formation of a Z ring perpendicular to the previous axis of cytokinesis.

the oscillation still occurs quite regularly in the majority of the cells and controls the placement of the Z ring.[51] In spherical cells the Z ring forms at 90° to the previous division plane. This reorientation is preceded by a switch in the oscillation of the Min proteins. It is likely that constriction of the Z ring results in a dividing cell in which the still attached newborn cells are not spherical. As a result a long axis is generated in the nascent daughter cells, which is perpendicular to the plane of division (Fig. 4). Min oscillation along this long axis would then be responsible for establishing a Z ring that would be perpendicular to the previous division plane.

Since the Min system is relatively easy to manipulate important features of the system were rapidly elucidated. Thus, expressing the proteins alone or in combination revealed their physiological roles.[8] The main role of MinE is to counteract the MinCD inhibitor and to remove the MinD polar zone. Additional observations have been made with various mutants that suggest a possible additional role for MinE. During the oscillation MinD appears in spirals, however, in the absence of MinE, MinD appears diffuse on the membrane without apparent spirals.[37,52] Also, a MinD mutant that binds MinE, but is not stimulated to undergo ATP hydrolysis (see below), forms spirals if MinE is present. However, if MinE is absent spirals are not present and the MinD mutant is diffuse on the membrane. These observations suggest that MinE promotes the formation of MinD spirals.[52] This remains an open question. Also, the expression of various MinE mutants has been examined in a wild type strain. Overproduction of various MinE mutants truncated for the domain required to stimulate the MinD ATPase have interesting effects. Production of MinE[22-88] causes minicell formation at low concentrations but inhibition of cell division at higher concentrations.[38,39] The latter observation is consistent with the truncated MinE forming heterodimers with the full length MinE that are inactive.[53] The induction of the minicells at low concentration has not been explained but is also observed with another truncation mutant. MinE[36-88] causes minicell formation but does not inhibit division when it is overproduced. Consistent with this last observation, it is unable to form heterodimers. How these truncated MinEs cause minicell formation is unclear.

Biochemistry of Min Proteins

For the oscillation to occur the Min proteins have to establish temporary residency at one pole, release and migrate to the other pole. How is this temporary residency established? The studies of the GFP fusions revealed that MinD localized to the membrane and was responsible for the membrane localization of MinC and MinE.[22,45,46] How does MinD bind to the membrane? MinD is a member of an interesting family of ATPases, called ParA, which contain a deviant Walker A motif involved in ATP hydrolysis.[25,26] The emerging theme of this family of proteins is that they dimerize in the presence of ATP, bind to a surface and subsequently interact with a partner protein that stimulates the ATPase activity.[26]

MinD binds to the membrane through a short C-terminal, amphipathic helix that inserts into the phospholipid bilayer[23,54] (Fig. 5). Investigations of MinD binding to phospholipid vesicles demonstrate that the binding requires ATP and is cooperative.[34,35] This ATP dependence immediately suggests how MinD binding to the membrane could be reversible as ATP hydrolysis would release it from the membrane. Also, MinD has a preference for anionic phospholipids, which may be important, as staining of *E. coli* cells with lipid specific dyes indicate that the distribution of lipids is not random.[55] Anionic phospholipids are enriched at the poles and at midcell.[56] In vivo studies indicate that the minimal unit for binding to the membrane is a dimer.[57] Furthermore, dimers undergo surface-assisted assembly in vitro to produce tubulated vesicles in which MinD polymers are wrapped around the vesicle.[35] This ability of MinD dimers to assemble into a polymer on a vesicle surface is likely responsible for the MinD spirals observed in vivo and presumably underlies the ability of MinD to undergo cooperative movement in vivo.

MinD is the only member of the ParA family that contains this C-terminal, amphipathic helix. At least several other members of the ParA family are observed to undergo oscillatory behavior in vivo but in these cases it occurs between nucleoids.[58,59] Such ParA proteins bind nonspecifically, but cooperatively to DNA instead of membrane. For these DNA-associated members to undergo oscillation they also need a partner protein that plays a similar role to MinE.

MinD has a basal ATPase activity that is stimulated ~10-fold by the addition of MinE in the presence of phospholipid vesicles.[60] This stimulation is critical for the oscillation to occur. MinE mutants that have reduced ability to stimulate the ATPase display an increase in the period indicating that the rate of the ATPase is a major determinant of the frequency of the oscillation. MinE mutants that have completely lost the ability to stimulate MinD have lost the ability to induce oscillation. Most of the mutations that affect the ability of MinE to stimulate the MinD ATPase lie within the N-terminal domain.[60,61] One possibility is that the N-terminal domain of MinE forms a α-helix upon binding to MinD and that one face of this helix is the primary binding site (Fig. 5). Consistent with this, most of the mutations that eliminate MinE interaction with MinD change residues that lie on one face of this putative helix.[61]

MinD is able to recruit MinC to vesicles in vitro in the presence of ATP.[32,34] In contrast, MinD is released from vesicles by MinE due to the ATPase stimulation (Fig. 5). In the presence of a nonhydrolyzable analogue of ATP MinD recruits either MinC or MinE to the vesicles, however, if both are added MinE is the preferred binding partner. This suggests that the binding sites for MinC and MinE overlap on MinD. This suggestion is supported by mutagenesis studies which reveal amino acid residues in MinD that are only essential for MinE binding, some essential only for MinC binding and some that are required for both.[27,62] Although the binding sites overlap MinC does not interfere with MinE's ability to stimulate the MinD ATPase.

Although some of the biochemistry of the Min proteins is quite clear, other issues, particularly the interplay of Min proteins and the membrane, have not been fully resolved. For example, it is not clear if MinD dimerizes and then binds to the membrane or if monomers have a weak affinity for the membrane and dimerization is promoted by the presence of the membrane which locks MinD on the membrane.[23,57] It is possible that the C-terminal tail of MinD interferes with dimerization and that the presence of a membrane aides dimerization by sequestering the tail. While it is clear that MinD can recruit MinC or MinE to the membrane, it is not clear if interaction between these components occurs in the cytoplasm or only on the membrane. Yeast 2-hybrid studies indicate that MinD lacking a membrane binding domain interacts with MinC and MinE although not well with itself.[23,63] Other evidence suggests that MinE and MinC only bind to the MinD dimer arguing that the critical event is MinD dimerization.

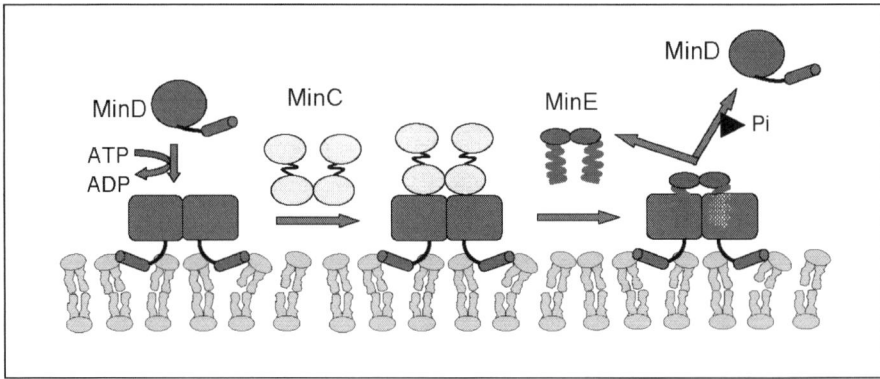

Figure 5. Dynamic interaction of the Min proteins with the membrane. MinD binds to the membrane as a dimer in the presence of ATP. The dimers further associate to form the spirals observed in vivo (not shown). MinC binds to MinD on the membrane but can be displaced by MinE. MinE induces the MinD ATPase causing MinD and MinE to be released from the membrane.

Models

The Min system is a relatively simple system with only a few components that have been relatively well characterized. Nonetheless, to fully understand the oscillation based simply upon the biochemistry of these few components is not possible. In an effort to try and understand the critical elements of this system needed to generate the dynamic behavior investigators have turned towards mathematical modeling. As models have been developed they have increased in complexity as new experimental details of the system are incorporated. Additionally, models are either stochastic or deterministic. In stochastic models individual molecules are accounted for whereas in the simpler deterministic models an average is assumed. In general the models generate oscillations based upon the concept of dynamic instability. Starting with a homogenous distribution small perturbations grow and ultimately lead to the oscillatory pattern. What are the features of the system necessary to achieve the oscillatory pattern? Recent reviews have aimed at bridging the gap between experimentalists and modelers.[64,65]

The initial models were attempts to explain the observations of the GFP fusions.[66-68] Reasonable assumptions about the activity of the various Min proteins were based upon the patterns observed following expression of the proteins alone or in various combinations. Subsequent models incorporated the biochemical activities, in particular the ability of the ATP form of MinD to bind the membrane and of MinE to stimulate the MinD ATPase.[69] These findings provided a molecular basis for the reversible association of the Min proteins with the membrane. Additional models have taken into account the observation that MinD is present in spirals during the oscillation.[70-73] There could be several explanations for spiral formation since many membrane associated proteins have been observed to form spirals when observed by fluorescence microscopy.[74,75] However, in the models it is assumed that MinD polymerizes. This assumption is supported by the ability of MinD to assemble on phospholipid vesicles in vitro and deform them.[35]

In general the models assume that the Min proteins move in the cytoplasm by diffusion and use reasonable rates of diffusion for MinD and MinE based upon in vivo measurements. Although there is increasing evidence that bacterial cells have an actin-like cytoskeleton that could potentially transport molecules it is clear that MinD oscillation works in the absence of this cytoskeleton.[51] It is also assumed that the membrane bound form of the proteins diffuse at a much lower rate. Direct measurements of the diffusion rates of MinD and MinE reveal two populations with different rates consistent with a cytoplasmic and membrane bound population.[76] Assuming that the molecules move by diffusion, it is more difficult to have a mechanism that drives the oscillation, particularly why MinD released from one pole binds to the opposite pole. Various models achieve this by different means.

In one of the initial models, as well as most subsequent models, it is assumed that MinD binds cooperatively to the membrane and recruits MinE which ultimately drives MinD off the membrane.[66] Subsequent measurements of MinD binding to vesicles found that it displayed cooperativity.[34] Also, FRET (fluorescence energy transfer and a measure of the interaction between fluorescently labeled proteins) was only observed between MinD molecules in the presence of phospholipid vesicles.[55] However, an oversight in this initial model was that MinD disappeared as it came off the membrane and had to be resynthesized.[66]

In another model that did not involve cooperative binding of MinD it was assumed that MinD binds anywhere on the membrane and that membrane bound MinD undergoes attraction resulting in MinD moving towards areas of higher concentrations of MinD.[67] The MinD then recruits MinE which causes the release of MinD and MinE. However, MinE comes off the membrane much slower than MinD. As a result MinD diffuses to regions of the cell not containing MinE producing the oscillation.

Huang et al produced the first model to incorporate the role of nucleotide hydrolysis and exchange in the oscillation.[69,77] In this model MinE stimulates MinD ATPase causing MinD to come off the membrane, however, MinD has to undergo nucleotide exchange before it can rebind to the membrane (Fig. 3B). The concentration of MinD-ATP in the cytoplasm near the occupied pole remains low. The reason for this is it binds cooperatively to membrane already containing MinD; the bound MinD acting as a sink. However, at the unoccupied pole the concentration of MinD-ATP has to rise before in can bind. Using a nucleotide hydrolysis rate that corresponds to the in vitro measured rate and a nucleotide exchange rate of 1 per second the oscillation was produced. This model was also utilized to explore the basis of the faster oscillation observed at higher temperatures.[47] Increasing the rate of ATPase, but not the nucleotide exchange rate, was sufficient to cause the observed decrease in the period and was the best candidate to explain the temperature effect. This model was also used to reproduce the oscillations observed in round cells.[78]

One of the important features to incorporate into the modeling is the number of molecules per cell. MinD is estimated at 2000 molecules per cell and MinE is estimated at about 1400 molecules per cell.[79] A problem with the above models is that this is a relatively small number of MinD molecules; certainly far less than necessary to occupy one half of the inner surface of the cell and have the molecules be in contact to generate cooperative behavior. As a result of this and the observation that MinD is present in spiral structures in vivo and on vesicles in vitro efforts have been made to introduce MinD polymerization into the models. Although the structure of MinD polymer is unresolved it is generally assumed to be a two stranded filament with the basic unit a MinD dimer. Such an assumption is consistent with this family of proteins dimerizing and then further associating on a surface.

Drew et al incorporated MinD polymerization into a deterministic model.[71] In order to achieve oscillation the polymers were nucleated at the poles. The pole playing a necessary role is not a feature required in other models. Also, a number of additional assumptions were required that are not supported by experimental evidence. Additional models that have incorporated polymers have been proposed but a three dimensional analysis of these did not reveal spirals, probably due to the short length distribution of the polymers.[72,73]

The most recent version of the polymer model is a variation of the model proposed by Drew et al. The model also includes nucleation of the polymers at the poles.[80] To restrict nucleation to the poles it is assumed that a MinD dimer binds anywhere in the cell but MinD bound at the pole is resistant to MinE leading to its persistence and preferred site for nucleation. There is no experimental evidence for this behavior, however, it was suggested that MinE may not activate the ATPase of MinD at the pole due to different stress on the membrane. Some interesting proposals are made for the orientation of subunits within the MinD polymer and for the interaction between MinE and MinD. Also, attempts are made to explain the behavior of the N-terminally truncated MinEs that are able to induce a minicell phenotype when overproduced in a wild type cell. This is the first attempt to explain these mutants but relies on mechanisms that have not been demonstrated. Some of these ideas can be experimentally tested.

Conclusions

The study of spatial regulation of cytokinesis in bacteria is focused on the mechanisms that are utilized by the cell to position the Z ring precisely at midcell. One of the key regulators of this process in model organisms such as *E. coli* is the Min system, whose components oscillate between the ends of the cell with a period that is much less than the generation time of the organism. Many of the details of the biochemistry of the Min proteins have been elucidated and these explain the dynamic interaction of the Min proteins with the membrane. However, more remains to be determined, particularly about MinD assembly on the membrane. What is the structure of the polymers formed and does MinE have any role? Certainly, the Min oscillatory system has proven to be an attractive problem for mathematical modeling and can explain behavior not anticipated from biochemical studies. One of the results of the modeling is the widespread appreciation that quite complex pattern formation can result from simple interactions among only a few molecules. Further understanding of the mechanism will likely come from continued oscillation between the experimental approach and mathematical modeling.

Acknowledgements

The author wishes to acknowledge the support of the National Institutes of Health.

References

1. Lutkenhaus J, Addinall SG. Bacterial cell division and the Z ring. Annu Rev Biochem 1997; 66:93-116.
2. Addinall SG, Lutkenhaus J. FtsZ-spirals and -arcs determine the shape of the invaginating septa in some mutants of Escherichia coli. Mol Microbiol 1996; 22:231-237.
3. Sun Q, Yu XC, Margolin W. Assembly of the FtsZ ring at the central division site in the absence of the chromosome. Mol Microbiol 1998; 29:491-503.
4. Woldringh CL, Mulder E, Huls PG et al. Toporegulation of bacterial division according to the nucleoid occlusion model. Res Microbiol 1991; 142:309-320.
5. Wu LJ, Errington J. Coordination of cell division and chromosome segregation by a nucleoid occlusion protein in Bacillus subtilis. Cell 2004; 117:915-925.
6. Bernhardt TG, de Boer PAJ. SlmA, a nucleoid-associated, FtsZ-binding protein required for blocking septal ring assmebly over chromosomes in E. coli. Mol Cell 2005; 555-564.
7. Adler HI, Fisher WD, Cohen A et al. Minature Escherichia coli cells deficient in DNA. Proc Natl Acad Sci USA 1967; 57:321-326.
8. de Boer PA, Crossley RE, Rothfield LI. A division inhibitor and a topological specificity factor coded for by the minicell locus determine proper placement of the division septum in E. coli. Cell 1989; 56:641-649.
9. Rothfield L, Taghbalout A, Shih YL. Spatial control of bacterial division-site placement. Nat Rev Microbiol 2005; 3:959-968.
10. Lutkenhaus J. Assembly dynamics of the bacterial MinCDE system and spatial regulation of the Z ring. Annu Rev Biochem 2007.
11. Pichoff S, Lutkenhaus J. Tethering the Z ring to the membrane through a conserved membrane targeting sequence in FtsA. Mol Microbiol 2005; 55:1722-1734.
12. Mukherjee A, Lutkenhaus J. Guanine nucleotide-dependent assembly of FtsZ into filaments. J Bacteriol 1994; 176:2754-2758.
13. Lowe J, Amos LA. Crystal structure of the bacterial cell-division protein FtsZ. Nature 1998; 391:203-206.
14. Mukherjee A, Lutkenhaus J. Dynamic assembly of FtsZ regulated by GTP hydrolysis. EMBO J 1998; 17:462-469.
15. Stricker J, Maddox P, Salmon ED et al. Rapid assembly dynamics of the Escherichia coli FtsZ-ring demonstrated by fluorescence recovery after photobleaching. Proc Natl Acad Sci USA 2002; 99:3171-3175.
16. Anderson DE, Gueiros-Filho FJ, Erickson HP. Assembly dynamics of FtsZ rings in Bacillus subtilis and Escherichia coli and effects of FtsZ-regulating proteins. J Bacteriol 2004; 186:5775-5781.
17. Desai A, Mitchison TJ. Microtubule polymerization dynamics. Annu Rev Cell Dev Biol 1997; 13:83-117.
18. Garner EC, Campbell CS, Mullins RD. Dynamic instability in a DNA-segregating prokaryotic actin homolog. Science 2004; 306:1021-1025.
19. Thanedar S, Margolin W. FtsZ exhibits rapid movement and oscillation waves in helix-like patterns in Escherichia coli. Curr Biol 2004; 14:1167-1173.
20. Yu XC, Margolin W. FtsZ ring clusters in min and partition mutants: Role of both the Min system and the nucleoid in regulating FtsZ ring localization. Mol Microbiol 1999; 32:315-326.
21. Bi E, Lutkenhaus J. Cell division inhibitors SulA and MinCD prevent formation of the FtsZ ring. J Bacteriol 1993; 175:1118-1125.
22. Hu Z, Mukherjee A, Pichoff S et al. The MinC component of the division site selection system in Escherichia coli interacts with FtsZ to prevent polymerization. Proc Natl Acad Sci USA 1999; 96:14819-14824.
23. Hu Z, Lutkenhaus J. A conserved sequence at the C-terminus of MinD is required for binding to the membrane and targeting MinC to the septum. Mol Microbiol 2003; 47:345-355.
24. de Boer PA, Crossley RE, Rothfield LI. Central role for the Escherichia coli minC gene product in two different cell division-inhibition systems. Proc Natl Acad Sci USA 1990; 87:1129-1133.
25. de Boer PA, Crossley RE, Hand AR et al. The MinD protein is a membrane ATPase required for the correct placement of the Escherichia coli division site. EMBO J 1991; 10:4371-4380.
26. Lutkenhaus J, Sundaramoorthy M. MinD and role of the deviant Walker A motif, dimerization and membrane binding in oscillation. Mol Microbiol 2003; 48:295-303.

27. Zhou H, Schulze R, Cox S et al. Analysis of MinD mutations reveals residues required for MinE stimulation of the MinD ATPase and residues required for MinC interaction. J Bacteriol 2005; 187:629-638.
28. Schindelin H, Kisker C, Schlessman JL et al. Structure of ADP x AIF4(-)-stabilized nitrogenase complex and its implications for signal transduction. Nature 1997; 387:370-376.
29. Cordell SC, Lowe J. Crystal structure of the bacterial cell division regulator MinD. FEBS Lett 2001; 492:160-165.
30. Sakai N, Yao M, Itou H et al. The three-dimensional structure of septum site-determining protein MinD from Pyrococcus horikoshii OT3 in complex with Mg-ADP. Structure 2001; 9:817-826.
31. Hayashi I, Oyama T, Morikawa K. Structural and functional studies of MinD ATPase: Implications for the molecular recognition of the bacterial cell division apparatus. EMBO J 2001; 20:1819-1828.
32. Hu Z, Saez C, Lutkenhaus J. Recruitment of MinC, an inhibitor of Z-ring formation, to the membrane in Escherichia coli: Role of MinD and MinE. J Bacteriol 2003; 185:196-203.
33. Leonard TA, Butler PJ, Lowe J. Bacterial chromosome segregation: Structure and DNA binding of the Soj dimer—A conserved biological switch. EMBO J 2005; 24:270-282.
34. Lackner LL, Raskin DM, de Boer PA. ATP-dependent interactions between Escherichia coli Min proteins and the phospholipid membrane in vitro. J Bacteriol 2003; 185:735-749.
35. Hu Z, Gogol EP, Lutkenhaus J. Dynamic assembly of MinD on phospholipid vesicles regulated by ATP and MinE. Proc Natl Acad Sci USA 2002; 99:6761-6716.
36. King GF, Shih YL, Maciejewski MW et al. Structural basis for the topological specificity function of MinE. Nat Struct Biol 2000; 7:1013-1017.
37. Shih YL, Le T, Rothfield L. Division site selection in Escherichia coli involves dynamic redistribution of Min proteins within coiled structures that extend between the two cell poles. Proc Natl Acad Sci USA 2003; 100:7865-7870.
38. Zhao CR, de Boer PA, Rothfield LI. Proper placement of the Escherichia coli division site requires two functions that are associated with different domains of the MinE protein. Proc Natl Acad Sci USA 1995; 92:4313-4317.
39. Pichoff S, Vollrath B, Touriol C et al. Deletion analysis of gene minE which encodes the topological specificity factor of cell division in Escherichia coli. Mol Microbiol 1995; 18:321-329.
40. Hu Z, Lutkenhaus J. Analysis of MinC reveals two independent domains involved in interaction with MinD and FtsZ. J Bacteriol 2000; 182:3965-3971.
41. Cordell SC, Anderson RE, Lowe J. Crystal structure of the bacterial cell division inhibitor MinC. EMBO J 2001; 20:2454-2461.
42. Shiomi D, Margolin W. The C-terminal domain of MinC inhibits assembly of the Z ring in Escherichia coli. J Bacteriol 2007; 189:236-243.
43. Hu Z, Lutkenhaus J. Topological regulation of cell division in Escherichia coli involves rapid pole to pole oscillation of the division inhibitor MinC under the control of MinD and MinE. Mol Microbiol 1999; 34:82-90.
44. Johnson JE, Lackner LL, de Boer PA. Targeting of (D)MinC/MinD and (D)MinC/DicB complexes to septal rings in Escherichia coli suggests a multistep mechanism for MinC-mediated destruction of nascent FtsZ rings. J Bacteriol 2002; 184:2951-2962.
45. Raskin DM, de Boer PA. MinDE-dependent pole-to-pole oscillation of division inhibitor MinC in Escherichia coli. J Bacteriol 1999; 181:6419-6424.
46. Raskin DM, de Boer PA. Rapid pole-to-pole oscillation of a protein required for directing division to the middle of Escherichia coli. Proc Natl Acad Sci USA 1999; 96:4971-4976.
47. Touhami A, Jericho M, Rutenberg AD. Temperature dependence of MinD oscillation in Escherichia coli: Running hot and fast. J Bacteriol 2006; 188:7661-7667.
48. Hale CA, Meinhardt H, de Boer PA. Dynamic localization cycle of the cell division regulator MinE in Escherichia coli. EMBO J 2001; 20:1563-1572.
49. Fu X, Shih YL, Zhang Y et al. The MinE ring required for proper placement of the division site is a mobile structure that changes its cellular location during the Escherichia coli division cycle. Proc Natl Acad Sci USA 2001; 98:980-985.
50. Corbin BD, Yu XC, Margolin W. Exploring intracellular space: Function of the Min system in round-shaped Escherichia coli. EMBO J 2002; 21:1998-2008.
51. Shih YL, Kawagishi I, Rothfield L. The MreB and Min cytoskeletal-like systems play independent roles in prokaryotic polar differentiation. Mol Microbiol 2005; 58:917-928.
52. Szeto J, Eng NF, Acharya S et al. A conserved polar region in the cell division site determinant MinD is required for responding to MinE-induced oscillation but not for localization within coiled arrays. Res Microbiol 2005; 156:17-29.

53. Zhang Y, Rowland S, King G et al. The relationship between hetero-oligomer formation and function of the topological specificity domain of the Escherichia coli MinE protein. Mol Microbiol 1998; 30:265-273.
54. Szeto TH, Rowland SL, Rothfield LI et al. Membrane localization of MinD is mediated by a C-terminal motif that is conserved across eubacteria, archaea, and chloroplasts. Proc Natl Acad Sci USA 2002; 99:15693-15698.
55. Mileykovskaya E, Fishov I, Fu X et al. Effects of phospholipid composition on MinD-membrane interactions in vitro and in vivo. J Biol Chem 2003; 278:22193-22198.
56. Mileykovskaya E, Dowhan W. Visualization of phospholipid domains in Escherichia coli by using the cardiolipin-specific fluorescent dye 10-N-nonyl acridine orange. J Bacteriol 2000; 182:1172-1175.
57. Szeto TH, Rowland SL, Habrukowich CL et al. The MinD membrane targeting sequence is a transplantable lipid-binding helix. J Biol Chem 2003; 278:40050-40056.
58. Marston AL, Errington J. Dynamic movement of the ParA-like Soj protein of B. subtilis and its dual role in nucleoid organization and developmental regulation. Mol Cell 1999; 4:673-682.
59. Ebersbach G, Gerdes K. Bacterial mitosis: Partitioning protein ParA oscillates in spiral-shaped structures and positions plasmids at mid-cell. Mol Microbiol 2004; 52:385-398.
60. Hu Z, Lutkenhaus J. Topological regulation of cell division in E. coli. spatiotemporal oscillation of MinD requires stimulation of its ATPase by MinE and phospholipid. Mol Cell 2001; 7:1337-1343.
61. Ma LY, King G, Rothfield L. Mapping the MinE site involved in interaction with the MinD division site selection protein of Escherichia coli. J Bacteriol 2003; 185:4948-4955.
62. Ma L, King GF, Rothfield L. Positioning of the MinE binding site on the MinD surface suggests a plausible mechanism for activation of the Escherichia coli MinD ATPase during division site selection. Mol Microbiol 2004; 54:99-108.
63. Taghbalout A, Ma L, Rothfield L. Role of MinD-membrane association in Min protein interactions. J Bacteriol 2006; 188:2993-3001.
64. Kruse K, Howard M, Margolin W. An experimentalist's guide to computational modeling of the Min system. Mol Microbiol 2007; 63:1279-1284.
65. Howard M, Kruse K. Cellular organization by self-organization: Mechanisms and models for Min protein dynamics. J Cell Biol 2005; 168:533-536.
66. Meinhardt H, de Boer PA. Pattern formation in Escherichia coli: A model for the pole-to-pole oscillations of Min proteins and the localization of the division site. Proc Natl Acad Sci USA 2001; 98:14202-14207.
67. Kruse K. A dynamic model for determining the middle of Escherichia coli. Biophys J 2002; 82:618-627.
68. Howard M, Rutenberg AD, de Vet S. Dynamic compartmentalization of bacteria: Accurate division in E. coli. Phys Rev Lett 2001; 87:278102.
69. Huang KC, Meir Y, Wingreen NS. Dynamic structures in Escherichia coli: Spontaneous formation of MinE rings and MinD polar zones. Proc Natl Acad Sci USA 2003; 100:12724-12728.
70. Kruse K, Julicher F. Self-organization and mechanical properties of active filament bundles. Phys Rev E Stat Nonlin Soft Matter Phys 2003; 67:051913.
71. Drew DA, Osborn MJ, Rothfield LI. A polymerization-depolymerization model that accurately generates the self-sustained oscillatory system involved in bacterial division site placement. Proc Natl Acad Sci USA 2005; 102:6114-6118.
72. Pavin N, Paljetak HC, Krstic V. Min-protein oscillations in Escherichia coli with spontaneous formation of two-stranded filaments in a three-dimensional stochastic reaction-diffusion model. Phys Rev E Stat Nonlin Soft Matter Phys 2006; 73:021904.
73. Tostevin F, Howard M. A stochastic model of Min oscillations in Escherichia coli and Min protein segregation during cell division. Phys Biol 2006; 3:1-12.
74. Taghbalout A, Rothfield L. RNaseE and the other constituents of the RNA degradosome are components of the bacterial cytoskeleton. Proc Natl Acad Sci USA 2007; 104:1667-1672.
75. Shiomi D, Yoshimoto M, Homma M et al. Helical distribution of the bacterial chemoreceptor via colocalization with the Sec protein translocation machinery. Mol Microbiol 2006; 60:894-906.
76. Meacci G, Ries J, Fischer-Friedrich E et al. Mobility of Min-proteins in Escherichia coli measured by fluorescence correlation spectroscopy. Phys Biol 2006; 3:255-263.
77. Kulkarni RV, Huang KC, Kloster M et al. Pattern formation within Escherichia coli: Diffusion, membrane attachment, and self-interaction of MinD molecules. Phys Rev Lett 2004; 93:228103.
78. Huang KC, Wingreen NS. Min-protein oscillations in round bacteria. Phys Biol 2004; 1:229-35.
79. Shih YL, Fu X, King GF et al. Division site placement in E. coli: Mutations that prevent formation of the MinE ring lead to loss of the normal midcell arrest of growth of polar MinD membrane domains. EMBO J 2002; 21:3347-3357.
80. Cytrynbaum EN, Marshall BDL. A Multi-stranded polymer model explains MinDE dynamics in E. coli cell division. Biophys J 2007; 93:1134-1150.

CHAPTER 5

Development on Time

Isabel Palmeirim, Sofia Rodrigues, J. Kim Dale and Miguel Maroto*

Abstract

Temporal control is considered the fourth dimension in embryonic development and it sets the pace to attain the correct molecular patterning of the developing embryo. In this chapter we review one of the best-studied time dependent events in embryogenesis, which is the formation of somites. Somites are the basis of the future segmented framework of the vertebrate adult body and their reiterated appearance during the early stages of embryo development establishes the proper temporal and physical template from where other structures will develop and consequently shape the segmentation pattern of the embryo. Several models have been proposed over the last few decades to explain the mechanism(s) regulating somite periodicity, but no molecular evidence seemed to back up any of the postulated models. Remarkably, in 1997 the first evidence that the formation of the somites depended on an intrinsic molecular clock was at last provided through the description of oscillating gene expression in the tissue from which somites are generated. Since then, a huge amount of data has been and continues to be provided that is gradually revealing the ever more complex molecular mechanism underlying this segmentation clock. We are also beginning to learn about embryonic structures other than the somites which exhibit oscillations of gene expression suggesting they too are dependent upon a segmentation-like clock. This is in itself the clearest evidence that there is still a long way to go before we unveil the myriad of molecular mechanisms that lead to the time control of embryonic development.

Somitogenesis Is a Strict Time-Controlled Embryonic Process

During the process of vertebrate fertilization, as soon as the sperm meets the egg a series of complex time-related mechanisms are initiated. It is no coincidence that some structures form before others and that some organs have a bigger size than others. The exact time at which embryological processes occur defines the sequence of molecular events that will determine the correct development of a properly shaped and sized vertebrate organism. Actually, time control during embryogenesis allows the establishment of the framework that defines when the foetus is ready to be born.

The importance of time control during embryonic development is particularly evident during the process of somitogenesis, i.e., the process of somite formation. Somites are transient embryonic structures that form from the paraxial mesoderm and they give rise to several segmented parts of the adult body such as vertebrae, intervertebral disks, ribs, skeletal bud muscles and limb tendons,[1] and they also impose a segmentation pattern to their surrounding structures such as the precursors of the peripheral nervous system. Thus, these early embryonic structures form the basis of the segmented pattern of vertebrate organisms and confer a high degree of mobility to the adult body.[2] This progressive process is initiated

*Corresponding Author: Miguel Maroto—College of Life Sciences, University of Dundee, Dow Street, Dundee DD1 5EH, Scotland, UK. Email: m.maroto@dundee.ac.uk

Cellular Oscillatory Mechanisms, edited by Miguel Maroto and Nicholas A.M. Monk. ©2008 Landes Bioscience and Springer Science+Business Media.

extremely early in development concomitant with gastrulation and the initiation of antero-posterior axis elongation of the embryo and it terminates with the formation of a species specific number of somites. Thus during gastrulation, prospective paraxial mesoderm cells in the epithelial epiblast involute through the primitive streak and undergo an epithelial to mesenchymal transition to form two rods of mesenchyme bilaterally located either side of the caudal neural plate. These mesenchymal rods form the presomitic mesoderm (PSM) and as development proceeds a pair of epithelial somites buds off at regular intervals from the most anterior tip of the PSM. Thereby the array of somites appears in an anterior (A) to posterior (P) sequential manner[3] (Fig. 1). The temporal periodicity of somite formation is remarkably precise and species specific. In the chick embryo a pair of somites forms every 90 minutes, while in mouse this takes 2 hours and in zebrafish embryos they appear every 30 minutes. Remarkably, this tight temporal control is an intrinsic characteristic of presomitic cells. Thus, embryonic manipulations performed in the avian embryo have demonstrated that when the PSM is either grafted at different AP locations or cultured as an isolated

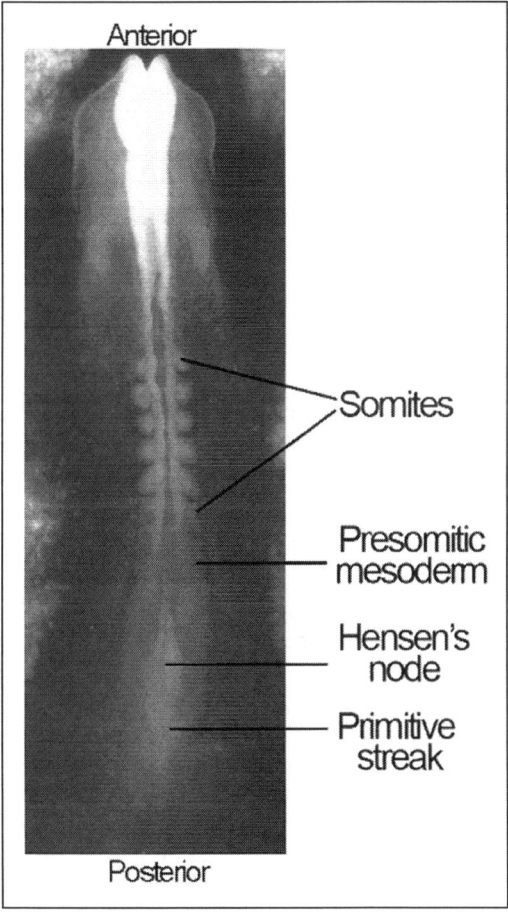

Figure 1. Somite formation in the chick embryo. Dorsal view of a 6-somite stage chick embryo: Epithelial somites arise from the rostral-most part of the presomitic mesoderm in an anterior to posterior direction. Concomitant with this process, the cells at Hensen's node/primitive streak region are constantly renovated as a consequence of gastrulation.

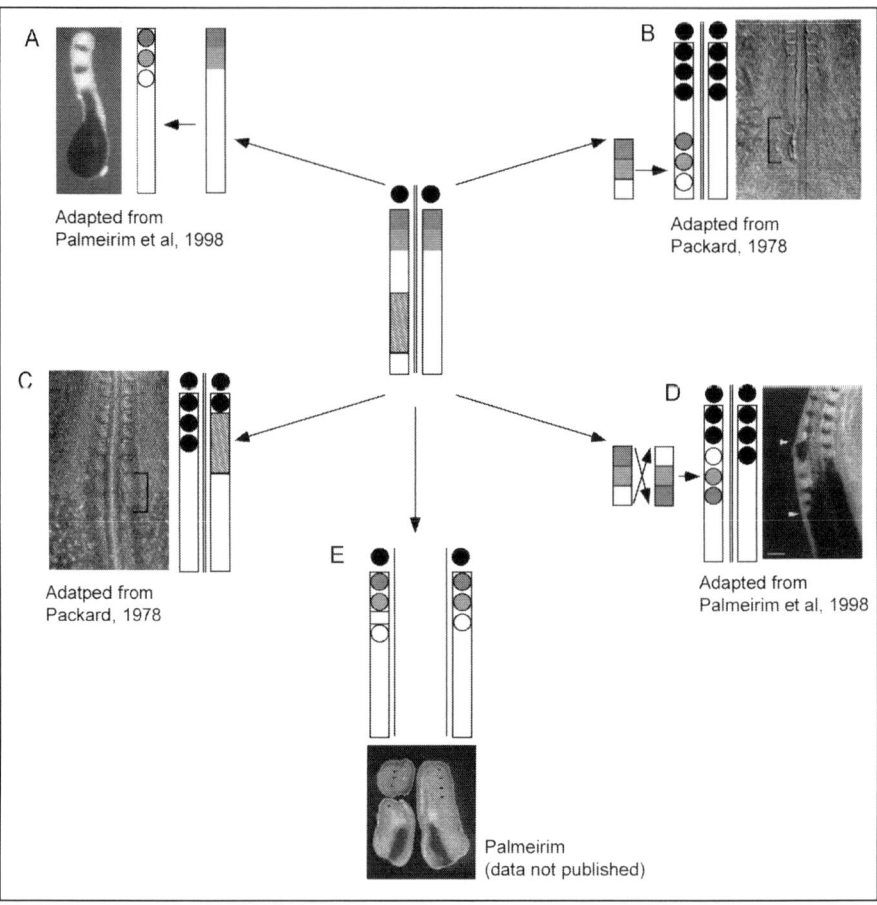

Figure 2. Somitogenesis following PSM grafting manipulations. This figure represents several PSM experimental manipulations that exemplify the intrinsic capacity of this tissue to segment. A) A PSM tissue isolated from its surroundings will form epithelial somites in an A to P direction, as it would in the intact embryo. This case is evidenced by the expression of the *delta1* gene in the experimental isolated PSM. B) When an anterior PSM fragment is grafted to a more posterior position, somites will wait to form according to their original schedule. C) Similarly, when a fragment of posterior PSM is grafted to a more anterior position it will not segment at the same time as the control PSM half, suggesting that it respects its intrinsic timing. D) If an anterior PSM fragment is AP reversed and then grafted to its original position, somites form in a P to A direction, respecting their predetermined timing. This can be clearly visualised by the unsegmented expression of *delta1* in the PSM of the experimental half (white arrow head). E) If an anteriormost fragment of the PSM is separated from the remaining posterior PSM, both fragments will segment according to their intrinsic schedule, as it is evidenced by the expression of *tbx6L* in the PSM explants. Images from Chick somite determination: the role of factors in young somites and the segmental plate, 203(2), 1978, 295-306 Packard DS, and Palmeirim et al. (1998) are reproduced with permission of Wiley-Liss, Inc., a subsidiary of John Wiley & Sons, Inc.

explant in vitro, somite segmentation invariably occurs according to the predetermined sequential schedule as exemplified by the donor embryo.[4-7] In addition, AP reversal of a PSM graft leads to the formation of somites in a P to A direction, clearly demonstrating that PSM cells respect the original sequence of AP somite formation[8,9] (Fig. 2).

Time Control during Somite Formation: The Segmentation Clock

The experiments described above strongly point to the existence of an intrinsic somitic segmentation programme that allows PSM cells to "know" when to form a somite and, consequently, the AP direction of this process. In agreement with these data, nine years ago, the first molecular evidence was provided for the existence of a molecular oscillator at work within the PSM cells.[10] This work showed that a batch of chick embryos with the same number of formed somites, i.e., synchronous in development with a maximum error of 90 minutes, displayed different PSM expression patterns of the *hairy1* gene, a basic Helix-Loop-Helix (bHLH) transcription repressor belonging to the Hairy/Enhancer-of-Split-1 (HES) superfamily of genes. Thus some embryos displayed *hairy1* mRNA expression in a broad caudal domain of the PSM while others showed mRNA expression of this gene in just a narrow anterior band in the rostral PSM. The authors were able to demonstrate that these different expression profiles were consecutive snapshots of a dynamic wave of mRNA expression which sweeps across the PSM in a posterior to anterior direction in a reiterative manner and stabilises as a narrow stripe in the anteriormost PSM. The periodicity of this cyclic expression corresponds to 90 minutes, which coincides with the formation time of a somite pair in the chick embryo. Embryonic manipulations in the chick have further verified that the autonomous PSM oscillations of the *hairy1* gene are independent of cell migration and do not rely on a diffusible signal travelling within the PSM tissue.[10] This kinematic "wave" of expression results from a slight asynchrony of the *hairy1* periodic expression that occurs between the PSM cells that are located at slightly different AP levels.

Additional experimental data on this subject has demonstrated that cyclic behaviour is initiated in prospective PSM cells, at the level of Hensen's node and the primitive streak region, as judged by cycles of expression of the *hairy1* gene aswell as other cyclic genes (detailed below).[11,12] Thus, this intrinsic property is bestowed upon paraxial mesoderm cells from the moment they gastrulate and take up a position in the primitive streak. Interestingly, explant culture experiments performed in Palmeirim's lab have also demonstrated that the lateral part of the PSM when isolated from its medial counterpart does not form somites and loses the expression of *hairy1* and other cyclic genes (see below) as well as presenting a downregulation of PSM markers such as *delta1*, *notch1* and *paraxis*.[11] In contrast, medial PSM explants isolated from the lateral PSM are able to form somites and retain the capacity to express all these molecular markers in a similar pattern to the intact control PSM.[11] Hence these experiments unveiled a marked difference between the medial and lateral regions of the PSM such that an intrinsic segmentation capacity and PSM identity is restricted to the medial PSM which then seems to impart this information to the lateral PSM.

Curiously, recent evidence has shown that dissociated PSM cells in vitro lose the ability to maintain synchronous oscillations. These findings imply that cell-cell communication or a community effect is essential for the synchronization of the normal cyclic gene expression in these cells.[13] Consistently, along with the in vivo visualization of the kinematic wave of mouse *hes1* expression in the PSM, Masamizu and collaborators also observed that dissociated PSM cells present individually with an unstable period and amplitude, reinforcing the idea that cell-cell communication is crucial to stabilize the cellular oscillator.[14]

The Genetic Complexity Underlying the Segmentation Clock

Following the discovery of the *hairy1* cycling gene in the chick embryo, many other genes were reported to exhibit a cyclic expression pattern at the level of the PSM and its prospective territory in the chick.[2] Furthermore, the molecular mechanisms underlying this process appear to be highly conserved among vertebrates, given that oscillatory gene transcription has also been reported in organisms such as the mouse, zebrafish, frog and medaka.[2] Until recently most of the genes exhibiting an oscillatory expression pattern in the PSM encode for Notch signalling pathway components which is consistent with the need for cell-cell communication since both the receptor and ligand in this pathway are transmembrane proteins. These Notch-related clock genes include the *hairy1, hairy2, lunatic fringe* and *hey2* in the chick;[10,15-18] *hes1, hes7, hey2, lunatic fringe* and the Notch intracellular domain (NICD) in the mouse;[15,18-23] *her1, her7, her11, her12, her15* and *deltaC* in zebrafish;[24-28] *esr9* in the frog[29] and *her7* in medaka.[30] This repertoire of cycling genes has since expanded and now includes three genes coding for regulators of the Wnt signalling pathway, namely *axin2, nkd1* and *dact1*, which have been shown to oscillate in the mouse PSM.[31-33]

An exhaustive study with mutant mice has further contributed to the understanding of the molecular complexity that underlies the process of somite formation. The authors showed that whereas Notch1/Notch2 or Notch1/Notch4 double mutants or Pofut1 mutants still form anterior somites, Presenilin1/Presenilin2 double mutants lack both anterior and posterior somite formation.[22,34-35] Consequently, this observation led to the conclusion that the formation of the rostral-most somites required an activity of the Presenilin protein which differs from its role as a γ-secretase and which is likely to be independent of Notch signalling.[22] Hence, this alternative Presenilin pathway is potentially another signalling pathway that adds to the molecular complexity controlling the process of somitogenesis.

Moreover, a very recent study using microarray technology has uncovered the existence of many more cycling genes in the mouse PSM, belonging not only to the Notch and Wnt signalling pathways but also to the FGF signalling pathway.[36] Interestingly, the authors show that the cycling genes may be classified into two main groups. The first group includes new oscillatory members of the Notch and FGF signalling pathways, and present the particularity of cycling in synchrony with the previously reported cycling genes belonging to the Notch pathway. Conversely, the second category of genes includes new cycling members of the Wnt signalling pathway which present oscillatory cycles that are out of phase with the members of the Notch and FGF signalling pathways. In agreement, this second group of genes exhibits an oscillatory cycle in synchrony with *axin2* that had already been reported to cycle with opposite phases to the *lunatic fringe* gene.[31] Taken together, these data open the possibility that many other cycling genes may exist, which indicates that complex genetic networks regulate the process of vertebrate segmentation, involving the interplay between several signalling pathways.[36] Clearly, it will be an important next step to investigate at what level this interplay exists between these different pathways.

Lastly, another recent study has reported a new class of cycling genes from the Snail superfamily of transcriptional repressors involved in epithelium-to-mesenchyme transitions, namely *Snail1* and *Snail2*. These genes present an oscillatory expression in the PSM of mouse and chick embryos, respectively.[37] The relevance of this work is that the cyclic expression of the *snail* genes seems to be Notch independent but Wnt and FGF signalling dependent. The authors suggest that these genes may be providing the link between the segmentation clock and the wavefront of differentiation (Fig. 3) (see below).

The "Clock and Wavefront" Model

An important theme that has attracted scientists in recent years is the molecular mechanism that underlies the conversion of an oscillatory temporal phenomenon, such as cyclic gene expression into a spatially periodic event such as the formation of a pair of somites every 90 minutes in the chick embryo. Experimental data gathered so far seems to support a well-known model called the 'clock and wavefront', which was the first theoretical model to postulate the existence of an intracellular oscillator intrinsic to PSM cells.[38] According to the 'clock and wavefront' model, periodicity and size of somite formation depends not only on an intrinsic cellular oscillator but also on a wavefront of maturation that travels along the AP axis of the embryo concomitant with the oscillator of the PSM cells.

As was previously described, experimental evidence for the existence of a molecular clock was provided with the discovery of the oscillatory expression of several so-called clock genes.[2] Likewise,

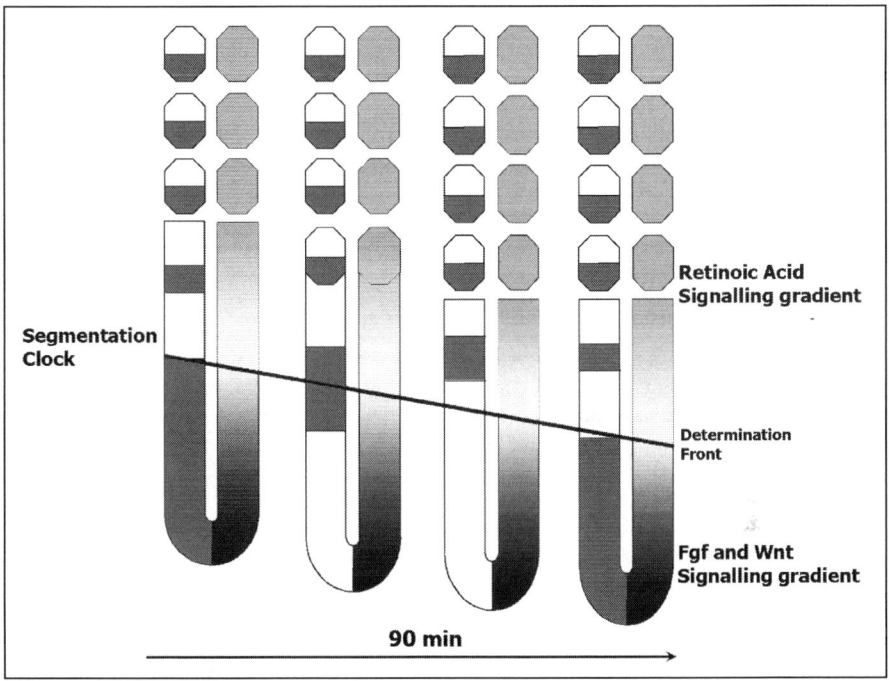

Segmentation Clock

Retinoic Acid Signalling gradient

Determination Front

Fgf and Wnt Signalling gradient

90 min

Figure 3. Representation of the segmentation clock and of the wavefront of differentiation that control somite formation in vertebrate embryos. The left side of this schematic diagram represents the oscillatory behaviour of the cycling genes (in dark orange) in the chick PSM. The cyclic expression of these genes appears as a caudal-to-rostral wave that crosses the PSM, every 90 minutes, which corresponds to the time required to form one pair of somites. This expression is stabilized at the level of the epithelial somites, once these are completely formed, and a new cycle of expression begins in the caudal PSM. The right side of the diagram represents the gradual displacement of the determination front (thick black line), whose position is defined by the opposing gradients of retinoic acid (in light orange) and FGF and Wnt (in black) signalling pathways. A color version of this figure is available online at www.eurekah.com.

a pioneer study in the chick embryo presented a putative molecular identity for the wavefront of maturation. This study showed that the PSM could be subdivided into two distinct regions: a mature and determined region with respect to segmentation located in the anterior third of the PSM and an immature and undetermined region located in its posterior part. The transition between these two regions is governed by a negative threshold of an *fgf8* gradient of expression whose anterior limit establishes a "determination front".[9] Snail acting downstream of FGF activity in the caudal PSM maintains cells in a mesenchymal state. With each pulse of the clock snail expression is temporarily downregulated in the caudal PSM, coincident with the determination of a group of cells as they cross the determination front, initiate epithelialisation and embark upon their segmentation programme. As the embryo grows and elongates, this front progressively regresses ensuring that epithelial somites form at constant periods, thus establishing a mechanism by which, the periodic oscillations of the cycling genes are converted into a reiterated spatial pattern along the PSM.[39] Subsequent studies in chick, mouse and zebrafish embryos have further demonstrated that the position of the determination front is regulated not only by FGF but, also by the Wnt and RA signalling pathways.[31,40,41] Since both assumptions of the clock-and-wavefront model have been demonstrated experimentally, it is currently accepted that this model is the most likely explanation for the mechanism by which the temporal and spatial regulation of somitogenesis is accomplished.

Temporal vs. Positional Information

Classical studies in chick and mouse embryos have established that the presomitic tissue contains 12 prospective somites within its extension.[42,43] Hence, when the molecular clock was first described the authors suggested that the PSM cells could be counting the number of oscillations of the cycling genes that they experienced. According to this idea only when 12 cycles had passed would the PSM cells undergo the mesenchymal to epithelial transition required for them to become incorporated into a somite.[10] It is now known that prospective PSM cells are already undergoing cyclic waves of expression prior to their incorporation into the PSM,[11,12] which indicates that these cells experience more than the 12 cycles of expression that they experience at the level of the PSM. Hence, a broadly accepted idea is that the main function of the segmentation clock is to provide AP positional information to PSM cells and their precursors, by imposing upon them a specific spatial organisation within the PSM prospective territory before they incorporate into a somite. Moreover, precise isotopic (same place) quail-chick grafts have determined that the most anterior cells within the prospective PSM territory will later be located in more medial PSM positions and more posterior cells will be located in more lateral PSM positions. Interestingly, since the 'wave' of expression of cycling genes spreads along the longitudinal axis of the PSM prospective territory, it implies that this 'wave' of gene expression also spreads along the future medial/lateral PSM axis. Hence, these findings imply that the segmentation clock provides the PSM cells with bidimensional positional information, not only along the AP but also along the medial-lateral axis.

The specific identity of a given somite along the AP axis of the body is controlled by the combinatorial expression of a group of genes that are denominated Hox genes. This class of transcription factors is known to confer positional identity along the AP body axis in a variety of tissues in vertebrate embryos by means of spatial and temporal colinearity. The term colinearity comprises the fact that within the four clusters of hox genes (Hox a-d) those genes located at the 3' end of the chromosomal clusters are expressed at an earlier developmental stage and in more rostral regions than the genes at the 5' end of the cluster, which are expressed later in progressively more posterior regions of the embryo.[44] This colinearity of expression is respected in the paraxial mesoderm.

A study performed in the mouse embryo has described that *Hoxd* genes present dynamic bursts of expression at the anterior part of the PSM just before a somite forms.[45] The authors of this work suggested the existence of an interaction between the segmentation clock and the sequential expression of the hox genes in the PSM. Hence, according to this hypothesis, a counting mechanism for AP segmental identity could be provided by the segmentation clock, which would ensure that the hox genes available in the cells of the next forming somite would be transcribed at every cycle of the clock. This mechanism would establish the correct coordination between sequential segment formation and AP regional identity.[45]

Interestingly, a study involving grafting and gain of function experiments in the chick embryo has recently shown that the sequential expression of Hox genes at the level of the primitive streak region is related with the order of migration of the somitic precursors.[46] The authors of this work demonstrated that the expression of more anterior *Hoxb* genes regulates the migration of somitic precursors that will give rise to more rostrally located somites. Conversely, the expression of more posterior *Hoxb* genes influences the migration of more caudally located somitic precursors. Hence it seems that the colinear activation of Hox genes at the level of the primitive streak regulates the timing of somitic precursor migration, so that their correct final positioning along the AP axis is achieved.[46]

Conclusions

Throughout this chapter we have provided data that indicate the existence of a conserved clock mechanism dictating the timing of segment formation. At this point, it is interesting to raise the question of whether this molecular oscillator operates elsewhere during embryogenesis.[47] On that note it is noteworthy that, as described above, onset of cyclic gene expression is first observed in the primitive streak as gastrulation is initiated. However, this dynamic expression is not restricted to PSM precursors but rather sweeps across the entire primitive streak and thus precursors of a wide variety of mesodermal tissues experience waves of cyclic gene expression before they migrate out to their respective positions in the developing embryo. It remains to be seen whether early exposure to this molecular oscillator plays a role in the timing of differentiation and or regionalisation of other primitive streak derived tissues. Moreover, a recent study has further unveiled that the *hairy2* gene is exhibiting cycles of expression in the chick limb bud suggesting that the clock mechanism may also control limb outgrowth.[48] The fascinating conclusion that comes out from this work is that different types of cells may be measuring time using a clock mechanism similar to the segmentation clock. Interestingly, a cell culture experiment performed with several mouse cell lines clearly showed that the hes1 mRNA and protein exhibit a 2h cyclic expression in these cultures following exposure to a serum shock.[49] These findings lead to the exciting possibility that a molecular oscillator may be providing cellular temporal information in many embryonic structures as a means of measuring developmental time, albeit with tissue-specific time periods.

Acknowledgements

We thank Tatiana Resende and Fernanda Bajanca for the critical reading of this chapter. IP is a member of the EU/FP6-Network of Excellence-Cells into Organs. JKD is a member of The Royal Society and is funded by an MRC Research Grant. MM is funded by the Muscle Dystrophy Association and an MRC Career Development Fellowship.

References

1. Hirsinger E, Jouve C, Dubrulle J et al. Somite formation and patterning. Int Rev Cytol 2000; 198:1-65.
2. Freitas C, Rodrigues S, Saude L et al. Running after the clock. Int J Dev Biol 2005; 49(2-3):317-324.
3. Gossler A, Hrabe de Angelis M. Somitogenesis. Curr Top Dev Biol 1998; 38:225-287.
4. Packard Jr DS. The influence of axial structures on chick somite formation. Dev Biol 1976; 53(1):36-48.
5. Packard Jr DS. Chick somite determination: The role of factors in young somites and the segmental plate. J Exp Zool 1978; 203(2):295-306.
6. Sandor S, Fazakas-Todea I. Researches on the formation of axial organs in the chick embryo. X. Further investigations on the role of ecto- and endoderm in somitogenesis. Morphol Embryol (Bucur) 1980; 26(1):29-32.
7. Palmeirim I, Dubrulle J, Henrique D et al. Uncoupling segmentation and somitogenesis in the chick presomitic mesoderm. Dev Genet 1998; 23(1):77-85.
8. Christ B, Jacob HJ, Jacob M. Somitogenesis in the chick embryo: Determination of the segmentation direction. Verh Anat Ges 1974; 68:573-579.
9. Dubrulle J, McGrew MJ, Pourquie O. FGF signaling controls somite boundary position and regulates segmentation clock control of spatiotemporal Hox gene activation. Cell 2001; 106(2):219-232.
10. Palmeirim I, Henrique D, Ish-Horowicz D et al. Avian hairy gene expression identifies a molecular clock linked to vertebrate segmentation and somitogenesis. Cell 1997; 91(5):639-648.
11. Freitas C, Rodrigues S, Charrier JB et al. Evidence for medial/lateral specification and positional information within the presomitic mesoderm. Development 2001; 128(24):5139-5147.
12. Jouve C, Iimura T, Pourquie O. Onset of the segmentation clock in the chick embryo: Evidence for oscillations in the somite precursors in the primitive streak. Development 2002; 129(5):1107-1117.
13. Maroto M, Dale JK, Dequeant ML et al. Synchronised cycling gene oscillations in presomitic mesoderm cells require cell-cell contact. Int J Dev Biol 2005; 49(2-3):309-315.

14. Masamizu Y, Ohtsuka T, Takashima Y et al. Real-time imaging of the somite segmentation clock: Revelation of unstable oscillators in the individual presomitic mesoderm cells. Proc Natl Acad Sci USA 2006; 103(5):1313-1318.
15. Jouve C, Palmeirim I, Henrique D et al. Notch signalling is required for cyclic expression of the hairy-like gene HES1 in the presomitic mesoderm. Development 2000; 127(7):1421-1429.
16. McGrew MJ, Dale JK, Fraboulet S et al. The lunatic fringe gene is a target of the molecular clock linked to somite segmentation in avian embryos. Curr Biol 1998; 8(17):979-982.
17. Aulehla A, Johnson RL. Dynamic expression of lunatic fringe suggests a link between notch signaling and an autonomous cellular oscillator driving somite segmentation. Dev Biol 1999; 207(1):49-61.
18. Leimeister C, Dale K, Fischer A et al. Oscillating expression of c-Hey2 in the presomitic mesoderm suggests that the segmentation clock may use combinatorial signaling through multiple interacting bHLH factors. Dev Biol 2000; 227(1):91-103.
19. Bessho Y, Sakata R, Komatsu S et al. Dynamic expression and essential functions of Hes7 in somite segmentation. Genes Dev 2001; 15(20):2642-2647.
20. Forsberg H, Crozet F, Brown NA. Waves of mouse Lunatic fringe expression, in four-hour cycles at two-hour intervals, precede somite boundary formation. Curr Biol 1998; 8(18):1027-1030.
21. Maruhashi M, Van De Putte T, Huylebroeck D et al. Involvement of SIP1 in positioning of somite boundaries in the mouse embryo. Dev Dyn 2005; 234(2):332-8.
22. Huppert SS, Ilagan MX, De Strooper B et al. Analysis of Notch function in presomitic mesoderm suggests a gamma-secretase-independent role for presenilins in somite differentiation. Dev Cell 2005; 8(5):677-688.
23. Morimoto M, Takahashi Y, Endo M et al. The Mesp2 transcription factor establishes segmental borders by suppressing Notch activity. Nature 2005; 435(7040):354-359.
24. Holley SA, Geisler R, Nusslein-Volhard C. Control of her1 expression during zebrafish somitogenesis by a delta-dependent oscillator and an independent wave-front activity. Genes Dev 2000; 14(13):1678-1690.
25. Oates AC, Ho RK. Hairy/E(spl)-related (Her) genes are central components of the segmentation oscillator and display redundancy with the Delta/Notch signaling pathway in the formation of anterior segmental boundaries in the zebrafish. Development 2002; 129(12):2929-2946.
26. Jiang YJ, Aerne BL, Smithers L et al. Notch signalling and the synchronization of the somite segmentation clock. Nature 2000; 408(6811):475-479.
27. Sieger D, Tautz D, Gajewski M. Her11 is involved in the somitogenesis clock in zebrafish. Dev Genes Evol 2004; 214:393-406.
28. Shankaran SS, Sieger D, Schroter C et al. Completing the set of h/E(spl) cyclic genes in zebrafish: Her12 and her15 reveal novel modes of expression and contribute to the segmentation clock. Dev Biol 2007.
29. Li Y, Fenger U, Niehrs C et al. Cyclic expression of esr9 gene in Xenopus presomitic mesoderm. Differentiation 2003; 71(1):83-89.
30. Elmasri H, Liedtke D, Lucking G et al. her7 and hey1, but not lunatic fringe show dynamic expression during somitogenesis in medaka (Oryzias latipes). Gene Expr Patterns 2004; 4(5):553-559.
31. Aulehla A, Wehrle C, Brand-Saberi B et al. Wnt3a plays a major role in the segmentation clock controlling somitogenesis. Dev Cell 2003; 4(3):395-406.
32. Ishikawa A, Kitajima S, Takahashi Y et al. Mouse Nkd1, a Wnt antagonist, exhibits oscillatory gene expression in the PSM under the control of Notch signaling. Mech Dev 2004; 121(12):1443-1453.
33. Suriben R, Fisher DA, Cheyette BN. Dact1 presomitic mesoderm expression oscillates in phase with Axin2 in the somitogenesis clock of mice. Dev Dyn 2006; 235(11):3177-3183.
34. Krebs LT, Xue Y, Norton CR et al. Genes Dev 2000; 14:1343-1352.
35. Shi S, Stanley P. Protein O-fucosyltransferase 1 is an essential component of Notch signaling pathways. Proc Natl Acad Sci USA 2003; 100(9):5234-9, (Epub 2003 Apr 15).
36. Dequeant ML, Glynn E, Gaudenz K et al. A complex oscillating network of signaling genes underlies the mouse segmentation clock. Science. 2006; 314(5805):1595-1598.
37. Dale JK, Malapert P, Chal J et al. Oscillations of the snail genes in the presomitic mesoderm coordinate segmental patterning and morphogenesis in vertebrate somitogenesis. Dev Cell 2006; 10(3):355-366.
38. Cooke J, Zeeman EC. A clock and wavefront model for control of the number of repeated structures during animal morphogenesis. J Theor Biol 1976; 58(2):455-476.
39. Pourquie O. The segmentation clock: Converting embryonic time into spatial pattern. Science 2003; 301(5631):328-330.
40. Sawada A, Shinya M, Jiang YJ et al. Fgf/MAPK signalling is a crucial positional cue in somite boundary formation. Development 2001; 128(23):4873-4880.

41. Diez del Corral R, Olivera-Martinez I, Goriely A et al. Opposing FGF and retinoid pathways control ventral neural pattern, neuronal differentiation, and segmentation during body axis extension. Neuron 2003; 40(1):65-79.

42. Packard Jr DS, Meier S. An experimental study of the somitomeric organization of the avian segmental plate. Dev Biol 1983; 97(1):191-202.

43. Tam PP. The control of somitogenesis in mouse embryos. J Embryol Exp Morphol 1981; 65(Suppl):103-128.

44. Deschamps J, van Nes J. Developmental regulation of the Hox genes during axial morphogenesis in the mouse. Development 2005; 132(13):2931-2942.

45. Zakany J, Kmita M, Alarcon P et al. Localized and transient transcription of Hox genes suggests a link between patterning and the segmentation clock. Cell 2001; 106(2):207-217.

46. Iimura T, Pourquie O. Collinear activation of Hoxb genes during gastrulation is linked to mesoderm cell ingression. Nature 2006; 442(7102):568-571.

47. Andrade RP, Pascoal S, Palmeirim I. Thinking clockwise. Brain Res Brain Res Rev 2005; 49(2):114-119.

48. 48. Pascoal S, Carvalho CR, Rodriguez-León J, Delphini MC, Duprez D, Thorsteinsdóttir S, Palmeirim I. A molecular clock operates during chick autopod proximal-distal outgrowth. J. Mol Biol. Apr 27 2007;368(2):303-9.

49. Hirata H, Yoshiura S, Ohtsuka T, et al. Oscillatory expression of the bHLH factor Hes1 regulated by a negative feedback loop. Science. Oct 25 2002;298(5594):840-843.

## CHAPTER 6

Oscillatory Expression of Hes Family Transcription Factors:
Insights from Mathematical Modelling

Hiroshi Momiji and Nicholas A.M. Monk*

Abstract

Oscillatory expression of the Hes family of transcription factors plays a central role in the segmentation of the vertebrate body during embryonic development. Analogous oscillations in cultured cells suggest that Hes oscillations may be important in other developmental processes, and provide an excellent opportunity to explore the origin of these oscillations in a relatively simple setting. Mathematical and computational modelling have been used in combination with quantitative mRNA and protein expression data to analyse the origin and properties of Hes oscillations, and have highlighted the important roles played by time delays in negative feedback circuits. In this chapter, we review recent theoretical and experimental results, and discuss how analysis of existing models suggests potential avenues for further study of delayed feedback oscillators.

Delay-Driven Oscillations in Cellular Signaling Systems

A primary response of cells to external stimuli is to regulate the transcriptional activity of target genes. Such transcriptional stimulus-response systems underlie a wide range of tissue-level processes such as physiological responses and the emergence of stable spatio-temporal patterns of cell fate during the development of multicellular organisms. The rapid responses characteristic of many physiological and developmental processes require key mRNA and protein targets to have short half-lives, and adaptive responses typically rely on negative feedback, which can operate at many different levels of the response pathway.[1] If the negative feedback involves transcriptional steps, then the time delays inherent in the processes of transcription and translation can play important roles in determining the dynamics of the signalling system. Delayed negative feedback often results in either transient or sustained oscillations, particularly when the total delay in the feedback circuit is comparable to the half lives of the key circuit components.

The propensity of delayed negative feedback to generate transcriptional oscillations has been recognised for many years (see, for example, refs. 2-3), but direct experimental evidence for such oscillations in cellular response systems has emerged only recently. These response oscillations are distinct from other well-studied intrinsic oscillators, such as those associated with the cell cycle[4] and circadian timekeeping,[5] in that they are initiated in response to extrinsic signals, involve a single transcriptional step and have quite short (ultradian) periods in the range of 2-3 hours. Notable examples are the NF-κB-IκB system,[6-8] the p53-Mdm2 system[8-10]

*Corresponding Author: Nicholas A.M. Monk—School of Mathematical Sciences, University of Nottingham, University Park, Nottingham, NG7 2RD, UK.
Email: nick.monk@nottingham.ac.uk

Cellular Oscillatory Mechanisms, edited by Miguel Maroto and Nicholas A.M. Monk.
©2008 Landes Bioscience and Springer Science+Business Media.

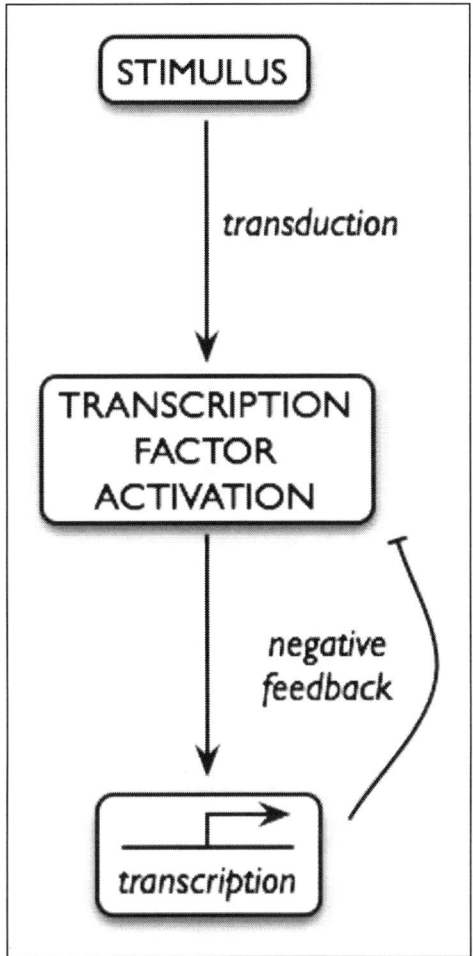

Figure 1. The basic logical structure of adaptive transcriptional response systems. Signal transduction converts an external stimulus into activation of one or more transcription factors. A feature of the transcriptional response is the production of one or more feedback inhibitors that act to suppress the response.

and the Hes1 system.[11-13] These systems share a common simple regulatory structure, centred around a rapid response to an external signal coupled to a negative feedback mediated by transcriptional regulation (Fig. 1).

The process of transcription introduces both irreducible and effective delays into the response network. Irreducible delays result from the limited speed of transcript elongation, which proceeds at a rate of around 1000-2000 nucleotide bases per minute in eukaryotes.[14] Transcription factors control the rate of initiation of transcripts, but it is only full length transcripts that can be used as templates for translation. Thus, the finite rate of transcript elongation introduces a delay between changes in regulatory input (rate of transcript initiation) and effective output (completion of mature transcript) that is proportional to the length of genomic sequence being transcribed. In addition to this irreducible delay, eukaryotic transcripts must undergo splicing, processing and export from the nucleus to the cytoplasm, introducing further effective delays between transcript initiation and appearance of mature translatable mRNA in the cytoplasm.[15,16] Taken together, these processes introduce a delay of around 15-20 minutes between initiation and completion of a 'typical' transcript,[17] although this delay can be much longer for large genes (the human dystrophin gene, for example, takes 16 hours to transcribe[18]). Similarly, the linear elongation of nascent proteins during translation (which proceeds at a rate of around 120 amino acids per minute[19]) introduces an additional irreducible delay into transcriptional regulation. Taken together with a regulatory logic centred on negative feedback, these delays play a significant role in generating the observed oscillatory dynamics of the cellular response systems centred on NF-κB, p53 and Hes1.[20-22]

In this chapter, we focus on the Hes family of basic helix-loop-helix transcription factors. The Hes family (whose members are referred to as Her in some species) are structurally related to the *Drosophila* hairy and Enhancer of split proteins, and play central roles in a range of key processes in vertebrate development.[23,24] Oscillatory expression has been observed for a number of Hes family members in vivo, and has been shown to play a central role during somitogenesis, the process by which the vertebrate body becomes overtly segmented during embryonic development.[25-31] In particular, we focus on the murine transcription factor Hes1, for which oscillations have been observed in a range of cultured cells and in cells isolated from the mouse presomitic mesoderm.[11-13] These culture systems present excellent opportunities for obtaining quantitative mRNA and protein expression data in a system that is much simpler than the network of oscillating factors underlying vertebrate somitogenesis.[32] We describe efforts to understand the origin of Hes1 oscillations using quantitative expression data together with mathematical and computational modelling, and discuss the insights that have been gained from these model-based studies.

Hes1 as a Cellular Oscillator

The Hes1 protein, and its corresponding mRNA, exhibit striking oscillatory expression with a period of around two hours in a number of different cell types during embryonic development, and these oscillations are believed to regulate the timing of other events in these cells.[11,12,24] Hes1 is a basic helix-loop-helix transcription factor that negatively regulates its own expression by binding directly (either as a homodimer or as a heterodimers with other Hes proteins) to at least four binding sites in the regulatory sequence of the *hes1* gene.[33] In the mouse embryo, Hes1 is only one of a large number of interacting factors that oscillate with a two hour period in the presomitic mesoderm.[34] The complexity of the resulting oscillatory network is further complicated by spatio-temporal coordination throughout the mesoderm, mediated by intercellular signalling. This complexity, which is only partially characterised, makes it difficult to infer the mechanistic details of oscillatory Hes1 regulation.

Fortunately, Hes1 oscillations can be studied in a much simpler system, since oscillatory Hes1 expression can be induced by serum stimulation of a range of murine cell types in culture.[11-13] Importantly, in cells such as fibroblasts, serum stimulation does not induce expression of many of the network components that interact with Hes1 in the embryo, increasing the likelihood that the oscillations are due to a network of interactions centred on Hes1 itself. Furthermore, in a population of induced cells the oscillations are at least initially in phase, making it possible to detect oscillations in mRNA and protein expression levels in samples drawn from a population at regular time intervals.[11,13] The fact that induced oscillations in cultured cells have a period that matches that of endogenous Hes1 during somitogenesis suggests that the same regulatory logic underlies both oscillations; this belief is further supported by the observation that expression of the human *HES1* gene has been observed to oscillate with a five hour period in a human mesenchymal stem/stromal cell model, which is consistent with the rate of somitogenesis in human.[13]

The ability to generate synchronous oscillations in cell culture makes it possible to obtain quantitative time-course data on the expression levels of both *Hes1* mRNA and Hes1 protein.

Hirata et al[11] used northern and western blots of fibroblasts harvested from culture at regular time intervals following serum treatment to show that mRNA and protein levels oscillate with a period of approximately 120 minutes. Additionally, these studies showed that the protein oscillation lags behind the mRNA oscillation by 15-20 minutes, and that the fold-difference amplitude (peak/trough ratio) of expression during oscillations is approximately 3 for mRNA and 3-6 for protein.[11] Recent analysis of oscillatory mRNA expression in mouse fibroblasts by quantitative PCR confirmed the period and amplitude of *Hes1* mRNA oscillations.[13] When assessed at the level of cell populations, Hes1 oscillations appear to be significantly damped after 6-12 hours.[11] However, live imaging of fibroblasts expressing a fluorescently-tagged Hes1 fusion protein shows that Hes1 oscillations persist for at least 48 hours.[12] These results suggest that the damping observed in cell populations is a result of a loss of synchrony within the population due to stochastic effects, rather than the damping of oscillations at the level of individual cells.[12]

The oscillatory dynamics exhibited by Hes1 depend on rapid turnover of mRNA and protein, whose concentrations must fall from maximum to minimum values in one hour. Pulse-chase experiments confirm this; both *Hes1* mRNA and Hes1 protein undergo approximately linear degradation, with half-lives of around 20-25 minutes in fibroblasts.[11] The short Hes1 protein half-life depends on ubiquitination of Hes1, followed by proteolysis; blockage of proteolysis increases the Hes1 half-life significantly and abolishes both mRNA and protein oscillations, highlighting the importance of both protein instability and Hes1-mediated negative feedback of *Hes1* transcription.[11] Further evidence of the importance of short protein half-lives for short period oscillations is provided by mouse Hes7, which also oscillates with a period of around two hours during somitogenesis as a result of direct self-inhibition.[26,27] Like Hes1, the Hes7 protein has a half-life of 22 minutes.[28] Strikingly, an increase in Hes7 half-life to 30 minutes results in the abolishment of Hes7 oscillations in the mouse presomitic mesoderm, with consequent severe disorganisation of the segmentation process.[28]

Mathematical Modelling of the Hes1 Oscillator

All available data—from genomic analysis, cell culture and studies of Hes oscillations in vertebrate embryos—suggest that oscillations depend critically on direct self-repression (autoregulation) of *Hes* transcription by Hes proteins. Furthermore, at least for Hes1 the main mode of repression is believed to be via direct binding of Hes1 dimers to specific DNA binding sites (N boxes) in the *Hes1* promoter, rather than competitive binding to transcriptional activators.[33] The resulting simple network topology is illustrated schematically in Figure 2.

The simplicity of the basic regulatory logic believed to underlie Hes1 oscillations in cultured cells, and the availability of quantitative oscillation and degradation data makes the Hes1 system an ideal subject for mathematical analysis. Assuming that Hes1 oscillations depend primarily on the negative autoregulation of Hes1, a simple differential equation model can be written in terms of two variables $M(t)$ and $P(t)$, representing the quantities of mRNA and protein in a cell, respectively:

$$\frac{dM}{dt} = k_M G\left[P\left(t - \tau_1\right)\right] - d_M M(t),$$

$$\frac{dP}{dt} = k_P M\left(t - \tau_2\right) - d_P P(t), \tag{1}$$

with

$$G\left[P(t)\right] = \frac{P_0^n}{P_0^n + P(t)^n}. \tag{2}$$

In this model, a specific form (a decreasing Hill function) has been chosen for the function representing the rate of transcription, and translation is assumed to be linear. However, other decreasing functions representing transcriptional repression would be equally appropriate. The

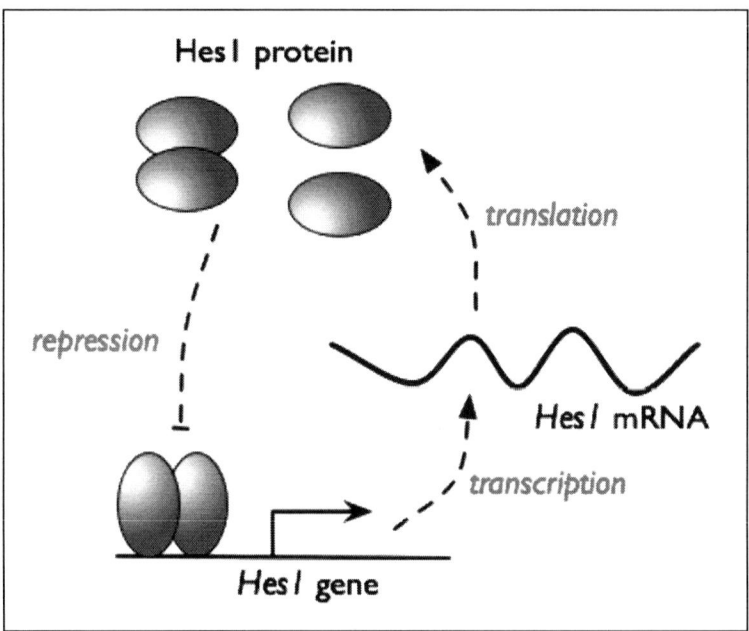

Figure 2. The basic feedback architecture of the Hes1 autoregulatory network. Hes1 protein can form homodimers that bind to a number of consensus DNA sequences in the *Hes1* promoter.

meanings of the parameters are as follows: kM is the maximal rate of *Hes1* transcription (in the absence of Hes1 protein); kP is the rate at which Hes1 protein is produced by translation from a single *Hes1* mRNA molecule; dM and dP are the linear degradation rates of *Hes1* mRNA and Hes1 protein, respectively; τ_1 and τ_2 are time delays representing the delays inherent in the transcription and translation processes, respectively; P_0 is the level of Hes1 protein for which *Hes1* transcription is reduced to half its maximal value (the repression threshold); n provides a measure of the sensitivity of the transcription rate to changes in the level of Hes1 protein (the sensitivity coefficient). Figure 3 illustrates the way in which the transcription function (a decreasing Hill function) depends on P_0 and n.

It is straightforward to show that if the transcription and translation delays are not included in this two-component model, then no sustained oscillatory solutions exist. This limitation was overcome by Hirata et al by the inclusion of a third, hypothetical, factor that interacted with Hes1 protein.[11] The resulting set of three ordinary (i.e., non-delayed) differential equations (ODEs) have sustained oscillatory solutions with properties in good agreement with the fibroblast expression data. However, as discussed above, the processes of transcription and translation introduce time delays into the regulatory feedback, which should be represented explicitly in the mathematical model as delays in the production terms for mRNA and protein, respectively. The *Hes1* gene has a length of 2440 nucleotides, indicating that the time required to produce a single nascent RNA transcript should be approximately 2 minutes. The Hes1 protein contains 282 amino acids, indicating a translation time also of approximately 2 minutes. While these figures suggest that the delays in the Hes1 system are rather small, comparison of the time-course of appearance of nascent and mature *Hes1* mRNA in fibroblasts using riboprobes directed against *Hes1* intronic sequences and mature mRNA indicates that there is an effective transcription delay of 15-20 minutes.[12] A similar transcription delay has been observed for Hes7.[27] A significant component of these delays could result from slow export of *Hes1* mRNA from the nucleus.[15]

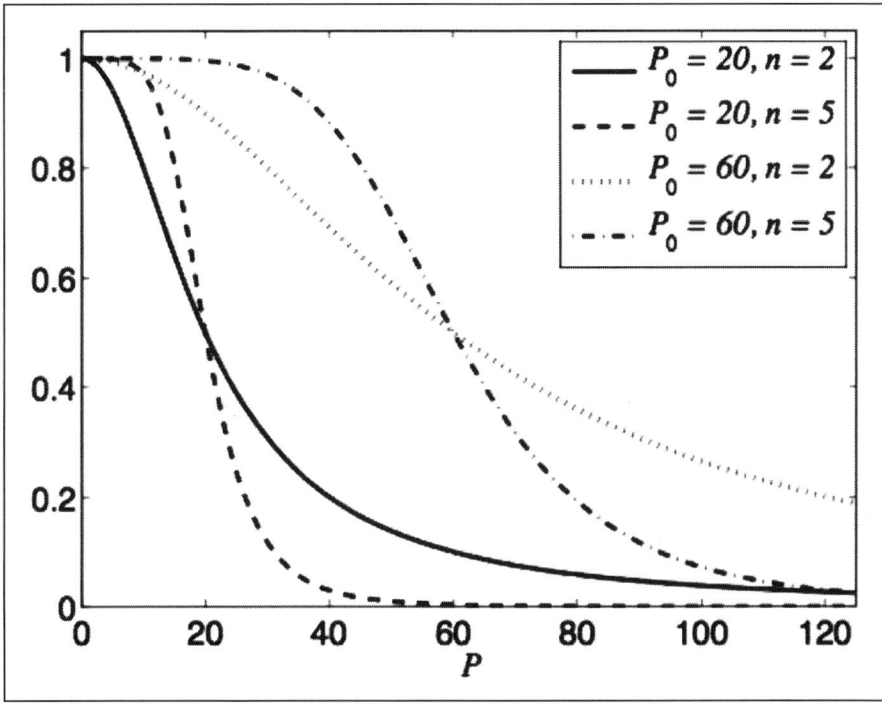

Figure 3. Illustration of the dependence of the form of the transcription rate Hill function $G(P) = P_0 n / (P_0 n + P n)$ on the parameters P_0 (the repression threshold) and n (the sensitivity coefficient).

Incorporation of non-zero transcription and translation delays in Equations (1) and (2) has a significant impact on the dynamical properties of solutions representing *Hes1* mRNA and Hes1 protein. Such delay differential equations (DDEs) are capable of generating sustained oscillations, even with only two components.[2,3,21,22,35] As the magnitude of the delays increases, critical values are reached for which the unique steady state of the system (which always exists) becomes unstable (the system goes through a Hopf bifurcation[36]). For delays above the critical values (which depend on the other model parameters), a stable limit cycle exists, corresponding to sustained oscillatory expression of mRNA and protein.

While the potential involvement of unknown components in addition to Hes1 mRNA and protein cannot be ruled out, the inclusion of transcription and translation delays opens up the possibility of accounting for the observed behaviour without them. To assess the ability of the delay model to account for the quantitative features of Hes1 oscillations in fibroblasts, it is important to determine the ways in which the solutions of the model depend on the model parameters. While the model encoded in Equations (1) and (2) appears to depend on eight parameters, the nature of the oscillatory solutions of the model actually depends on only 6 independent parameters. Furthermore, the forms of the expression profiles of mRNA and protein, considered separately, depend on only five parameters (the sixth affects only the relative timing of the two profiles).

Since the absolute expression levels of mRNA and protein cannot be determined from existing data, the mRNA and protein variables can be rescaled:

$$m(t) = \frac{M(t)}{k_M}, \ p(t) = \frac{P(t)}{k_M k_P},$$

yielding the following form of the model equations:

$$\frac{dm}{dt} = \frac{p_0^n}{p_0^n + p(t - \tau_1)^n} - d_M m(t)$$

$$\frac{dp}{dt} = m(t - \tau_2) - d_P p(t),$$

(3)

where $p_0 = P_0/(kMkP)$ is the scaled repression threshold. This simple rescaling shows immediately that the three parameters P_0, kM and kP do not act independently, but rather in the specific combination $p_0 = P_0/(kMkP)$. It is this effective parameter that determines the form of the mRNA and protein expression profiles (modulo unknown absolute scales). Furthermore, by introducing a time-shifted mRNA variable $x(t) = m(t - \tau_2)$, it can be seen that

$$\frac{dx}{dt} = \frac{p_0^n}{p_0^n + p(t - \tau)^n} - d_M x(t)$$

$$\frac{dp}{dt} = x(t) - d_P p(t),$$

(4)

where $\tau = \tau_1 + \tau_2$. The only effect of this time shift is to change the relative timing of the mRNA and protein profiles by an amount τ_2. Since $\tau_2 \approx 2$ minutes for Hes1, and the available expression data give little information on these relative timings, the model encoded in Equation (4) can be used to investigate the parameter-dependence of model solutions.[22]

Properties of Delay-Driven Oscillations

The experimentally determined half-lives of 20-25 minutes for *Hes1* mRNA and Hes1 protein correspond to linear degradation rates $dM = dP = 0.03/\text{min}$. Given these parameter values, the model depends only on three free parameters—the total delay τ, the Hill function threshold p_0 and the sensitivity coefficient n. The observed oscillatory period can be used to impose constraints on these parameter values, since the oscillatory period at the Hopf bifurcation must be at most 120 minutes. For a wide range of values of the threshold p_0, the Hopf bifurcation period meets this criterion only if the Hill sensitivity coefficient n is greater than approximately 4.5 (Fig. 4). For $n = 5$, oscillations with a period of 120 minutes are generated by a total delay of approximately 20 minutes, in good agreement with experimental data (Fig. 5).[22]

The two-component DDE model for Hes1 thus predicts that the repression of *Hes1* transcription by Hes1 protein must be highly sensitive. Put another way, this implies that there must be significant cooperativity in the action of Hes1 on the *Hes1* promoter. This result does not depend critically on the precise form of the function used to represent transcriptional repression, but only on the steepness of this function for physiological expression levels of Hes1 protein. The model reveals a further striking property of the delay-driven oscillations: the period of oscillation is almost totally insensitive to the value of the repression threshold p_0 (Fig. 6).[22,35] Recalling that p_0 is a combination of three basic model parameters, including the basal transcription and translation rates, this result shows that variation of these parameters (resulting, for example, from changes in the *Hes1* gene dosage or from the presence or absence of transcriptional activators of *Hes1* transcription) should have no measurable effect on the period of Hes1 oscillations. Thus, at least in a simple DDE model, the period of oscillations is strikingly robust to variation in maximal transcription rate, translation rate and in the binding affinity of Hes1 protein to the *Hes1* promoter. Since the two-component model is incapable of generating sustained oscillations without inclusion of delays, it is difficult to assess the extent to which this robustness depends on the inclusion of delays in the model. However, comparison of higher-dimensional DDE models and their ODE equivalents suggests that when both can generate sustained oscillations, the robustness

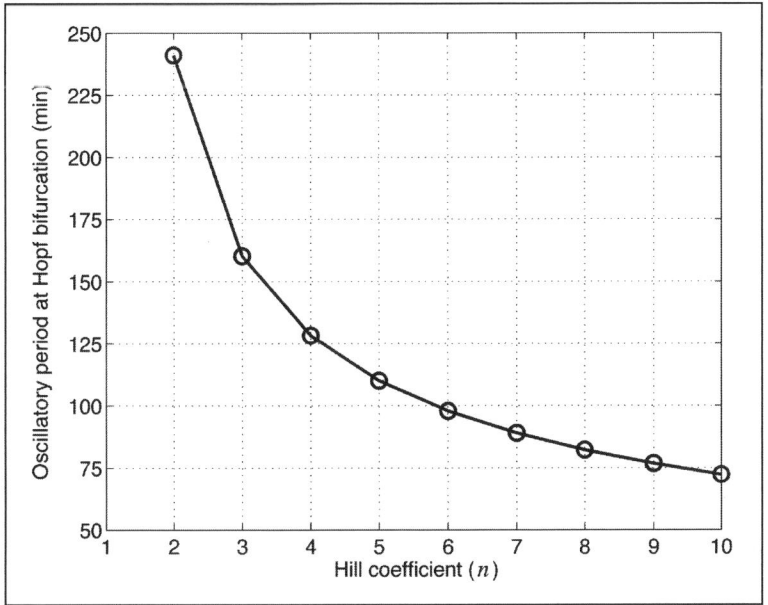

Figure 4. Dependence of the oscillatory period at Hopf bifurcation on the Hill sensitivity coefficient n, for $dM = 0.03$/min, $dP = 0.03$/min. Sustained oscillations with a period of 120 minutes are possible only for n greater than approximately 4.5. The Hopf bifurcation period is approximately independent of the (biologically plausible) values of the parameters kM, kP and P_0.

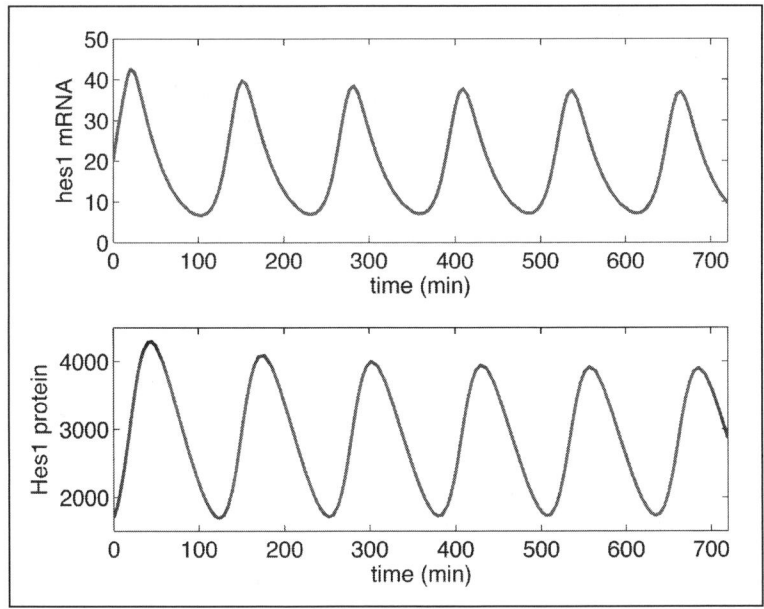

Figure 5. A typical oscillatory solution of the two-component Hes1 delay model described by Equations (1) and (2). Parameters used: $kM = 33$/min, $kP = 4.5$/min per mRNA molecule, $dM = 0.03$/min, $dP = 0.03$/min, $\tau_1 = 16.2$ min, $\tau_2 = 2$ min, $n = 5$, $P_0 = 1000$ molecules.

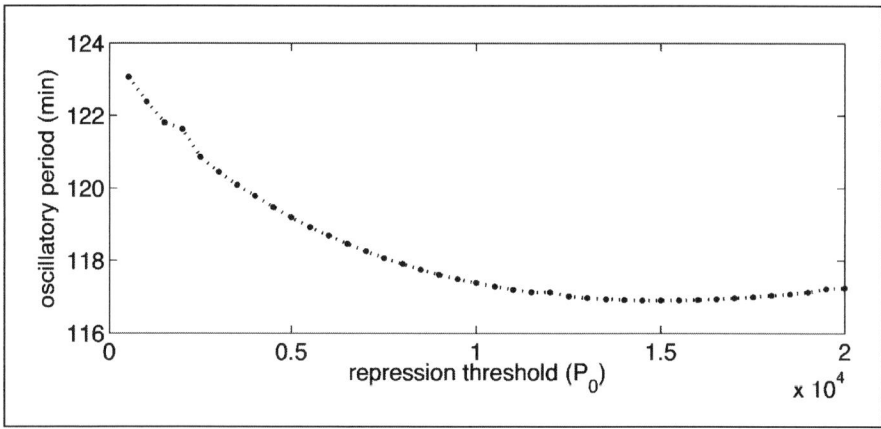

Figure 6. Insensitivity of the period of Hes1 oscillations to changes in the repression threshold P_0. The period (determined by numerical simulation of Equations (1) and (2)) varies by only 5% around its mean value of 120 min for values of P_0 ranging from 500 to 20000 molecules. Numerical simulation performed using the following parameter values: $kM = 33$/min, $kP = 4.5$/ min per mRNA molecule, $dM = 0.03$/min, $dP = 0.03$/min, $\tau_1 = 16.2$ min, $\tau_2 = 2$ min, $n = 5$.

of the oscillatory period to changes in maximal production rates is enhanced significantly by transcription and translation delays (N. Monk, unpublished data).

While the two-component DDE model (Equations (1) and (2)) has oscillatory solutions with a period and mRNA-protein expression lag that agree well with experimental data, the amplitude of the oscillations (measured as the ratio of maximum to minimum expression levels) does not match that observed in the data. In particular, oscillatory model solutions have protein expression ratios that are significantly lower than the corresponding mRNA expression ratios (see Fig. 5). This is in sharp contrast to the quantitative expression data, for which the protein ration is at least as large as the mRNA ratio.[11] It can be seen from a simple argument that this property results directly from the mathematical form adopted for the terms in Equation (1) that represent Hes1 translation and degradation. Assuming that both translation and degradation depend linearly on their substrates (mRNA and protein, respectively), the equation describing the dynamics of Hes1 protein expression is

$$\frac{dP}{dt} = k_P M(t - \tau_2) - d_P P(t). \tag{5}$$

P takes its maximum and minimum values, P_{max} and P_{min}, when $dP/dt = 0$. If adjacent maxima and minima occur at times t_1 and t_2, respectively (see Fig. 7), then the ratio of maximal to minimal protein expression, RP is given by

$$R_P = \frac{P_{max}}{P_{min}} = \frac{M(t_1 - \tau_2)}{M(t_2 - \tau_2)}. \tag{6}$$

Since the translation delay τ_2 is always less than the time lag between the mRNA and protein expression profiles (and the protein profile must always follow the mRNA profile in time), the mRNA expression levels in the numerator and denominator of Equation (6) are less than and greater than the maximal and minimal mRNA expression levels, respectively. It therefore follows directly that $RP < RM$.

This argument rests only on the assumption that translation and protein degradation can be described by linear functions. While there is no reason to assume that translation of *Hes1* mRNA should deviate significantly from linearity, and experimental data fit well with linear

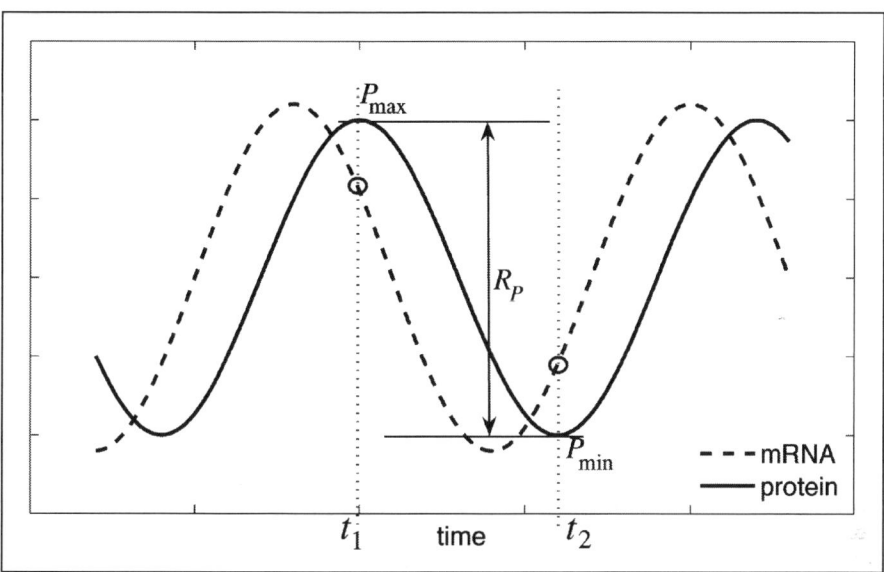

Figure 7. Schematic illustration of the relationship between oscillatory mRNA and protein expression. Adjacent maxima and minima of the protein expression profile occur at times t_1 and t_2. Because the protein expression profile lags that of the mRNA, the fold-difference in mRNA expression levels at these times is less than the maximal fold difference in the mRNA profile.

protein degradation,[11] the equation describing the dynamics of protein expression can be generalised to include nonlinearity in these two processes:

$$\frac{dP}{dt} = k_P(M)M(t - \tau_2) - d_P(P)P(t),$$ (7)

where the proportional translation and degradation rates now depend on the mRNA and protein expression levels, respectively (rather than being constant values as before). In this case, Equation (6) becomes

$$R_P = \frac{P_{max}}{P_{min}} = \frac{k_P\big(M(t_1 - \tau_2)\big)\, d_P(t_2)\, M(t_1 - \tau_2)}{k_P\big(M(t_2 - \tau_2)\big)\, d_P(t_1)\, M(t_2 - \tau_2)}$$ (8)

The magnitude of RP relative to RM can thus be increased in two ways:

1. The proportional translation rate (rate of protein production per mRNA molecule per unit time) increases as the overall number of mRNA molecules in a cell increases (i.e., translation is self-enhancing).
2. The proportional Hes1 degradation rate (i.e., rate of decay per protein molecule per unit time) decreases as the overall number of protein molecules in a cell increases (i.e., the stability of Hes1 is an increasing function of its concentration).

While self-enhanced translation of Hes1 cannot be ruled out, there is certainly no compelling evidence to suggest that this plays a significant role in generating the high amplitude oscillations observed in cell culture. Furthermore, existing protein degradation data constrain the degree of nonlinearity of the proportional protein degradation rate.[11] Notwithstanding this constraint, a possible mechanism that could result in a proportional degradation rate for Hes1 protein that decreases with Hes1 concentration depends on the differential stability of the monomeric and dimeric forms of Hes1. A number of bacterial transcription factors that operate as dimers have been reported to be more stable in dimeric form than in monomeric form, and mathematical modelling confirms that such nonlinear degradation can increase the amplitude of protein oscillations.[37] Extension of the two-component DDE model to include dimerisation of Hes1, with differential degradation rates of monomeric and dimeric forms of Hes1 can enhance the amplitude of Hes1 protein oscillations, but it remains difficult to obtain a good quantitative fit between model simulations and experimental data (H. Momiji and N. Monk, unpublished data).

Extended Models of Hes1 Regulation

The failure of a simple model of Hes1 regulation to generate oscillations with appropriate amplitudes could result from at least two possible shortcomings of the model. First, it could be that the network operating in cell culture contains components other than *hes1* mRNA and Hes1 protein that are important in generating high-amplitude oscillations. Alternatively, it might be that the two components are actually capable of generating higher-amplitude oscillations, but that the level of mechanistic detail in the current model is insufficient.

One possible extension to the Hes1 network centres on the inclusion in the network model of a transcriptional corepressor protein Groucho/TLE1. Gro/TLE1 is a necessary corepressor for Hes1, and can be activated by Hes1-induced hyperphosphoryllation under certain circumstances.[38] Addition of a variable representing Gro/TLE1 to the two-component DDE model for Hes1 results in a model that generates oscillations with an appropriate period and mRNA-protein expression lag.[39] The principal mathematical effect of adding Gro/TLE1 to the two-component model is to increase the effective sensitivity coefficient of the transcriptional response of *Hes1* mRNA to Hes1 protein. Simulations suggest that while the inclusion of Gro/TLE1 can increase the amplitude of Hes1 protein oscillations above that seen in the

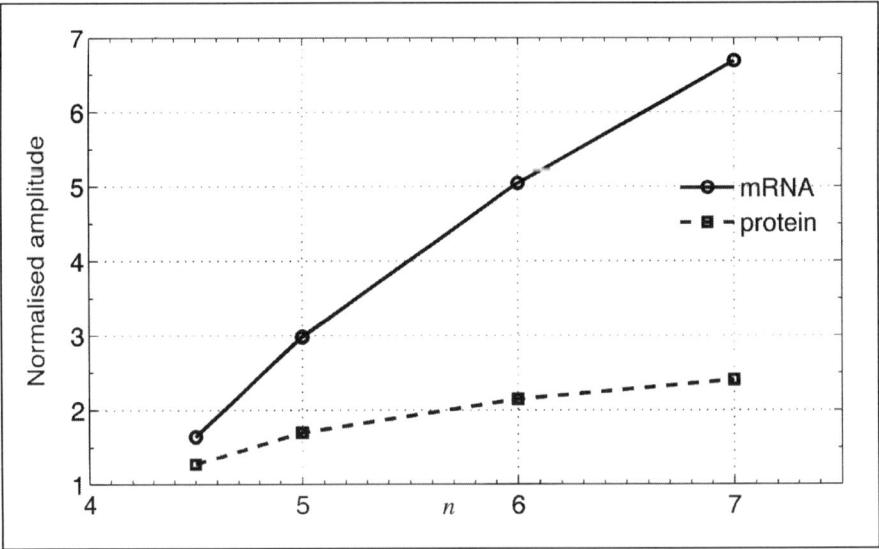

Figure 8. Dependence of the normalised amplitudes (max/min ratios) of mRNA (*RM*) and protein (*RP*) oscillations on the Hill sensitivity coefficient (*n*). Note that sustained oscillations are possible only for *n* > 4, and that as *n* increases above this value, *RM* increases faster than *RP*. Results obtained with the model described in Equations (1) and (2) with the following parameters: *kM* = 7/min, *kP* = 7/min per mRNA molecule, *dM* = 0.03/min, *dP* = 0.03/min, P_0 = 2500 molecules. The delay is tuned to generate oscillations with a period of 120 minutes (the magnitude of delay required is a decreasing function of *n*).

two-component model, this results primarily from the increase in transcriptional sensitivity. As would be expected, enhanced sensitivity also increases the amplitude of mRNA oscillations. Indeed, an increase in transcriptional sensitivity (as measured by the Hill coefficient *n*) results in a larger increase in the mRNA amplitude than in the protein amplitude (Fig. 8).

These results suggest that increases in the transcription sensitivity, whether due to direct interaction of Hes1 with the *Hes1* promoter or due to the effects of cofactors, will only exacerbate the discrepancy between the amplitude of model oscillations and those observed in cell culture. Furthermore, arguments based on consideration of the binding of Hes factors to multiple DNA binding sites in a promoter suggest that the effective Hill coefficient should be around 2.4 (ref. 40), which is much lower than the value required to achieve oscillations for Hes1 under the experimentally-imposed constraints on the mRNA and protein degradation rates.

The second possibility—that the level of mechanistic detail in the current models is insufficient—can be explored through the analysis of more detailed mechanistic models of the Hes1 network, incorporating explicit representations of basic biochemical mechanisms known to be involved, such as Hes1 dimerisation and nucleo-cytoplasmic shuttling. As discussed above, an extension of the Hes1 model to include explicit Hes1 dimerisation (with differential stability) can go some way towards addressing the mismatch between model behaviour and experimental observations. Inclusion of homo- and hetero-dimerisation of Hes factors has been considered in models of Her1/Her7 oscillations in zebrafish somitogenesis.[35,41] The somitogenesis clock in zebrafish runs significantly faster than that in mouse, with Her oscillatory periods of around 20-30 minutes.[29-31] Reproduction of such fast oscillations in delayed feedback models requires the specification of *her* mRNA half-lives that are much smaller than those measured for Hes1 in mouse.[35,41] Consequently, the forms of oscillations produced by zebrafish models are significantly different to those obtained in the experimentally-constrained mouse models. In particular, the fact that in these models the total feedback delay is significantly greater than the mRNA half-life makes it possible to generate large amplitude model oscillations with a transcription Hill coefficient $n = 2$.[35,41] Direct validation of these models awaits detailed quantitative expression data for zebrafish Her1 and Her7.

The observed variability of Hes1 oscillations in isolated cells shows clearly that the Hes1 circuit is operating in a noisy stochastic environment.[12] A number of stochastic models of biochemical systems have been shown to support oscillatory solutions for values of kinetic parameters for which equivalent deterministic models are non-oscillatory (see, for example, ref. 42). This raises the possibility that stochastic models of the Hes1 feedback circuit may exhibit more pronounced oscillations than deterministic DDE equivalents. A discrete and stochastic model of the Hes1 circuit based on the model in Equations (1) and (2) has been developed by Barrio et al,[43] who employ an extension of the Gillespie algorithm for stochastic simulation of chemical kinetics,[44] The stochastic model produces oscillations that have similar overall features (period and average amplitude) to those produced in the deterministic models.[43] Furthermore, the average behaviour of a population of individual stochastic oscillators corresponds well to the damped oscillations observed in populations of cultured mouse fibroblasts.[11] Stochastic simulation models have also been developed for Her oscillations in zebrafish.[35,41,45] As for the stochastic simulations of mouse Hes1, the overall properties of the resulting oscillations do not differ markedly from those resulting from deterministic equivalents. While the behaviour of stochastic delay models remains to be explored fully, results obtained to date suggest that for parameter values that support sustained oscillations in deterministic models, the oscillatory behaviour of stochastic equivalents does not differ markedly.

The models described above, both deterministic and stochastic, assume that the delay involved in transcriptional feedback always takes a discrete, well-defined single value (termed a discrete delay). The more realistic assumption that the delays for each instance of transcription and translation are drawn from a statistical distribution has been studied both for the two-component Hes1 model[22,46] and for the Hes1-Gro/TLE1 model.[46] The effects of including a distributed delay depend on the form of distribution used. Distributions that have finite support (i.e., for which finite minimum and maximum delays are specified) appear to have little effect on the dynamical behaviour of oscillatory model solutions.[22] However, distributions that have infinite support (so that the delay can take any non-zero value) can result in a failure to support sustained oscillations for large average delays, even though sustained oscillations can be generated for smaller average delays.[46] Such a "reverse" Hopf bifurcation has yet to be observed in a real biological system, and the possibility of an upper limit on the period of delay-driven oscillations deserves further theoretical investigation.

Spatio-Temporal Coordination of Oscillatory Dynamics

The models outlined above provide insight into the origin and properties of cell autonomous Hes oscillations. In reality, however, cells undergoing sustained oscillations (such as the cells in the presomitic mesoderm during somitogenesis) communicate their state to their neighbours by intercellular signalling. While sustained Hes1 oscillations can be observed in dissociated cells, the oscillations show a significant degree of stochasticity that is not captured by the deterministic models discussed so far.[12] Furthermore, the robust spatial coordination of Hes oscillations observed in the presomitic mesoderm suggests that intercellular signalling, which is likely to be mediated by the Notch pathway, can have a significant impact on the form of Hes oscillations.

A number of models have been developed that incorporate intercellular signalling between cells that are capable of generating autonomous Hes factor oscillations, with a specific emphasis on the short-period oscillations in Her1 and Her7 in zebrafish somitogenesis.[35,41,45] Signalling between nearest neighbour cells is mediated through the Notch signalling pathway, which lies both upstream and downstream of Her activity. These models show that coupling between cells can lead to synchronisation and phase-coupling, both for deterministic and stochastic models of oscillators in individual cells.

Discussion

Following the observation of Hes1 oscillations in a range of mouse cultured cell lines,[11] a number of different mathematical models have been developed to explore both the Hes1 regulatory network and that of the related proteins Hes7 (in mouse) and Her1 and Her7 in zebrafish. These models are summarised in (Table 1). These studies have served to highlight the dynamical importance of time delays in the production of mature mRNA and protein, and of tight regulation of mRNA and protein stability. Furthermore, the models have revealed a striking potential insensitivity of delay-driven feedback oscillations to transcription and translation rates and to the affinity of Hes/Her proteins for their DNA binding sites in the promoters of *Hes/her* target genes.

The models of Hes1 oscillations in mouse cultured cell lines are tightly constrained by quantitative measurements of mRNA and protein half-lives. The inability of simple models that satisfy these constraints to account for the observed large amplitude Hes1 oscillations poses both experimental and modelling challenges. Further careful quantification of Hes1 oscillatory expression would clarify the seriousness of the mismatch between data and models. Quite general arguments presented here suggest that autonomous feedback oscillators have the property that mRNA oscillation amplitudes are greater than protein oscillation amplitudes. If further experimental studies confirm that this property does not hold for Hes/Her oscillations, then this will pose a serious challenge to existing pictures of the regulatory circuitry that underlies these oscillations.

Existing models ignore basic biochemical processes such as movement of mRNA and proteins between the nucleus and cytoplasm, which have been shown to be important features of other oscillatory networks.[6-8] As models become more realistic by incorporating more biochemical species and associated processes, the number of unknown model parameters increases rapidly. This can make it difficult to identify the link between basic cellular processes and specific features of the resulting oscillations. This question has been addressed for oscillatory

Table 1. Summary of mathematical and computational models for Hes/Her transcriptional oscillations

Model	Components	Model Type	Spatial Coupling
Hirata et al[11]	*Hes1*, Hes1, X (unknown)	dODE	no
Jensen et al[21]	*Hes1*, Hes1	dDDE	no
Monk[22]	*Hes1*, Hes1	distributed dDDE	no
Lewis[35]	*her1*, Her1, *her7*, Her7, *deltaC*, DeltaC	dDDE; sDDE	two cells
Hirata et al[28]; Zeiser et al[40]	*hes7*, Hes7	dDDE	no
Bernard et al[39]	Hes1, Gro/TLE1	dDDE	no
Barrio et al[43]	*Hes1*, Hes1; Hes1, Gro/TLE1	stochastic simulation	no
Rateitschak and Wolkenhauer[46]	*Hes1*, Hes1; Hes1, Gro/TLE1	distributed dDDE	no
Horikawa et al[45]	*her1*, Her1, *her7*, Her7, *deltaC*, DeltaC	dDDE; sDDE	1-d array
Cinquin[41]	*her1*, Her1, *her7*, Her7, her13.2, Her13.2, *deltaC*, DeltaC	dDDE; stochastic simulation	1-d array

Model abbreviations: dODE, deterministic ordinary differential equations; dDDE, deterministic delay differential equations; distributed dDDE, dDDE with distributed delay; sDDE, stochastic DDE.

dynamics of the NF-κB-IκB system by performing a systematic sensitivity analysis.[47] A similar detailed study of Hes/Her oscillations would provide valuable insight into delay-driven oscillations. The inclusion of delays in models of genetic regulatory networks significantly reduces their mathematical tractability. While this is not a significant problem for simple networks, analysis of the potential dynamical effects of delays in more complex networks is challenging. A recently developed graph-theoretic approach that provides conditions for a delay-induced instability in networks of arbitrary complexity should prove invaluable in this regard.[48]

An exciting avenue for future research is the development of models of the multiple interlocked feedback loops that underlie somitogenesis.[32] Recent models have made steps towards this goal by incorporating spatial coupling and imposed positional information in 1-dimensional arrays of delay-driven cell autonomous oscillators.[41,45] The increasing availability of quantitative time-course expression data for this highly dynamic developmental event makes this extremely fertile ground for an integrative approach based on complementary experimental and theoretical studies.

Acknowledgements

This work was funded by the UK Biotechnology and Biological Sciences Research Council (grant number BB/D014840).

References

1. Freeman M. Feedback control of intercellular signalling in development. Nature 2000; 408:313-319.
2. Mahaffy JM, Pao CV. Models of genetic control by repression with time delays and spatial effects. J Math Biol 1984; 20:39-57.
3. Mahaffy JM. Genetic control models with diffusion and delays. Math Biosci 1988; 90:519-533.
4. Csikász-Nagy A, Novák B, Tyson JJ. Reverse engineering models of cell cycle regulation. In: Maroto M, Monk NAM. Cellular Oscillatory Mechanisms. Austin: Landes Bioscience, 2008.

5. Rougemont J, Naef F. Stochastic phase oscillator models for circadian clocks. In: Maroto M, Monk NAM. Cellular Oscillatory Mechanisms. Austin: Landes Bioscience, 2008.
6. Hoffmann A, Levchenko A, Scott ML et al. The IκB-NF-κB signaling module: Temporal control and selective gene activation. Science 2002; 298:1241-1245.
7. Nelson DE, Ihekwaba AEC, Elliott M et al. Oscillations in NF-κB signaling control the dynamics of gene expression. Science 2004; 306:704-708.
8. Lev Bar-Or R, Maya R, Segel LA et al. Generation of oscillations by the p53-Mdm2 feedback loop: A theoretical and experimental study. Proc Natl Acad Sci USA 2000; 97:11250-11255.
9. Lahav G, Rosenfeld N, Sigal A et al. Dynamics of the p53-Mdm2 feedback loop in individual cells. Nat Genet 2004; 36:147-150.
10. Lahav G. Oscillations by the p53-Mdm2 feedback loop. In: Maroto M, Monk NAM. Cellular Oscillatory Mechanisms. Austin: Landes Bioscience, 2008.
11. Hirata H, Yoshiura S, Ohtsuka T et al. Oscillatory expression of the bHLH factor Hes1 regulated by a negative feedback loop. Science 2002; 298:840-843.
12. Masamizu Y, Ohtsuka, T, Takashima Y et al. Real-time imaging of the somite segmentation clock: Revelation of unstable oscillators in the individual presomitic mesoderm cells. Proc Natl Acad Sci USA 2006; 103:1313-1318.
13. William DA, Saitta B, Gibson JD et al. Identification of oscillatory genes in somitogenesis from functional genomic analysis of a human mesenchymal stem cell model. Dev Biol 2007; 305:172-186.
14. Uptain SM, Kane CM, Chamberlin MJ. Basic mechanisms of transcript elongation and its regulation. Annu Rev Biochem 1997; 66:117-172.
15. Darzacq X, Singer RH, Shav-Tal Y. Dynamics of transcription and mRNA export. Curr Opin Cell Biol 2005; 17:332-339.
16. Audibert A, Weil D, Dautry F. In vitro kinetics of mRNA splicing and transport in mammalian cells. Mol Cell Biol 2002; 22:6706-6718.
17. Lewin B. Genes VII. Oxford: Oxford University Press, 2000.
18. Tennyson CN, Klamut HJ, Worton RG. The human dystrophin gene requires 16 hours to be transcribed and is cotranscriptionally spliced. Nat Genet 1995; 9:184-190.
19. Alberts B, Johnson A, Lewis J et al. Molecular Biology of the Cell. 4th ed. New York: Garland/ Taylor and Francis, 2002.
20. Tiana G, Jensen MH, Sneppen K. Time delay is a key to apoptosis induction in the p53 network. Eur Phys J B 2002; 29:135-140.
21. Jensen MH, Sneppen K, Tiana G. Sustained oscillations and time delays in gene expression of protein Hes1. FEBS Lett 2003; 541:176-177.
22. Monk NAM. Oscillatory expression of Hes1, p53, and NF-κB driven by transcriptional time delays. Curr Biol 2003; 13:1409-1413.
23. Davis RL, Turner DL. Vertebrate hairy and Enhancer of split related proteins: Transcriptional repressors regulating cellular differentiation and embryonic patterning. Oncogene 2001; 20:8342-8357.
24. Kageyama R, Ohtsuka T, Kobayashi T. The Hes gene family: Repressors and oscillators that orchestrate embryogenesis. Development 2007; 134:1243-1251.
25. Palmeirim I, Henrique D, Ish-Horowicz D et al. Avian hairy gene expression identifies a molecular clock linked to vertebrate segmentation and somitogenesis. Cell 1997; 91:639-648.
26. Bessho Y, Sakata R, Komatsu S et al. Dynamic expression and essential functions of Hes7 in somite segmentation. Genes Dev 2001; 15:2642-2647.
27. Bessho Y, Hirata H, Masamizu Y et al. Periodic repression by the bHLH factor Hes7 is an essential mechanism for the somite segmentation clock. Genes Dev 2003; 17:1451-1456.
28. Hirata H, Bessho Y, Kokubu H et al. Instability of Hes7 protein is crucial for the somite segmentation clock. Nat Genet 2004; 36:750-754.
29. Holley SA, Julich D, Rauch GJ et al. Her1 and the Notch pathway function within the oscillator mechanism that regulates zebrafish somitogenesis. Development 2002; 129:1175-1183.
30. Oates AC, Ho RK. Hairy/E(spl)-related (Her) genes are central components of the segmentation oscillator and display redundancy with the Delta/Notch signalling pathway in the formation of anterior segmental boundaries in the zebrafish. Development 2002; 129:2929-2946.
31. Pasini A, Jiang YJ, Wilkinson DG. The zebrafish Hairy/Enhancer-of-split-related genes, her6 and her4, are required to maintain the coordination of cyclic gene expression in the presomitic mesoderm. Development 2004; 131:1529-1541.
32. Palmeirim I, Rodrigues S, Dale JK, Maroto M. Development on Time. In: Maroto M, Monk NAM. Cellular Oscillatory Mechanisms. Austin: Landes Bioscience, 2008.
33. Takebayashi K, Sasai Y, Sakai Y et al. Structure, chromosomal locus, and promoter analysis of the gene encoding the mouse helix-loop-helix factor Hes-1. J Biol Chem 1994; 269:5150-5156.

34. Dequéant ML, Glynn E, Gaudenz K et al. A complex oscillating network of signaling genes underlies the mouse segmentation clock. Science 2006; 314:1595-1598.

35. Lewis J. Autoinhibition with transcriptional delay: A simple mechanism for the zebrafish somitogenesis oscillator. Curr Biol 2003; 13:1398-1408.

36. Verdugo A, Rand R. Hopf bifurcation in a DDE model of gene expression. Commun Nonlinear Sci Numer Simulat 2006, (doi:10.1016/j.cnsns.2006.05.001).

37. Buchler NE, Gerland U, Hwa T. Nonlinear protein degradation and the function of genetic circuits. Proc Natl Acad Sci USA 2005; 102:9559-9564.

38. Nuthall HN, Husain J, McLarren KW et al. Role for Hes1-induced phosphoryllation in Groucho-mediated transcriptional repression. Mol Cell Biol 2002; 22:389-399.

39. Bernard S, Cajavec B, Pujo-Menjouet L et al. Modelling transcriptional feedback loops: The role of Gro/TLE1 in Hes1 oscillations. Phil Trans R Soc A 2006; 364:1155-1170.

40. Zeiser S, Liebscher HV, Tiedemann H et al. Number of active transcription factor binding sites is essential for the Hes7 oscillator. Theor Biol Med Modelling 2006; 3:11.

41. Cinquin O. Repressor dimerization in the zebrafish somitogenesis clock. PLoS Comput Biol 2007; 3(2):e32.

42. McKane AJ, Nagy JD, Newman TJ et al. Amplified biochemical oscillations in cellular systems. J Stat Phys 2007, (in press).

43. Barrio M, Burrage K, Leier A et al. Oscillatory regulation of Hes1: Discrete stochastic delay modelling and simulation. PLoS Comput Biol 2006; 2(9):e117.

44. Gillespie DT. Exact stochastic simulation of coupled chemical reactions. J Phys Chem 1997; 81:2340-2361.

45. Horikawa K, Ishimatsu K, Yoshimoto E et al. Noise-resistant and synchronized oscillation of the segmentation clock. Nature 2006; 441:719-723.

46. Rateitschak K, Wolkenhauer O. Intracellular delay limits cyclic changes in gene expression. Math Biosci 2007; 205:163-179.

47. Ihekwaba AEC, Broomhead DS, Grimley RL et al. Sensitivity analysis of parameters controlling oscillatory signalling in the NF-κB pathway: The roles of IKK and IκBα. Syst Biol 2004; 1:93-103.

48. Mincheva M, Roussel M. Graph-theoretic methods for the analysis of chemical and biochemical networks. II. Oscillations in networks with delays. J Math Biol 2007; 55:87-104.

## CHAPTER 7

Reverse Engineering Models of Cell Cycle Regulation

Attila Csikász-Nagy,* Béla Novák and John J. Tyson

Abstract

From general considerations of the basic physiological properties of the cell division cycle, we deduce what the dynamical properties of the underlying molecular control system must be. Then, taking a few hints from the biochemistry of cyclin-dependent kinases (the master regulators of the eukaryotic cell cycle), we guess what molecular mechanisms must be operating to produce the desired dynamical properties of the control system.

Bottom-Up Modeling and Reverse Engineering

The physiological characteristics of living cells-their abilities to grow and divide, to respond to external stimuli, to move around, to find food or sexual partners-are regulated ultimately by networks of interacting genes and proteins. Molecular geneticists have been very successful in identifying the genetic components of these control systems and their molecular interactions, and a new field of molecular systems biology has arisen to assemble the pieces into comprehensive mechanisms that accurately reflect cell behavior, that predict new aspects of the control systems, and that provide intellectually satisfying explanations of how cells work. A major component of this systems approach is the construction of mathematical models that capture the intricacies of complicated networks and reliably simulate their properties. Most examples of successful models- slime mold signaling,[1] bacterial chemotaxis,[2] viral lysogeny,[3] cell cycle regulation,[4] circadian rhythms[5]-have been built from the bottom up, working from a detailed molecular mechanism to an appropriate mathematical description, to computer simulations of signal-response characteristics of the model, to careful comparisons with the observed behavior of cells. At least, that is the way the story is told in scientific publications. But, in actual fact, modelers often work in the reverse direction, from observed physiological properties to the state transitions that must underlie the signal-response curves, to speculate about mechanisms that can produce these transitions and are consistent with the chemical properties of proteins known to participate in the control system.

We call this approach reverse engineering, as in trying to figure out how a complex piece of electromechanical equipment works without having access to the design documents. Our case study is the eukaryotic cell cycle, and the 'story' we tell here is actually closer to how we developed our models than the highly contrived bottom-up description in our publications.

---

*Corresponding Author: Attila Csikász-Nagy—Materials Structure and Modeling Research Group of the Hungarian Academy of Sciences and Department of Applied Biotechnology and Food Science, Budapest University of Technology and Economics, Gellért tér 4, H-1521 Budapest, Hungary. Email: csikasz@mail.bme.hu

Cellular Oscillatory Mechanisms, edited by Miguel Maroto and Nicholas A.M. Monk.
©2008 Landes Bioscience and Springer Science+Business Media.

Physiology of the Cell Cycle

The cell division cycle is the sequence of events by which cells reproduce themselves. The most important events are DNA replication and partitioning of sister chromosomes (identical DNA molecules) to daughter cells at division. In eukaryotic cells, these events are separated in time: DNA synthesis (S phase) alternating with sister chromosome separation (mitosis, or M phase). The alternation of S and M phases is crucial to keeping the genome intact from one generation to the next.[6]

The time required to copy and segregate chromosomes is largely independent of the nutritional conditions under which a cell is growing, which determine, of course, the rate of synthesis of most cytoplasmic constituents.[7] In general, S and M phases can be completed much faster than the time needed to double the mass of a cell. Hence, cell growth is the rate limiting process in cellular reproduction, and eukaryotic cells have to slow down the DNA replication-division cycle by inserting gaps (G1 and G2) between S and M phases (Fig. 1). 'Balanced growth and division' is the general rule: interdivision time = mass doubling time.[8,9] Were these two times not equal, then cells would become progressively larger or smaller from one division cycle to the next!

Cells can adjust their interdivision time to their mass doubling time because certain cell cycle transitions are dependent on reaching a critical cell size (Fig. 1), as is well documented for single-celled eukaryotes.[10] For example, the duration of G1 phase in budding yeast is longer for small newborn cells than for large newborn cells, suggesting that the G1→S transition is executed when cells reach a critical size.[7] Fission yeast cells adjust their cycle time to the mass doubling time of the culture by varying the length of G2 phase.[11]

A third characteristic feature of the eukaryotic cell cycle are the checkpoint mechanisms that block a cell cycle transition if some previous necessary event has not yet been completed.[12] There are three primary checkpoints. At the G1→S transition, cells check

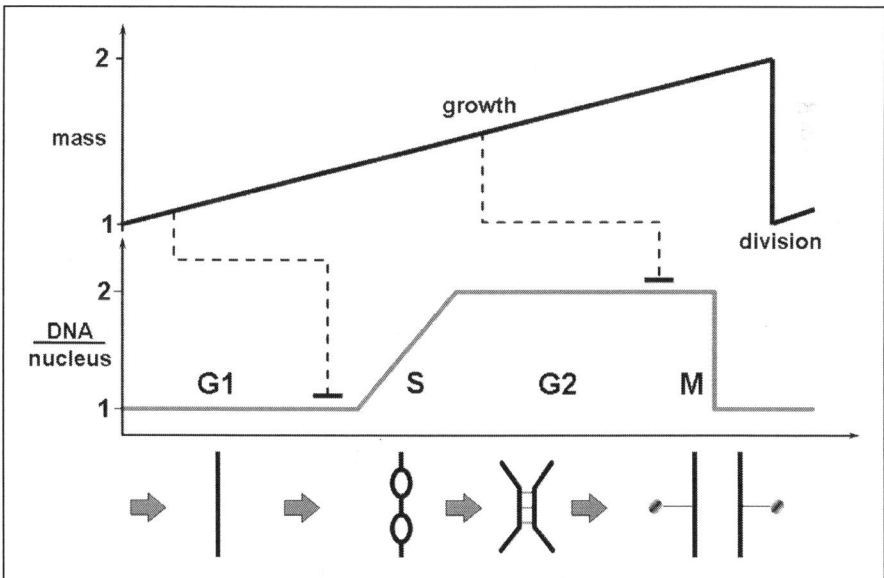

Figure 1. Coupling between the growth-division cycle (upper) and the chromosome replication-segregation cycle (lower). Cells have to grow to a critical mass in G1 phase before inducing DNA replication (S-phase). A second mass checkpoint may work in G2 phase, delaying M-phase until the cell grows large enough. After mitosis the cell divides, which sets cell mass back to the initial condition.

nutritional conditions to decide if the environment is suitable for another round of DNA replication. They also check for signaling molecules in the environment (e.g., pheromones, hormones) to see if there are good 'reasons' why they may or may not want to proceed with mitotic reproduction.[13] At the G2→M checkpoint, cells verify if DNA replication has finished properly.[14] At the metaphase checkpoint, a cell makes sure that all its chromosomes are properly aligned on the mitotic spindle; even one misaligned chromosome is enough to block further progression through mitosis.[15]

Alternation of S and M phases, balanced growth and division, and checkpoint controls are the three major characteristics of the eukaryotic cell cycle. Let's not fuss over the exceptions to these 'rules'. Our job is to reverse engineer a mechanism that will account for these basic physiological features and is consistent with the little bit of molecular and genetic information that was available in the early 1990s, when the models were being built.

Three Cell Cycle States and Three Cell Cycle Transitions

We can easily imagine the existence of a master regulator protein (R) whose state (concentration or functional activity) changes abruptly at the major transitions of the cell cycle (Fig. 2). The lowest state of R corresponds to G1 phase (uncommitted to replication). At the G1→S transition, R increases to an intermediate state, and the cell commits to a new round of DNA synthesis and division. We call this intermediate level of R the 'S/G2' state, because this state begins with DNA replication (S phase) and continues into G2 phase. (S and G2 differ only in terms of whether DNA synthesis is ongoing or finished, but not in terms of cell cycle regulation.) At the G2→M transition, R increases again, to a state that is sufficiently high to drive the major reorganization of cell structure and metabolism required by mitosis and cell division. The M-state of the master regulator is 'unstable' (dashed line in Fig. 2) because cells do not normally linger in M phase. As cells leave M phase and return to G1, R must decrease back to the low G1-state. In the early 1990s, ideas like these were floating around the cell-cycle community. The master regulator was guessed to be a protein kinase (called cdc2) in combination with a regulatory subunit (called cyclin), and the three-state model in Figure 2 was explicitly described in a review article by Stern and Nurse in 1996 (ref. 16).

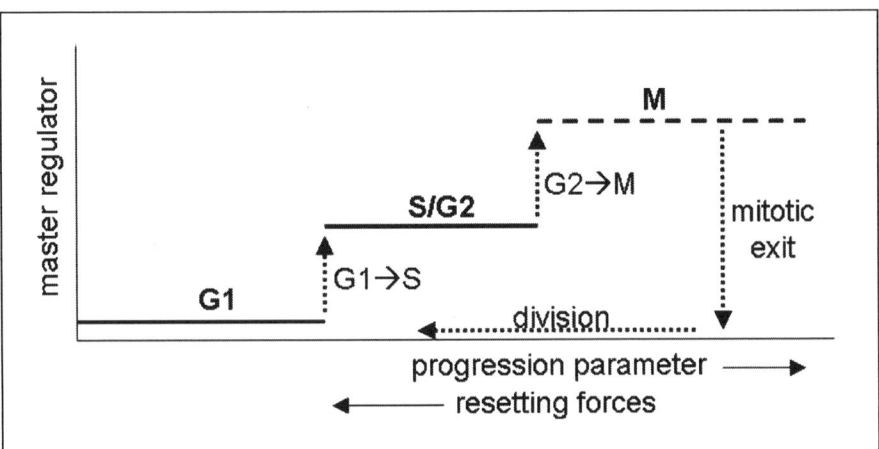

Figure 2. Three critical cell cycle transitions are driven by a master regulator. In G1 phase the master regulator is present at very low level. At the G1→S transition, the master regulator jumps to a higher stable state (S/G2). At the G2→M transition, the activity of the master regulator increases further, but only transiently. The M state is unstable, and the master regulator drops precipitously as the cell exits mitosis. The 'progression parameter' is likely cell size, in which case cell division is the resetting force that switches the system back to the initial state.

Although it is tempting to interpret the 'progression parameter' in Figure 2 as time since birth, it is not cell age that drives cells through the replication-division cycle but rather cell size. In order to achieve balanced growth and division, the state of the master regulator must be sensitive to the cell's mass-to-DNA ratio. Hence, in Figure 2, we interpret the horizontal axis as cell size. At cell division, cell size is reset birth size = 0.5*(division size). If birth size is less than the critical size for the G1→S transition (as is the case for budding yeast), then R will captured by the stable G1 state, and the cell will linger in G1 phase until it grows large enough to make the transition into S phase. If birth size is larger than the critical size for the G1→S transition (as is the case for fission yeast), then the cell will visit G1 phase only transiently, as R makes its way to the stable S/G2 state. In this case, the cell will linger in G2 phase until it grows large enough to make the transition into M phase.[11] This is one of the characteristic differences between the yeasts: size control operates at the G1→S transition in budding yeast and at the G2→M transition in fission yeast.[10]

In this view there are three characteristic cell cycle states, based on the activity of the master regulator, and three irreversible transitions between them. Two of the transitions (G1→S and G2→M) are governed by an increase in cell size, whereas the third (exit from mitosis) is 'automatic' because the mitotic state is fundamentally unstable (entry into mitosis sets the stage for exit from mitosis). If a vital cell cycle event is not completed properly, then a checkpoint signal is generated to postpone the next cell cycle transition.[17] For example, if DNA replication is blocked, then the S/G2-state is stabilized and the G2→M transition is pushed off to very large size. Or, if chromosomes fail to align properly on the mitotic spindle, then the M-state is stabilized and exit from mitosis is blocked.

Cell Cycle Transitions and Bifurcation Points

To an applied mathematician, Figure 2 looks suspiciously like a bifurcation diagram. In dynamical systems theory,[18,19] a bifurcation point is a specific parameter value where the steady state solutions of a nonlinear differential equation change in number and/or stability. Bifurcations can be visualized on a diagram where one plots the possible steady state values of a relevant variable of the system as functions of the 'bifurcation' parameter. In our case, the relevant dynamical variable is R and the crucial bifurcation parameter is cell mass.

The G1→S and G2→M transitions both correspond to an abrupt change from one steady state to another, which is the signature of a saddle-node (SN) bifurcation. For example, the G1→S transition appears to happen when the stable G1 state coalesces with an unstable saddle point at a generic SN bifurcation point (Fig. 3A). Past the SN point, both the node (the G1 state) and the saddle disappear, and R must jump to the upper branch of stable steady states (the S/G2 state). This transition occurs at a critical size, namely the location of the SN bifurcation point. The G2→M transition is regulated by a similar saddle-node bifurcation, at a larger critical size (Fig. 3A), where the S/G2 state disappears and R must jump to a still higher steady state (the M state).

Unlike G1 and G2, the M phase of the cell cycle appears to be unstable: entry into M phase sets the stage for an abrupt inactivation of R as the cell exits mitosis. In Figure 3A we propose that this basic instability of the M state is characterized by a Hopf bifurcation (HB), where a stable steady state loses stability and is replaced by stable limit cycle oscillations. In Figure 3A, these oscillatory solutions are denoted by heavy black dots which mark the maximum and minimum values of R over the course of an oscillation at fixed cell size. In this case, the activation of R, which drives the cell into mitosis, turns on processes that destroy R activity and drive the cell out of mitosis. The control system is not able to settle on a stable steady state of balanced R activity. Instead it oscillates repeatedly between transient states of high and low activity.

Checkpoints can prevent cell cycle transitions by pushing the bifurcation points to much larger cell size.[17] If S phase needs to be delayed, then the G1 state can be stabilized by pushing the SN point to larger mass (Fig. 3A, lower right, grey curve). If DNA replication is blocked,

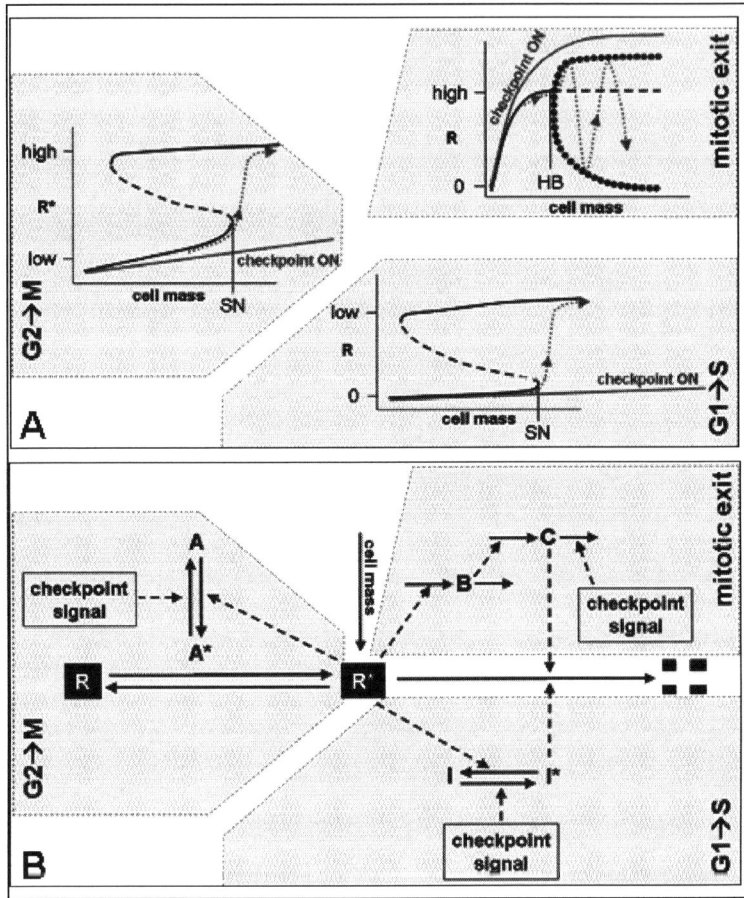

Figure 3. Modules of the cell cycle regulatory network. A) Schematic bifurcation diagrams of the three cell cycle transitions (solid lines—stable steady states, dashed lines—unstable steady states, dots—max and min of oscillations). Saddle-node bifurcations (SN) regulate the **G1→S** and **G2→M** transitions, while **mitotic exit** is governed by an oscillator created at a Hopf bifurcation (HB). B) The proposed underlying molecular network. (* notes the active form of a protein.) The three reaction modules correspond to the three bifurcation diagrams in part A. **G1→S**—R and I are mutually antagonistic. **G2→M**—R and A are mutual activators. **Mitotic exit**—R, B and C are involved in a negative feedback loop. Each transition can be inhibited by checkpoint signals. The solid grey curves in part A show the checkpoints might alter the bifurcation diagrams.

then the G2 state can be stabilized in a similar fashion. If chromosomes fail to align properly on the mitotic spindle, then the M state can be stabilized by pushing the HB point to larger mass (Fig. 3A, upper right, gray curve).

By this sort of reasoning, we are able to deduce what must be the fundamental bifurcation diagrams ('signal-response' curves) underlying progression through the cell cycle, in order to account for the three fundamental characteristics of the cell cycle: alternation of S and M phases, balanced growth and division, and checkpoint delays. Our next job is to guess what sort of molecular mechanisms might govern the master regulator in order to create these bifurcation diagrams.

Reverse Engineering the Molecular Regulatory Network

To reverse engineer the network we need a few clues about the master regulator R (also known as MPF, M-phase promoting factor). By 1989 it was known that MPF is a dimer of cdc2 and cyclin B.[20,21] The level of cdc2 in cells is constant, but its cyclin partner comes and goes. MPF activity is abruptly lost at the M→G1 transition, because cyclin subunits are rapidly degraded. Degradation was known to depend on ubiquitinylation of cyclin by a complex 'machine' called the APC. A crucial experiment by Felix et al[22] suggested that the APC is activated by MPF, after a significant time delay. In addition, it was known that, during S and G2 phases, MPF is kept in a less active, tyrosine-phosphorylated form by the action of a tyrosine kinase (wee1). At the G2→M transition, MPF is rapidly activated by a tyrosine phosphatase (cdc25).[23] How can we build bifurcation diagrams like Figure 3A from these bits and pieces?

We start with the M-state oscillator in the upper right of Figure 3A. It is quite reasonable to assume that the oscillator is created by a delayed negative feedback loop[24]: MPF → intermediate → cyclin degradation —‖ MPF. This module, drawn in the upper right of Figure 3B, can be described by the differential equations:

$$\frac{dR}{dt} = m - \alpha \cdot R \cdot \frac{C^n}{1 + C^n} \tag{1}$$

$$\frac{dB}{dt} = R - \beta \cdot B \tag{2}$$

$$\frac{dC}{dt} = B - \gamma \cdot C \tag{3}$$

Synthesis of the master regulator (R) depends on cell mass (m) and degradation depends on the activity of the APC (C). The intermediate B is needed to delay the signal from MPF to the APC. For appropriate choices of parameter values (in particular, n must be > 8),[24] this system of differential equations will generate oscillations for m between two HB points. (For example, for $\alpha = 10$, $\beta = \gamma = 0.5$ and $n = 12$, Eqs. (1)-(3) oscillate for $0.024 < m < 0.30$). In general, these oscillations are lost, and the M-state becomes stable if β or γ are increased, which is likely how the mitotic checkpoint works.

Next we need a module that will stabilize a G1-state with very low MPF activity. It is reasonable to expect that cyclin level is very low in G1 phase because cyclin subunits continue to be rapidly degraded in G1. But the APC, as modeled in Eqs. (1-3), turns off after the cell leaves mitosis. We need a new component, call it I, to carry on cyclin degradation in G1 phase after C turns off. Furthermore, we want the R-I interaction to create a bistable system with saddle-node bifurcations as in Figure 3A, lower right. Mutual antagonism between R and I will do the trick, as in Figure 3B, lower right. The module can be described by the differential equations:

$$\frac{dR}{dt} = m - \rho \cdot R \cdot \frac{\varepsilon + I^{*p}}{1 + I^{*p}} \tag{4}$$

$$\frac{dI^*}{dt} = \kappa \cdot \left(1 - I^*\right) - \sigma \cdot R \cdot I^* \tag{5}$$

The inhibitor I can exist in an active form (denoted by *) and an inactive form (with $I^* + I = 1$), and R converts the inhibitor to its inactive form. The G1→S transition can easily be delayed by increasing the value of κ, making it harder for R to inactivate I. The inhibitor in Eq. (4) is functioning as another route of cyclin degradation, secondary to the mitotic-exit form of APC. Alternatively, I could be a stoichiometric inhibitor of cyc2/cyclin dimers, in which case Eq. (4) would have to be written differently.

In S/G2 phase, the master regulator is in a less active, tyrosine-phosphorylated form, and it is switched abruptly to the more active, dephosphorylated form at the G2→M transition by the action of an activatory phosphatase (call it A). The transition will be governed by a bistable switch if R and A are involved in a mutually activatory feedback loop, as in Figure 3B left side. The governing differential equations for R^* and A^*, the more active forms of the proteins, might be:

$$\frac{dR^*}{dt} = A^* \cdot R - \lambda \cdot R^* \tag{6}$$

$$\frac{dA^*}{dt} = \frac{\left(\delta_1 \cdot R + \delta_2 \cdot R^*\right) \cdot \left(1 - A^*\right)}{J + 1 - A^*} - \frac{\omega \cdot A^*}{J + A^*} \tag{7}$$

In Eq. (7), $R + R^* = R_{total}$ and $A + A^* = 1$. Also, $\delta_1 < \delta_2$, since R is less active than R^*. Activation of A is written as a Goldbeter-Koshland zero-order ultrasensitive switch.[25] That is, the activation and inactivation rates of A are described by Michaelis-Menten rate laws, under conditions where the enzymes are usually substrate-saturated ($J \ll 1$). In this case, A^* responds to R^* in a steeply sigmoidal fashion, and it is easy to find parameter values that give the desired bistability. The easiest way for a checkpoint to arrest cells in G2 is to elevate the value of ω, making it harder for R to activate A.

The Complete Bifurcation Diagram

Putting together Eqs. (1-7) and choosing appropriate parameter values (see appendix), we can create a complete model of the eukaryotic cell cycle, with irreversible transitions, balanced growth and division, and reasonable checkpoint controls. For this mathematical model, we can plot the full bifurcation diagram (Fig. 4), which looks very similar to the imagined 'physiological state diagram' in Figure 2. The likeness is expected because the model was specifically engineered to reproduce the physiological properties of the cell cycle.

Nonetheless, there is a significant difference between Figures 2 and 4. The cell cycle states (G1, S/G2 and M) are overlapping in Figure 4 but not so in Figure 2. The mathematical model predicts that the cell cycle control system should exhibit regions of bistability, where two stable steady states coexist under identical conditions. This behavior, predicted by us in 1993,[4] ran completely counter to the intuition of the molecular biologists studying cell cycle controls in the gene-cloning heyday (1985-1995). Bistability was confirmed only ten years later, in budding yeast[26] and frog embryos.[27,28]

The grey dotted line in Figure 4 follows the trajectory of a cell from very small initial size, say a germinating yeast spore. At first the cell-cycle control system is attracted by the stable G1 steady state. When cell mass reaches a critical value (close to 2 arbitrary units—a. u.) this stable steady state disappears and the control system moves to the stable S/G2 steady state with higher activity of the master regulator. This transition happens at a saddle-node bifurcation. The cell stays in S/G2 phase until it grows to a size of about 4 a.u., where another bifurcation takes place. Here the stable S/G2 state disappears and the control system is attracted to a stable oscillation around an unstable M state. The cell goes into M phase and then exits from mitosis, as the master regulator is destroyed. This is the signal for cell division, which resets cell mass to a value just above the region of existence of the G1 steady state. These newly divided cells skip G1 and proceed directly into S phase. This sequence of events is an accurate account of the cell cycle progression of wild-type fission yeast cells.

Cell Cycles and Limit Cycles

The reverse engineering approach suggests that the molecular machinery regulating the eukaryotic cell cycle is composed of two bistable switches and an oscillator (Fig. 3). As a cell progresses through the cell cycle, it halts in one stable steady state (G1) or the other (S/G2)

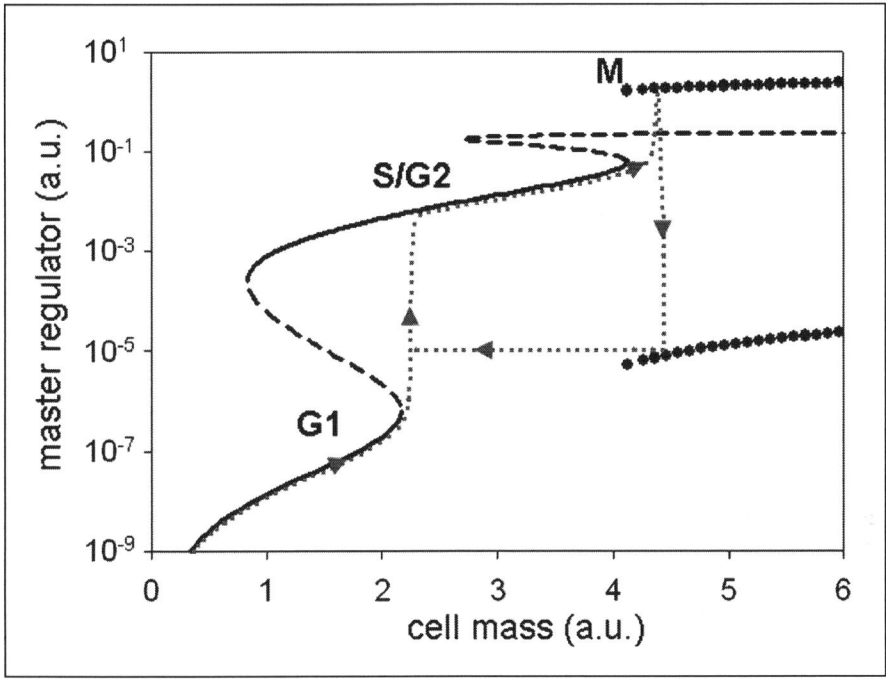

Figure 4. Bifurcation diagram of the proposed cell cycle regulatory network. Cells can visit any of three steady state regimes with characteristically different values of R, corresponding to the three basic phases of the cell cycle (G1, S/G2, and M). These three basic states are separated by unstable saddle points. Cell cycle transitions correspond to bifurcation points on the diagram. The grey dotted line shows the trajectory of a cell starting from very small size (see text). Parameter values: $\alpha = 10$, $n = 12$, $\beta = 0.5$, $\gamma = 0.5$, $\rho = 100$, $\varepsilon = 0.01$, $p = 6$, $\kappa = 4$, $\sigma = 10$, $\lambda = 0.2$, $\delta_1 = 0.1$, $\delta_2 = 4$, $\omega = 1$, $J = 0.01$.

just long enough to match its interdivision time to its mass doubling time. This balancing of growth and division is essential to cell viability. In general, it is not correct or helpful to think of the cell cycle as a limit cycle oscillator, because the period of a limit cycle is set by the rate constants of its constituent reactions and bears no obvious relation to the mass doubling time of a growing cell (set by the nutritional conditions presented to the cell). To coordinate these two kinetically unrelated processes, the cell cycle must halt somewhere to give growth processes a chance to catch up.

This general rule of balanced growth and division is proved by its exceptions. In the laboratory, a yeast cell can be forced to grow exceptionally large without dividing, putting it at a cell mass >> 6 a.u. on the bifurcation diagram (Fig. 4). When the division-block is released, the cell finds itself in the limit cycle regime and proceeds to divide very rapidly (at the period of the underlying limit cycle). Dividing faster than it is growing, the cell gets smaller and smaller each generation, until its birth mass drops below 4 a.u., the bifurcation point for losing the stable S/G2 state. At this size, the cell cycle control system can finally put a 'pause' in the division cycle and equalize the interdivision time to the mass doubling time.

Under natural conditions, the limit-cycle mode of operation of the cell cycle control system is clearly evident only in fertilized eggs. The oocyte is programmed to grow very large, without cell division, in order to stockpile all the goodies necessary for future embryonic development. After fertilization, the embryo's first job is to run through a series of rapid mitotic cycles, to divide the large egg into ~4000 small cells with one nucleus each. These rapid early embryonic cell cycles are taking place in the limit cycle regime of Figure 4, until cell size is brought down to the typical size of somatic cells (~4 a.u. on Fig. 4). At this point, called the midblastula transition, the rapid size-reducing division cycles cease abruptly, and more typical size-controlled division cycles commence.

Conclusion

Working backwards from the fundamental physiological characteristics of eukaryotic cell cycle controls, and using only the sort of molecular information available in the early 1990s, we have shown how one could have reverse engineered the basic control mechanism. The set of differential equations we derived and the parameter values we chose (see appendix) are incorrect in hindsight, but the bifurcation diagram they generate (Fig. 4) is qualitatively correct, according to our best current understanding.[29] Of course, we were not so insightful in the mid 1990s to get the full qualitative picture correct on our first try, as we imagine in this story. As a matter of fact, the details were worked out over many years by a messy process of trial and error, proceeding simultaneously in both bottom-up and top-down directions.

For more complete and more traditional bottom-up accounts of cell cycle regulation, one should consult Tyson and Novak[30] for an introduction and Csikasz-Nagy et al[29] for the full story.

Acknowledgements

ACN is a Bolyai fellow of the Hungarian Academy of Sciences. Work done in the authors' laboratory is supported by the James S. McDonnell Foundation (21002050), the European Commission (COMBIO: LSHG-CT-2004-503568) and OTKA (F-60414).

Appendix: ODE File for the Model

```
# ODE file for the chapter: Reverse Engineering Models of Cell Cycle Regulation
# You can simulate the model by running it in XPP-AUT
# (http://www.math.pitt.edu/~bard/xpp/xpp.html)
# initial conditions
init Rtot=0.4, R=0.08, B=1, C=1.3, I=0.8, A=0.01
#differential equations
Rtot'=m - alpha*Rtot*(c^n/(1+c^n)) - rho*Rtot*((epsilon+I^p)/(1+I^p))
R'= alpha*R*(c^n/(1+c^n)) - rho*R*((epsilon+I^p)/(1+I^p)) + A*(Rtot-R) - lamda*R
B'=R - beta*B
C'=B - gamma*C
I'=kappa*(1-I) - sigma*Rtot*I
A'=((delta1*(Rtot-R) + delta2*R)*(1-A))/(J+1-A) - omega*A/(J+A)
# parameters
param alpha=10, beta=0.5, gamma=0.5, rho=100, epsilon=0.01, kappa=4, sigma=10
param lamda=0.2, delta1=0.1, delta2=4, omega=1, n=12, p=6, J=0.01
# the next 4 lines have to be replaced by: "param m=2.2"
# to run bifurcation analysis on the model
init m=2.2
m'=m*mu
global -1 {r-0.1} {m=0.5*m}
param mu=0.005776
# definition of simulation method
@ Maxstore=100000, bound=2000, dt=0.5
@ Meth=Stiff, total=500, xplot=t, yplot=R, xlo=0, xhi=500, ylo=0, yhi=2
done
```

References

1. Goldbeter A, Segel LA. Unified mechanism for relay and oscillation of cyclic AMP in Dictyostelium discoideum. Proc Natl Acad Sci USA 1977; 74:1543-1547.
2. Bray D, Bourret RB, Simon MI. Computer simulation of the phosphorylation cascade controlling bacterial chemotaxis. Mol Biol Cell 1993; 4:469-482.
3. Arkin A, Ross J, McAdams HH. Stochastic kinetic analysis of developmental pathway bifurcation in phage lambda-infected Escherichia coli cells. Genetics 1998; 149:1633-1648.
4. Novak B, Tyson JJ. Numerical analysis of a comprehensive model of M-phase control in Xenopus oocyte extracts and intact embryos. J Cell Sci 1993; 106:1153-1168.
5. Forger DB, Peskin CS. A detailed predictive model of the mammalian circadian clock. Proc Natl Acad Sci USA 2003; 100:14806-14811.
6. Murray A, Hunt T. The Cell Cycle: An Introduction. New York: W.H. Freeman and Co., 1993.
7. Johnston GC, Pringle JR, Hartwell LH. Coordination of growth with cell division in the yeast Saccharomyces cerevisiae. Exp Cell Res 1977; 105:79-98.
8. Cooper S. A unifying model for the G1 period in prokaryotes and eukaryotes. Nature 1979; 280:17-19.
9. Tyson JJ. The coordination of cell growth and division—Intentional or incidental? Bioessays 1985; 2:72-77.
10. Rupes I. Checking cell size in yeast. Trends Genet 2002; 18:479-485.
11. Fantes P, Nurse P. Control of cell size at division in fission yeast by a growth-modulated size control over nuclear division. Exp Cell Res 1977; 107:377-386.
12. Hartwell LH, Weinert TA. Checkpoints: Controls that ensure the order of cell cycle events. Science 1989; 246:629-634.
13. Murray AW. The genetics of cell cycle checkpoints. Curr Biol 1995; 5:5-11.
14. Rhind N, Russell P. Mitotic DNA damage and replication checkpoints in yeast. Curr Opin Cell Biol 1998; 10:749-758.
15. Amon A. The spindle checkpoint. Curr Opin Genet Dev 1999; 9:69-75.
16. Stern B, Nurse P. A quantitative model for the cdc2 control of S phase and mitosis in fission yeast. Trends Genet 1996; 12:345-350.
17. Tyson JJ, Csikasz-Nagy A, Novak B. The dynamics of cell cycle regulation. Bioessays 2002; 24:1095-1109.
18. Kuznetsov YA. Elements of Applied Bifurcation Theory. New York: Springer Verlag, 1995.
19. Strogatz SH. Nonlinear Dynamics and Chaos. Reading: Addison-Wesley Co., 1994.
20. Draetta G, Luca F, Westendorf J et al. Cdc2 protein kinase is complexed with both cyclin A and B: Evidence for proteolytic inactivation of MPF. Cell 1989; 56:829-838.
21. Gautier J, Norbury C, Lohka M et al. Purified maturation-promoting factor contains the product of a Xenopus homolog of the fission yeast cell cycle control gene cdc2+. Cell 1988; 54:433-439.
22. Felix MA, Labbe JC, Doree M et al. Triggering of cyclin degradation in interphase extracts of amphibian eggs by cdc2 kinase. Nature 1990; 346:379-382.
23. Coleman TR, Dunphy WG. Cdc2 regulatory factors. Curr Opin Cell Biol 1994; 6:877-882.
24. Griffith JS. Mathematics of cellular control processes. I. Negative feedback to one gene. J Theor Biol 1968; 20:202-208.
25. Goldbeter A, Koshland Jr DE. An amplified sensitivity arising from covalent modification in biological systems. Proc Natl Acad Sci USA 1981; 78:6840-6844.
26. Cross FR, Archambault V, Miller M et al. Testing a mathematical model for the yeast cell cycle. Mol Biol Cell 2002; 13:52-70.
27. Sha W, Moore J, Chen K et al. Hysteresis drives cell-cycle transitions in Xenopus laevis egg extracts. Proc Natl Acad Sci USA 2003; 100:975-980.
28. Pomerening JR, Sontag ED, Ferrell Jr JE. Building a cell cycle oscillator: Hysteresis and bistability in the activation of Cdc2. Nat Cell Biol 2003; 5:346-351.
29. Csikasz-Nagy A, Battogtokh D, Chen KC et al. Analysis of a generic model of eukaryotic cell-cycle regulation. Biophys J 2006; 90(12):4361-4379.
30. Tyson JJ, Novak B. Regulation of the eukaryotic cell cycle: Molecular antagonism, hysteresis and irreversible transitions. J Theor Biol 2001; 210:249-263.

Mitochondrial Oscillations in Physiology and Pathophysiology

Miguel A. Aon, Sonia Cortassa and Brian O'Rourke*

Abstract

O scillations in chemical reactions and metabolic pathways have historically served as prototypes for understanding the dynamics of complex nonlinear systems. This chapter reviews the oscillatory behavior of mitochondria, with a focus on the mitochondrial oscillator dependent on reactive oxygen species (ROS), as first described in heart cells. Experimental and theoretical evidence now indicates that mitochondrial energetic variables oscillate autonomously as part of a network of coupled oscillators under both physiological and pathological conditions. The physiological domain is characterized by small-amplitude oscillations in mitochondrial membrane potential ($\Delta\Psi_m$) showing correlated behavior over a wide range of frequencies, as determined using Power Spectral Analysis and Relative Dispersion Analysis of long term recordings of $\Delta\Psi_m$. Under metabolic stress, when the balance between ROS generation and ROS scavenging is perturbed, the mitochondrial network throughout the cell locks to one main low-frequency, high-amplitude oscillatory mode. This behavior has major pathological implications because the energy dissipation and cellular redox changes that occur during $\Delta\Psi_m$ depolarization result in suppression of electrical excitability and Ca^{2+} handling, the two main functions of the cardiac cell. In an ischemia/reperfusion scenario these alterations scale up to the level of the whole organ, giving rise to fatal arrhythmias.

Introduction

The study of oscillatory phenomena in physics, chemistry and biology has fascinated scientists for centuries. For example, the synchronization of pendulum clocks as coupled oscillators was described by Huygens in 1665, and in biological systems, Kaempfler wrote of the synchronized blinking of fireflies that he had observed on a visit to Siam in 1680 (see refs. 1,2 for historical reviews). In the 20th century, Van der Pol modeled the electrophysiological properties of the heart as collection of coupled relaxation oscillators[3] and other examples of electrical, biochemical, and ionic oscillators in physiology abound.[4-7]

The Russian scientist B.P. Belousov demonstrated that complex temporal and spatial dynamics can be observed in the simple chemical reaction of citric acid/bromate/cerium. He had difficulty publishing the work when first submitted in 1951,[8] but after Zhabotinsky repeated Belousov's experiments,[9] the Belousov-Zhabotinsky reaction grew to became a prototype for the theoretical and experimental study of oscillators. In the same era, oscillations in enzyme-catalyzed biochemical pathways were reported. Duysens and Amesz[10] published the

*Corresponding Author: Brian O'Rourke—The Johns Hopkins University, Institute of Molecular Cardiobiology, 720 Rutland Avenue, 1059 Ross Building, Baltimore, MD 21205-2195, USA. Email: bor@jhmi.edu

Cellular Oscillatory Mechanisms, edited by Miguel Maroto and Nicholas A.M. Monk. ©2008 Landes Bioscience and Springer Science+Business Media.

first observation of biochemical oscillations of reduced pyridine nucleotides in intact cells and these findings were followed by the elucidation of a glycolytic oscillator in yeast[11,12] and in cell-free extracts from various sources.[13-18] This triggered an explosion of interest in the elucidation of the mechanism(s) of biological oscillators (see refs. 4 and 19 for early reviews, see Lloyd, D, this volume). In yeast, this interest has continued throughout the years with new exciting findings.[7,20-22]

Oscillations in ion fluxes, respiration, and mitochondrial volume were noted 40 years ago in several laboratories[23-25] and Chance and Yoshioka[26] demonstrated that they could be sustained over many cycles. Others have also observed mitochondrial oscillations triggered by divalent cations.[27-30] In these earlier studies, the oscillations were typically induced by an increase in cation cycling (e.g., by adding valinomycin) in isolated energized mitochondria and usually took the form of damped sinusoidal oscillations, the damping corresponding to a loss of synchrony among mitochondria in the population over time.[31-33]

In 1994, our laboratory reported that substrate deprivation could induce spontaneous low frequency oscillations in sarcolemmal K^+ currents, action potential duration and excitation-contraction coupling in adult cardiomyocytes.[34] These oscillations were associated with cycles of oxidation and reduction of the intracellular NADH pool. At the time, we proposed that the mechanism could involve the well-known glycolytic oscillator, which could entrain oxidative phosphorylation, but we could not exclude mitochondria as the source of oscillation. Subsequent investigations revealed that the oscillations were associated with mitochondrial flavoprotein redox transients and waves of mitochondrial membrane potential ($\Delta\Psi_m$) depolarization,[35] which shifted our view to a mitochondrial mechanism. More recently, we have investigated in detail the mechanisms involved in triggering and maintaining synchronized, self-sustaining oscillations of bioenergetics in the mitochondrial network of intact cardiac cells, aided by the discovery that they could be reproducibly triggered by laser-induced depolarization of just a few mitochondria in the cell.[36]

Here, we review the properties of mitochondrial oscillators described previously and present a comprehensive account of our theoretical and experimental studies of the reactive oxygen species (ROS)-dependent mitochondrial oscillator induced by metabolic stress in heart cells. Moreover, we put forward the idea, based on relative dispersion and power spectral analysis that coupled oscillation is an inherent property of the mitochondrial network under physiological conditions as well. Understanding the basic mechanism of mitochondrial oscillation is shown to provide fundamental new insights into the origins of post-ischemic electrical and contractile dysfunction in the whole heart and also suggests a novel frequency- and amplitude-encoded ROS signalling function for mitochondria.

Early Descriptions of Mitochondrial Ionic Oscillations

Oscillations in ion flux across the inner membrane of isolated liver or heart mitochondria have been known since the 1960s (reviewed in ref. 32). Chance and Yoshioka reported persistent sinusoidal oscillations of H^+ and K^+ induced by valinomycin in the presence of oxygen, monitored with ion-selective glass electrodes.[26] Initially, K^+ is taken up by the mitochondria (seen as a decrease of K^+ in the medium) and this is then accompanied by H^+ extrusion. The K^+ uptake results in mitochondrial swelling, as judged photometrically and by electron microscopy.[31] Oscillations come to a halt after oxygen in the medium depletes and the ionic changes reverse, i.e., H^+ concentration outside the mitochondria decreases and the K^+ concentration increases.[26,31] The damping of the ionic oscillations in isolated mitochondria is a function of the external pH, the K^+/H^+ ratio, and ADP, and the F_1F_o ATPase is required, since oligomycin blunts the oscillations.[26,31]

Subsequent work on mitochondrial suspensions showed that the addition of a pulse of Sr^{2+} (a Ca^{2+} analogue that is efficiently transported across mitochondrial membranes) could trigger sustained oscillations in fluxes of divalent ions (reviewed in ref. 27). The shape, amplitude and frequency of oscillation were sensitive to the type of substrate. The oscillatory period ranged from 20 s up to 3 min, depending on the substrate, or from 15 s up to 10 min as a function of the amount of Ca^{2+} or Sr^{2+} added.[27] Further experimentation demonstrated the existence of mitochondrial Ca^{2+}-induced oscillations in permeabilized protozoa[37] and in Erhlich ascites tumor cells.[38]

Mitochondrial Oscillations in Intact Cells and Tissues

While the phenomena described above clearly show the potential for autonomous synchronized oscillation of mitochondria in suspension, only recently have oscillations in mitochondrial parameters been observed in intact cells, and it becomes more difficult to determine whether the oscillatory mechanism is intrinsic or extrinsic to the mitochondrial network. For example, mitochondria have been shown to respond to oscillatory Ca^{2+} signals evoked by signal transduction pathways[39] and have been implicated in the mechanism of bursting patterns of insulin release in pancreatic cells[40-42] and ultradian rhythms in yeast.[43] However, it is still not clear whether the mitochondria are a fundamental component of the oscillatory mechanism or are entrained by extramitochondrial factors, including cyclical changes in the plasma membrane electrical potential or Ca^{2+}.

In excitable cells, in which cyclical changes in plasmalemmal membrane potential and Ca^{2+} handling may occur, it becomes even more difficult to separate cause and effect when oscillatory behavior is observed. For instance, oscillations in mitochondrial variables in neurons from the brainstem respiratory center have been reported.[44] Measurements of FAD and NADH autofluorescence, $\Delta\Psi_m$ (Rhodamine123) and mitochondrial Ca^{2+}, Ca^{2+}_m (Rhod-2), were performed in slice preparations of the preBötzinger complex (pBC) and in the hypoglossal (XII) nucleus. The neural activity of the pBC is essential for maintaining rhythmic respiratory activity in brainstem neurons in vivo and in vitro. Rhythmic respiration was functionally correlated with oscillations in NADH, FAD, $\Delta\Psi_m$ and Ca^{2+}_m. These oscillations in mitochondrial variables were reversibly abolished by brief hypoxia (2-4 min) and, in parallel, ATP-sensitive K^+ channels were activated and respiratory output was depressed. These authors proposed that respiratory function was modulated by spontaneous activity in the mitochondrial network.

Adult cardiac ventricular myocytes are a good example of a cell-type containing multiple oscillators. However, since an external pacemaker normally entrains them, their mitochondria can be studied in the quiescent (noncontracting) state. Under such conditions, individual mitochondria have been observed to undergo spontaneous transient depolarization-repolarization cycles. This was first observed in 1982 by Berns et al[45] in myocytes loaded with fluorescent $\Delta\Psi_m$ sensors using focal laser excitation. Again, cause and effect become blurred when the mitochondrial depolarization is associated with the spontaneous local discharge of the intracellular Ca^{2+} store, as was reported for mitochondrial "flickers" in cardiac myocytes.[46] Similar transient mitochondrial depolarizations were also observed in cultured neurons[47,48] and in smooth muscle cells;[49] in the latter case, they were found to be independent of sarcoplasmic reticular Ca^{2+} release.[50] In addition, spontaneous $\Delta\Psi_m$ fluctuations can be observed in individual isolated mitochondria.[51-54] With respect to Ca^{2+}-induced ionic oscillations in mitochondria, a Ca^{2+}-induced Ca^{2+}-release mechanism[30] involving the permeability transition pore (PTP) has been proposed[46,51,52] and may be responsible for fast mitochondrial Ca^{2+} release in cells;[55] however, in many of the examples mentioned above, the phenomenon is insensitive to cyclosporin A, calling into question the conclusion that the PTP is involved.[48,53]

Another important consideration is whether or not the method of observation of $\Delta\Psi_m$ depolarization is actually contributing to the perceived "spontaneous" event. In the original work of Berns et al,[45] the fluorescence oscillations depended on the type of dye used, suggesting that photosensitization played a role, and it is now well-recognized that even low levels of fluorescence excitation can generate enough free radicals to cause mitochondrial depolarization. This effect of laser-induced radical generation was used to great advantage by Zorov and Sollott[56,57] in describing mitochondrial ROS-induced ROS release in rat cardiomyocytes.

Metabolic Oscillations in Substrate-Deprived Heart Cells

We previously observed that cardiomyocytes subjected to energetic stress by substrate deprivation display spontaneous oscillations (period ~1-3 min) in sarcolemmal currents that were attributed to the cyclical activation and deactivation of ATP-sensitive potassium current $(I_{K,ATP})$.[34] The activation of $I_{K,ATP}$ was correlated with, and slightly preceded by, oxidation of the intracellular NADH/NAD$^+$ redox couple (Fig. 1A), indicating that large changes in energy metabolism were occurring. In addition to $I_{K,ATP}$ activation, the amplitude of the Ca^{2+} transient was suppressed, highlighting the global effects of metabolic oscillation on the integrated function of the cell. This was also illustrated by the shortening and suppression of the action potential of myocytes undergoing oscillations in $I_{K,ATP}$ (Fig. 1B), leading us to propose that this mechanism may be of pathophysiological relevance as a trigger of arrhythmias related to ischemia-reperfusion injury (refs. 34,58 and see discussion below).

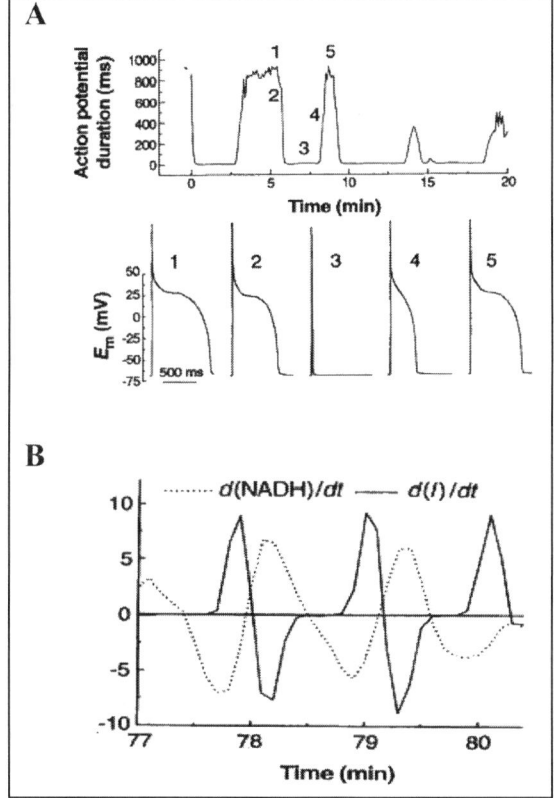

Figure 1. Oscillations of membrane current, excitability and redox pool in substrate-deprived isolated cardiomyocytes. A) Effects of metabolic oscillations on electrical excitability. Upper panel, the action potential duration (90% repolarization time) for a series of action potentials (APs) evoked by brief current injections in a current-clamped cardiomyocyte. Lower panel, selected APs recorded at the time points indicated by the numbers on the upper panel. The brief depolarization in 3 is the stimulus artifact. E_m is the cell membrane potential. B) Phase shift between the first derivative plots of NADH (dashed line) and membrane current (solid line). Reprinted with permission from O'Rourke, Ramza and Marban. Oscillations of membrane current and excitability driven by metabolic oscillations in heart cells. Science 1994; 265(5174):962-966. Copyright ©1994 AAAS.

Since the period and amplitude of the $I_{K,ATP}$ oscillations were the same in electrically-stimulated or quiescent cells, a Ca^{2+}- or plasma membrane potential-dependent source of oscillation was ruled out. On the other hand, manipulation of substrate supply (by increasing glucose availability or inhibiting glycolysis), temporarily uncoupling mitochondria, or photolytically releasing ADP within the cell, strongly influenced the oscillator, suggesting that the underlying driver was metabolism itself. Hence, we proposed that the well-studied glycolytic oscillator, previously demonstrated in cell-free heart extracts, could be the source of oscillation;[59] however, we could not rule out a mitochondrial origin.

The evidence for the mitochondria being the source of oscillation was subsequently reinforced by demonstrating that the redox potential of mitochondrial flavoproteins rapidly cycles between the oxidized and reduced state in association with depolarization and repolarization of $\Delta\Psi_m$.[35] Confocal imaging experiments revealed that flavoprotein oxidation could either involve the entire cell or clusters of mitochondria, and that redox waves could propagate from one myocyte to another through the intercalated disc,[35,59] emphasizing the role of synchronization of the mitochondrial network in the response. Moreover, the findings suggested the presence of a putative low molecular weight messenger responsible for the propagation of redox waves. Importantly, it was shown that neither Ca^{2+}, nor the permeability transition pore were likely to be involved in the mechanism of the oscillator in substrate-deprived cells. Alternatively, a mechanism involving the mitochondrial benzodiazepine receptor and the inner membrane anion channel (IMAC) was proposed.[58]

The Mitochondrial Oscillator of Heart Cells: The Pathophysiological Domain

Focal Oxidative Stress as a Trigger

Since it was difficult to predict when or how the oscillations in metabolism could be initiated in substrate-deprived cells, the detailed study of the oscillatory mechanism was greatly facilitated by the discovery that they could be triggered by oxidative stress.[36] Unlike the earlier studies of direct laser-induced mitochondrial depolarization mentioned in the introduction, we found that focal excitation of a small portion of the mitochondrial network of an adult cardiomyocyte can induce autonomous oscillations in $\Delta\Psi_m$ and mitochondrial redox potential in the whole cell. This provided a tool for studying the mitochondrial oscillator under controlled and highly reproducible conditions, allowing us to elucidate the mechanism in the context of pathophysiology.[36]

$\Delta\Psi_m$ depolarization and local mitochondrial ROS generation were initiated using a two-photon laser to generate free radicals in a small volume of the cell (a "flash"), affecting only a few mitochondria (~50; Fig. 2A). In contrast to the rapid and sustained effect of the laser within the flashed region (Fig. 2A), the remainder of the mitochondrial network was initially unaffected; however, after a variable latency period (43 seconds on average), ROS levels abruptly increased and $\Delta\Psi_m$ collapsed throughout the cell (Fig. 2A, top right). This was followed by synchronized and self-sustained mitochondrial oscillations in $\Delta\Psi_m$, NADH, ROS (Fig. 2B),[36] as well as reduced glutathione.[60]

The important role of intracellular ROS in the mechanism of cell-wide oscillations was suggested by the observation that cells showing the oscillatory behavior always had ROS levels exceeding a threshold of ~20% above baseline. In addition, scavenging ROS with TMPyP (Mn(III)tetrakis(1-methyl-4-pyridil)porphyrin pentachloride), a superoxide dismutase mimetic, or N-acetyl cysteine (NAC), a thiol modifier, decreased ROS levels below threshold and prevented oscillations (Figs. 3C,D).

Mitochondrial Respiration as the Source of ROS Production

Acute application of mitochondrial electron transport inhibitors could immediately stop the oscillations in $\Delta\Psi_m$ and could also prevent the accumulation of ROS to the threshold for

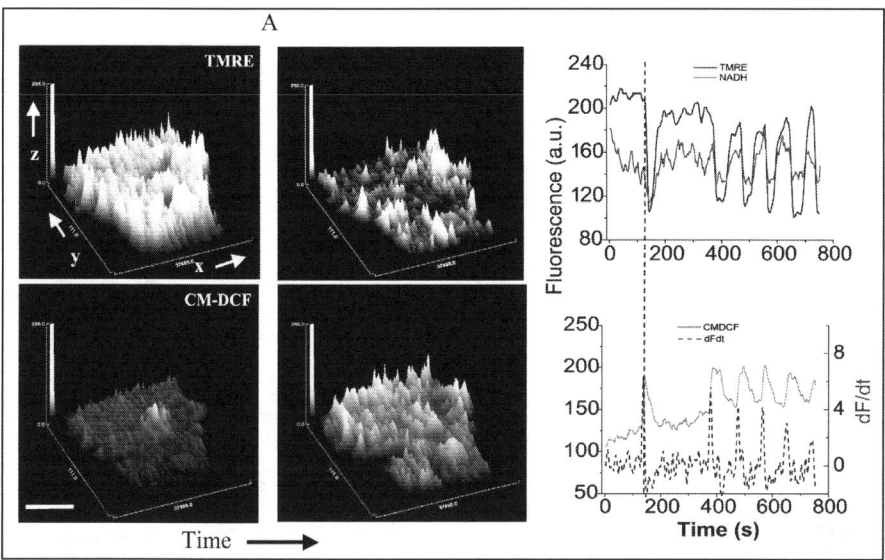

Figure 2. Whole-cell oscillations in mitochondrial metabolism triggered by a local perturbation. A) Top panels, surface plot of mitochondrial membrane potential ($\Delta\Psi_m$) in a TMRE-loaded cardiomyocyte during the flash (white arrow, top left panel) showing the local $\Delta\Psi_m$ depolarization, and the cell-wide $\Delta\Psi_m$ collapse (top right panel) ~40s (on average) after the flash. Bottom panels, surface plot of the fluorescence intensity of the ROS-sensitive fluorophore CM-H_2DCF during the flash showing the local (bottom left panel) and the cell-wide (bottom right panel) increase in ROS generation associated with the $\Delta\Psi_m$ collapse. x, y, z, in the axes of the surface plot correspond to the transversal and longitudinal axes of the cell, respectively, and the fluorescence intensity of TMRE (top panels) or CM-DCF (bottom panels). Bar ~ 20μm. B) The first cell-wide $\Delta\Psi_m$ collapse was followed by synchronized oscillations in mitochondrial energetics. Simultaneous recordings of the time course of average whole-cell fluorescence of TMRE and NADH (top panel) and CM-DCF and the derivative of CM-DCF signals (dF/dt, dashed line) (bottom panel). The precise phase relationship between all signals can be clearly appreciated from the vertical reference line drawn. (Panel B is reproduced from Aon, Cortassa, Marban and O'Rourke. J Biol Chem 2003; 278, 44735, with permission of the American Society for Biochemistry and Molecular Biology).

depolarization (Fig. 3A,B). This experimental evidence directly implicated mitochondrial respiration as the source of ROS in the oscillatory mechanism. Thus, we next addressed the question of which site(s) of the electron transport chain were responsible for the ROS produced. Our findings, obtained in living cardiomyocytes under quiescent conditions and unrestricted access to oxygen, pointed to complex III as the source of superoxide anion (O_2^-). Our attempts to halt respiration with inhibitors of complex I (rotenone) and complex IV (cyanide) caused a reduction in ROS, indicating that ROS generation did not correspond to a highly reduced, high $\Delta\Psi_m$ state, which can cause ROS prodution in isolated mitochondria. At the level of complex III, O_2^- production was enhanced only when ubisemiquinone accumulated in the presence of antimycin A, but not when the oxidation of ubiquinol to ubisemiquinone and electron transfer to the FeSIII center of complex III was prevented with myxothiazol.[36]

The main site of ROS production in the respiratory chain of living cells is unclear see also Appendix in (ref. 60) for a detailed discussion of this topic); however, in isolated mitochondria, there is evidence for ROS production by several different sites. Depending upon conditions, superoxide can be generated either at complex I or complex III (from the Q cycle). ROS production from complex I appears to be favored at high $\Delta\Psi_m$ and highly reduced redox potentials

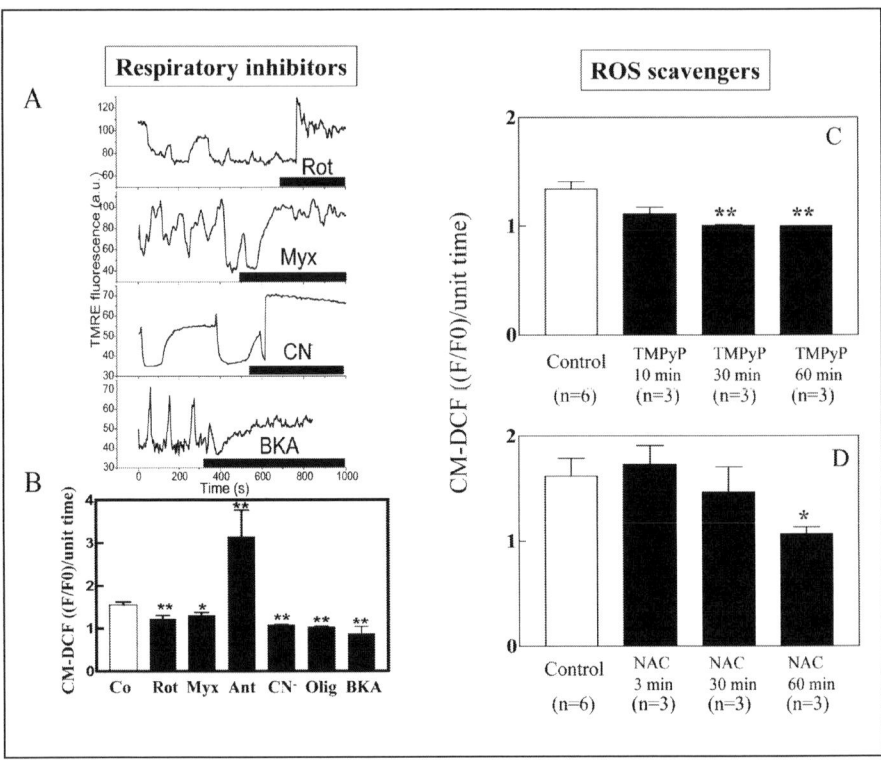

Figure 3. Effect of respiratory inhibitors and ROS scavengers on mitochondrial oscillations. A) TMRE traces of myocytes showing cell-wide mitochondrial oscillations after a laser flash and, subsequently, being subjected to an acute addition of rotenone (15 μM, Rot) (see also B), myxothiazol (5 μM, Myx), NaCN (5 mM, CN⁻) or bongkrekic acid (25 μM, BKA) while the image acquisition was briefly paused. After imaging resumed (within ~3 min of inhibitor addition), the oscillations were abolished. Thick line in each panel indicates presence of inhibitor. B) The effect of the different inhibitors on ROS production as measured by the normalized CM-DCF signal per unit time. Antimycin (Ant) and oligomycin (Olig) concentrations were 6 μM and 10 μg/ml whereas the other inhibitor concentrations were as described in (A). ROS production following a flash was quantified for cells preincubated in the presence of each inhibitor. Under these conditions, the cells did not exhibit oscillations after the laser flash. $*p < 0.05$, $**p < 0.01$ vs. control. C) The SOD mimetic TMPyP (250 or 500 μM) or (D) the ROS scavenger N-acetyl-L-cysteine (NAC, 4 mM) was acutely added to myocytes. Prolonged incubation (1h) with the scavengers completely suppressed the synchronized oscillations.[36] The control corresponds to cells exhibiting cell-wide mitochondrial oscillations before addition of the scavenger. The time-dependent effect of TMPyP and NAC to suppress oscillations correlated with a significant decrease of ROS production to basal levels. Panels A and B are reproduced from Aon, Cortassa, Marban and O'Rourke (2003) J. Biol. Chem. 278, 44735, with permission of the American Society for Biochemistry and Molecular Biology © 2003.

(>-390mV), usually achieved when respiration is inhibited (e.g., with rotenone). ROS production from complex III in isolated mitochondria is promoted by treatment with antimycin A, which promotes the accumulation of ubisemiquinone on the outer aspect of the mitochondrial inner membrane. We showed that this treatment can cause massive ROS accumulation and the collapse of $\Delta\Psi_m$ in myocytes subjected to the flash protocol, complementing the evidence using inhibitors that complex III is the main source of ROS in intact cells. This model would be consistent with the proportionality between complex III-derived ROS production and respiration reported previously.

The key question is whether ROS production is mainly controlled by $\Delta\Psi_m$ or flux through the electron transport chain. Cyanide inhibition of the respiratory flux and, concomitantly, of ROS levels, suggested that electron transport was necessary for mitochondrial ROS production. Taking mitochondria to state 4 and slowing down the electron flux should also decrease ROS production. This was done in our experimental system by inhibiting the F_1F_0 ATPase with oligomycin, or the adenine nucleotide translocator with bongkrekic acid (BKA). Both inhibitors decreased ROS levels below threshold and suppressed oscillations pointing out that mitochondrial electron transport is necessary for ROS production and, consequently, oscillations.

The Role of Mitochondrial Ion Channels in the Oscillatory Mechanism

The asymmetry of the $\Delta\Psi_m$ depolarization-repolarization cycle is consistent with the behavior exhibited by relaxation oscillators that possess slow and fast components.[60] The sudden depolarization phase of $\Delta\Psi_m$ during the oscillations suggests that an energy dissipating ion channel is opening, causing rapid uncoupling of oxidative phosphorylation.

An obvious candidate for rapid depolarization of $\Delta\Psi_m$ was the PTP, which can be activated by various toxic agents or metabolic changes associated with necrosis and/or apoptosis. Ca^{2+} overload is one cofactor in the opening of the PTP (see ref. 61,62 for reviews) and a model of Ca^{2+}-induced Ca^{2+} release from the mitochondrial matrix through the PTP has been proposed.

We investigated whether or not the PTP and/or Ca^{2+} was involved in the mechanism of whole-cell $\Delta\Psi_m$ oscillation. Several lines of evidence ruled out both the PTP and Ca^{2+} as playing a role in the mitochondrial oscillations observed in heart cells. With regard to Ca^{2+}, as we have previously reported: (i) the myocytes were studied under quiescent, minimally Ca^{2+}-loaded conditions, and no sarcomere shortening was evident; (ii) suppression of sarcoplasmic reticulum (SR) or mitochondrial Ca^{2+} handling did not influence flash-induced mitochondrial oscillations; (iii) extensive buffering of intracellular Ca^{2+} with 1 mM EGTA did not affect flash-induced oscillations. The possible contribution of the PTP was ruled out by the following evidence: (i) cyclosporin A (CsA) did not block the transitions, and (ii) small (600 MW) fluorophores were not lost from the mitochondrial matrix upon depolarization. Bongkrekic acid inhibited the oscillations and stabilized $\Delta\Psi_m$. This compound is often used as a PTP blocker because it is assumed that the adenine nucleotide translocase is a component of the PTP. However, since the effects of BKA were similar to those of other inhibitors of electron transport such as cyanide, our interpretation was that this compound's main effect, to inhibit the distal electron transport chain, causes a decrease in mitochondrial ROS production by putting the mitochondria in state 4.[36]

Other ion channels have been described on the mitochondrial inner membrane, and could be candidates for fast mitochondrial depolarization. An IMAC was described in isolated mitochondria and was shown to be inhibited by cationic amphiphiles including peripheral (mitochondrial) benzodiazepine receptor (mBzR) ligands.[63-65] Subsequently, single channel patch-clamp studies of mitoplasts have provided evidence that anion channels are present on the inner membrane, the most common being the outwardly rectifying 108 pS (or "centum-picosiemen") anion channel which is inhibited by mBzR antagonists. We showed that PK11195, an isoquinoline carboxamide mBzR ligand, could acutely inhibit mitochondrial $\Delta\Psi_m$ oscillations, initiated either by substrate deprivation or laser flash, in a reversible manner. Mitochondrial oscillations were also abolished by a structurally different mBzR ligand, 4'-chlorodiazepam (4'Cl-DZP) (Ro5-4864) or by the anion transport inhibitor DIDS.[36,58] These inhibitors prevented ROS accumulation in the mitochondrial network, but actually potentiated ROS accumulation in the small laser-flashed region of the cell, leading to the proposal that IMAC might also be an efflux pathway for superoxide anion from the matrix, since O_2^- is membrane impermeable. Moreover, induction of mitochondrial $\Delta\Psi_m$ depolarization by FGIN-1-27, an agonist that binds selectively to the mBzR, reinforced the idea that this receptor, which is thought to be present on the mitochondrial outer membrane, may be modulating IMAC. Taken together, the data are consistent with a role for IMAC, rather than PTP, in both $\Delta\Psi_m$ depolarization and O_2^- efflux, forming the mechanistic basis for our theoretical model of the mitochondrial oscillator.

The Theoretical Approach

An Integrated Computational Model of the Mitochondrial Oscillator

An integrated model of mitochondrial energetics and Ca^{2+} handling was extended to describe the key features of the proposed mechanism of mitochondrial oscillations based on our experimental findings.[36] These included incorporating a shunt of electrons of the respiratory chain toward the generation of O_2^-, a ROS scavenging system, and an outwardly rectifying IMAC modeled after the centum pS channel. The normal anion permeability of IMAC would permit the passage of O_2^- from the matrix to the cytoplasmic side of the inner membrane. In addition, the IMAC opening probability was assumed to be increased by O_2^- at an external site. The scheme of the integrated model is shown in (Fig. 4A).

Model simulations show the ability to reproduce the oscillatory period and the phase relationship between $\Delta\Psi_m$ and NADH observed experimentally (see Fig. 2B). According to the model, a burst in cytoplasmic ROS accompanies $\Delta\Psi_m$ depolarization as a result of a mixed process of accelerated O_2^- production (due to an increase in the rate of mitochondrial respiration during uncoupling) and a transient increase in O_2^- release (as a result of the self-amplifying effect of IMAC opening on anion transport (Fig. 4B)). Thus, a pulse of cytoplasmic $O_2^-{}_i$ is released when the buffering capacity of superoxide dismutase (SOD) is exceeded. This pulse subsides because of several factors, including (i) a decrease in O_2^- efflux when the electrochemical driving force for anions is diminished by $\Delta\Psi_m$ depolarization, (ii) an increase in SOD-mediated O_2^-removal, and (iii) a decrease in respiration as the NADH is consumed.

The model was able to reproduce the major experimental findings, including the requirement for ROS to cross a threshold to trigger fast $\Delta\Psi_m$ depolarization, the suppressive effect of inhibitors of the electron transport chain, ANT and the F_1F_O ATPase on ROS production and $\Delta\Psi_m$ oscillation, the effects of anion channel inhibitors, and the sensitivity of the oscillator to the levels of ROS scavengers. The model also predicted oscillations in reduced glutathione that could be demonstrated experimentally.[60]

Figure 4, figure viewed on following page. Model of mitochondrial energetics coupled to ROS production, transport, and scavenging. A) The IMAC and the ROS scavenging system were incorporated into an integrated model of mitochondrial energetics and Ca^{2+} handling.[60,73] The model postulates that superoxide anion in the mitochondrial matrix ($O_2^-{}_m$) is transported through the IMAC whose opening probability is activated by cytoplasmic (intermembrane) superoxide anion ($O_2^-{}_i$). The integrated computational model of mitochondrial energetics incorporates IMAC, ROS production, and ROS scavenging. See (ref. 60) for a description of the parameters utilized in the simulations. B) Simulation of the 100 s period oscillations observed experimentally (see Fig. 2) using the integrated computational model of mitochondrial energetics with incorporated IMAC, ROS production, and ROS scavenging (panel A). Represented are the oscillations in $O_2^-{}_m$, and the O_2 consumption flux. See (ref. 60) for a description of the parameters utilized in the simulations. C) Bifurcation diagram of $\Delta\Psi_m$ as a function of ROS production and scavenging. The dynamic behavior of the computational model shows an upper branch of steady states in which $\Delta\Psi_m$ is predominantly polarized, and a lower branch, in which $\Delta\Psi_m$ is mainly depolarized. Transitions between both branches happen at arrowheads 3 and 4. Thick lines indicate domains of stable steady-state behavior whereas thin lines denote either unstable or oscillatory states. A stable oscillatory domain, embedded within the upper branch, emerges as SOD concentration increases. Arrowheads 1 and 2 in the upper branch indicate Hopf bifurcations delimiting the oscillatory region (thin line). Key to abbreviations: im, inner mitochondrial membrane; IMAC, inner membrane anion channel; CAT, catalase; SOD, Cu,Zn superoxide dismutase; GPX, glutathione peroxidase. (Panels A and C are reproduced from Cortassa, Aon, Winslow and O'Rourke (2004) Biophys. J. 87, 2060, with permission of the Biophysical Society © 2004).

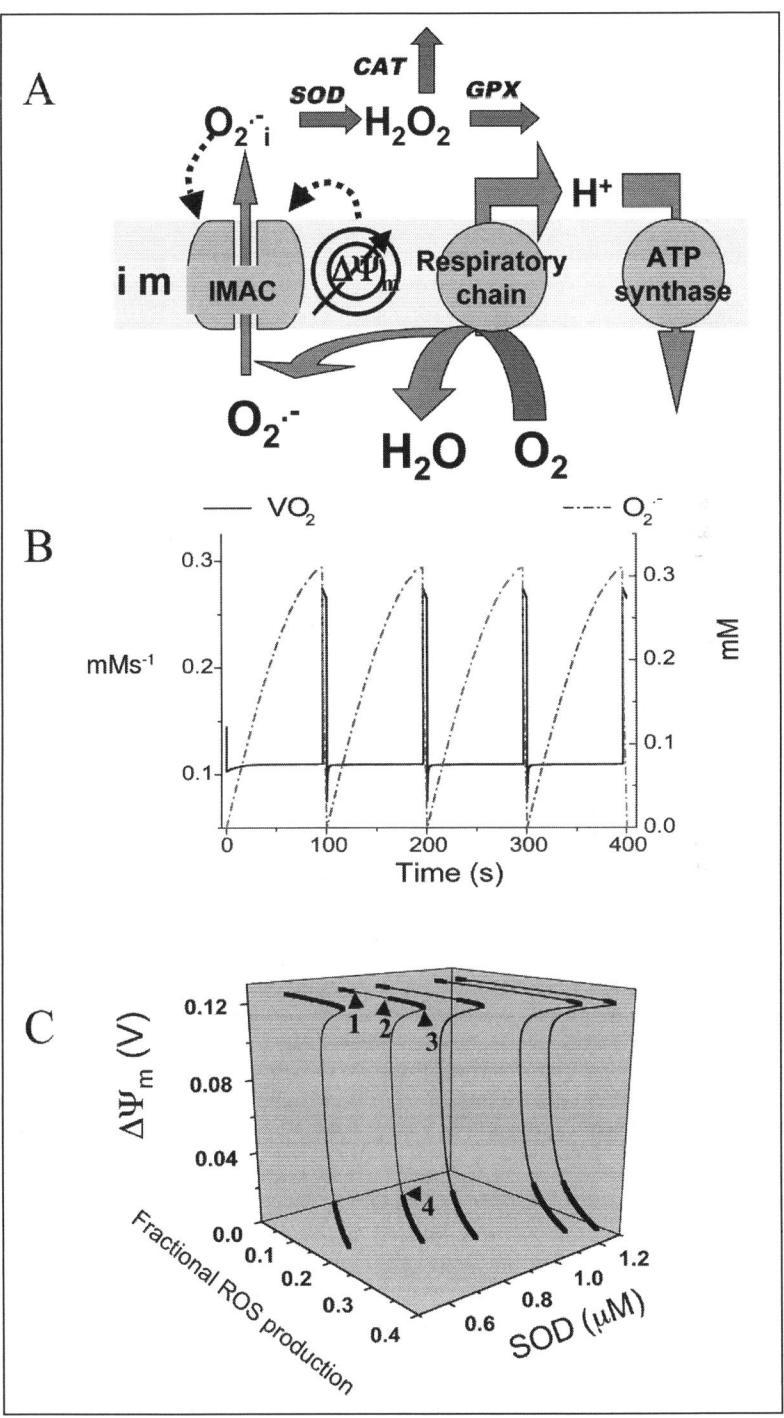

Figure 4, legend viewed on previous page.

Predicting the High Frequency Domain of the Mitochondrial Oscillator

Stability analysis of the model confirmed the presence of Hopf bifurcations, a signature of the existence of limit cycles, visualized as sustained oscillations (Fig. 4C). The bifurcation diagrams have the typical S-shape that describes the behavior of systems exhibiting bistability, and show an unstable region (thin lines) between the upper (polarized) and lower (depolarized) branches of steady states (thick lines in Fig. 4C). This diagram illustrates the importance of the balance between mitochondrial ROS generation and ROS buffering since the oscillatory domain, flanked by Hopf bifurcations, appears within the upper branch of the curve as the concentration of ROS scavenger increases. This domain gradually expands at higher SOD concentrations (from left to right in Fig. 4C) until the limit between the upper or lower branch, where the model behavior changes precipitously and $\Delta\Psi_m$ jumps from polarized to depolarized steady states or vice versa (see Fig. 4C).

At each oscillatory cycle, the computational model predicts a burst of respiration (Fig. 4B) triggered by the rapid membrane uncoupling and the concomitant oxidation of the mitochondrial NADH pool together with the rapid release of $O_2^{\cdot-}$ to the mitochondrial intermembrane space (Fig. 4B).

An intriguing finding in the model simulations was that the frequency and amplitude of the stable oscillations could be modulated over several orders of magnitude (milliseconds to hours) by simply changing (as little as) one parameter, e.g., the SOD concentration. From the physiological point of view, the observation that fast oscillations in ROS could be generated by the mitochondria with minimal energetic consequences (i.e., only μV to mV changes in $\Delta\Psi_m$) led us to propose that the ROS-dependent mitochondrial oscillator could represent a frequency- and/or amplitude-modulated signaling mechanism that could connect bioenergetics to ROS-activated signal transduction pathways, including those responsible for regulating gene transcription.[66]

These computational studies motivated experiments to determine if small amplitude fluctuations in $\Delta\Psi_m$ could be detected in cardiomyocytes under physiological conditions, described in the next section.

The Mitochondrial Oscillator in the Physiological Domain

As mentioned in the Introduction, mitochondria in various cell types, including neurons, smooth muscle cells and cardiomyocytes, have been observed to undergo spontaneous transient depolarizations or flickers of $\Delta\Psi_m$. These observations suggest that individual, or small clusters of mitochondria may be able to oscillate autonomously in intact cells. However, the results discussed above indicate that pathological conditions appear to induce synchronized, coupled oscillations across the mitochondrial network of the cardiac myocyte. The computational studies of the mitochondrial oscillator suggested two fundamentally different views to explain this self-organization process for large amplitude oscillations in $\Delta\Psi_m$. The first possibility was that mitochondria in the "normal" state are in a dynamic steady-state and metabolic stress pushes the system towards a bifurcation point and oscillation. The second possibility was suggested by the parametric analysis, which showed that low-amplitude, high-frequency oscillations were possible. We hypothesized that if mitochondria behaved as high-frequency oscillators under physiological conditions, small fluctuations in $\Delta\Psi_m$ may be detectable by correlation analysis of long time series recordings of $\Delta\Psi_m$.

In the absence of metabolic stress, cardiomyocytes loaded with tetramethylrhodamine methyl ester (TMRM), a fluorescent reporter of mitochondrial membrane potential, display stable $\Delta\Psi_m$ for more than an hour. Using two-photon laser scanning fluorescence microscopy, cells were imaged every ~100ms and the average fluorescence for the whole cell was calculated (Fig. 5). By applying Relative Dispersional Analysis (RDA) and Power Spectral Analysis (PSA) to the data, we found that collectively, cardiac mitochondria behave as a highly correlated network of oscillators.[66] According to RDA, the fluorescence time series exhibit long-term memory quantitatively characterized by an inverse power law with a fractal dimension, D_f, of approximately 1.0. This behavior, characteristic of self-similar fractal processes, is distinct from

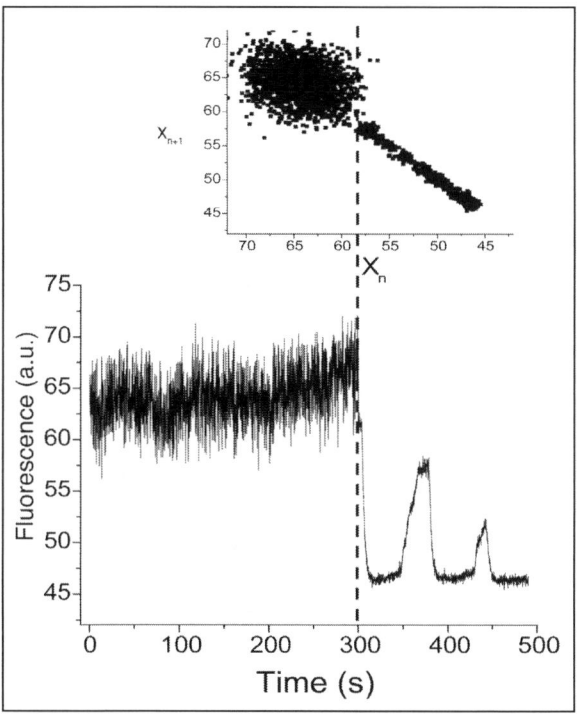

Figure 5. Physiological and pathophysiological behaviors of the mitochondrial network in heart cells in the presence of glucose. The main panel shows the time series of TMRM fluorescence of a freshly isolated ventricular cardiomyocyte, imaged by two photon microscopy (150ms time resolution). Before the mitochondrial network reaches criticality,[74-76] the $\Delta\Psi_m$ (as measured by TMRM) oscillates at high frequencies and small amplitudes. After criticality, the network behavior evolves into "pathophysiological" behavior characterized by low-frequency, high-amplitude oscillations.[36,60] The inset shows a return plot of the time series, the dashed line separating the richness of high frequency-low amplitude oscillations present in the physiological as opposed to the low frequency-high amplitude oscillations present in the pathophysiological regime. (Reproduced from Aon, Cortassa and O'Rourke (2006) Biophys. J. 91, 4317-4327, with permission of the Biophysical Society © 2006).

processes without memory that show completely random behavior (white or brown noise), which are characterized by an exponential (Poisson) law with a slope corresponding to $D_f = 1.5$.

Self-similar scaling was also revealed by PSA after applying Fast Fourier Transform (FFT) to the TMRM fluorescence time series. The power spectrum followed an homogenous inverse power law of the form $1/f^\beta$ with with $\beta \sim 1.7$. These results pointed out that mitochondrial oscillations exhibit a broad frequency distribution spanning at least three orders of magnitude (from milliseconds to a few minutes).

The results indicate that collective behavior of the mitochondrial network is a statistically fractal, self-similar, process characterized by a large number of frequencies in multiple time scales, rather than an inherent "characteristic" frequency. We propose that these mitochondrial oscillators are weakly coupled by low levels of mitochondrial ROS in the physiological state but that an increase in ROS production under metabolic stress can reach a threshold that results in strong coupling through mitochondrial ROS-induced ROS release, and organization of the network into a synchronized cluster spanning the whole cell. A dominant low-frequency high-amplitude oscillation ensues.

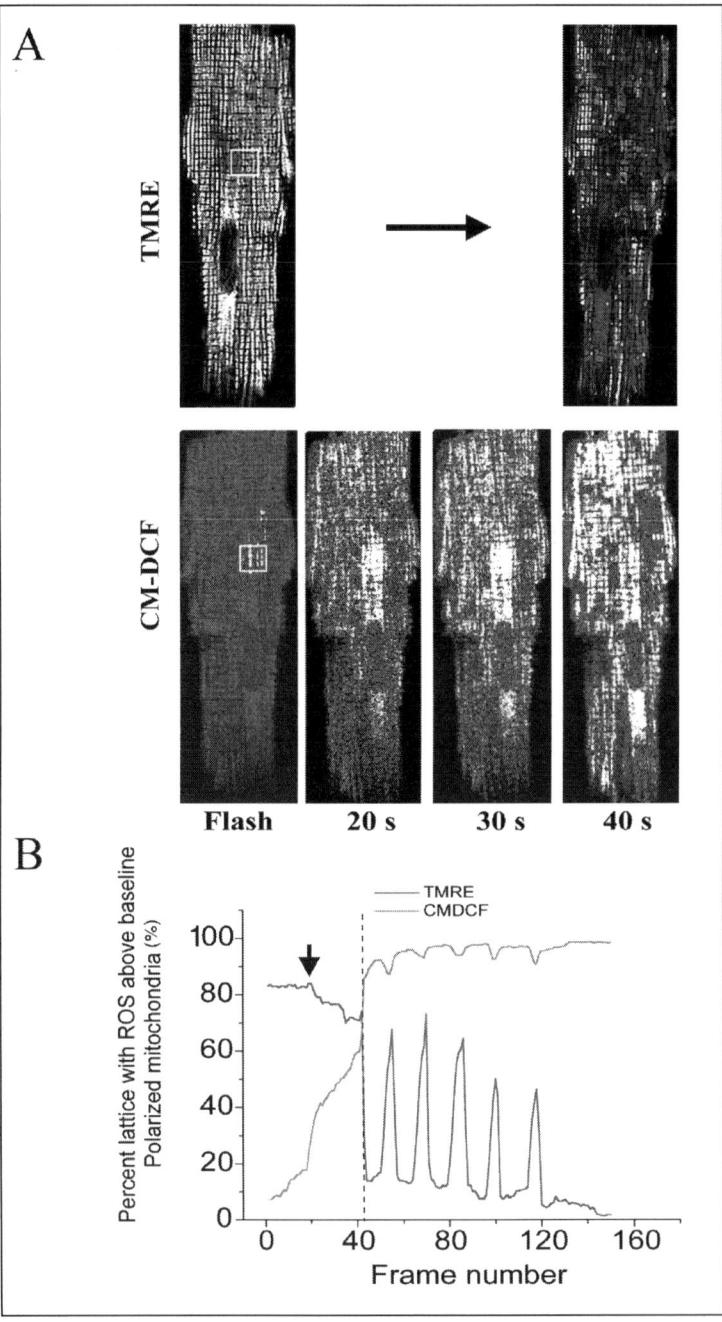

Figure 6. Time course of the mitochondrial cluster formation. A) Sustained oscillations in $\Delta\Psi_m$ happening beyond criticality are depicted. Arrow indicates the timing of the flash. B) At criticality, a cell-wide $\Delta\Psi_m$ depolarization (TMRE, top right) occurs in a cluster encompassing about 60% of the mitochondria with ROS levels above baseline (CM-DCF, bottom). Adapted from Aon, Cortassa and O'Rourke (2004) Proc Natl Acad Sci USA 1018, 4447).

Spatial Aspects: ROS and Mitochondrial Criticality

The transition between the physiological and pathophysiological domains of mitochondrial oscillation is a clear example of emergent self-organization in both time (limit cycle oscillation) and space (synchronization across the mitochondrial network) (Fig. 5). With respect to the spatial organization, we have applied percolation theory to explain how a local interaction among mitochondria organized in a lattice can lead to a widespread change in the state of energization of the system. The mitochondria of the heart cell are particularly amenable to this analysis because they are organized almost as a cubic lattice, with a spacing of ~0.2-1 μm between elements. In two-dimensional images of a single focal plane of the myocyte, we measured $\Delta\Psi_m$ and ROS accumulation after a local laser flash, and determined the percentage of the mitochondria showing a ROS signal above a certain threshold level (20% above baseline fluorescence) as a function of time after the flash (Fig. 6A). At the point in time just before the first cell-wide collapse of $\Delta\Psi_m$, which we referred to as "criticality", we found that ~ 60% of the mitochondrial network had ROS levels at or near threshold (Fig. 6A), and this cluster of mitochondria spanned the whole cell (i.e., a "spanning cluster" was evident) (Fig. 6B). This number is very close to the theoretical prediction for systems at a percolation threshold ($p_c = 0.59$).[67,68] Moreover, fractal analysis of the shape of the spanning cluster was also consistent with percolation theory.[69]

The significance of this characterization of the mitochondrial network as a percolation process is that it helps to explain why $\Delta\Psi_m$ depolarization occurs in a synchronized manner throughout the cell and where it will occur. Only those mitochondria belonging to the spanning cluster take part in the global limit cycle oscillation, explaining why some mitochondria appear to resist oscillation even though they are surrounded by depolarized mitochondria (Fig. 2A). Furthermore, it explains why there does not seem to be a single point in the cluster (for example, the flashed area) from which each cycle originates—the system at criticality is susceptible to small perturbations anywhere in the spanning cluster to initiate a transition.

With faster time resolution, or by slowing the kinetics of the oscillator (e.g., with submaximal oligomycin concentrations), the $\Delta\Psi_m$ depolarization wave can often be resolved. This wave travels at a speed of 22 μm/s, corresponding to a total time for global depolarization of about 4s (see Fig. 6B) (considering an average myocyte length of 100 μm), in agreement with the experimental data. Although the $\Delta\Psi_m$ depolarization is global (Fig. 6B), the interaction between mitochondria is local. The short lifetime of the O_2^- radical and the presence of fast scavenger systems prevents long range diffusion, but in our mechanistic model, O_2^- liberated from a mitochondrion in the spanning cluster must only diffuse to its neighbors. The second criterion is that the neighbor must also be a member of the spanning cluster (i.e., be close to the threshold for depolarization). According to percolation theory, a p_c of 0.59 corresponds to a coordination number of four, again emphasizing that each mitochondrion is influencing its nearest neighbors in the network. These results also explain why the speed of the depolarization wave is faster than it would be if sustained by diffusion of the chemical messenger (O_2^-) alone.

From Mitochondrial Dynamics to Whole Heart Arrhythmias

Coupling of Mitochondrial Oscillations to Cellular Electrical Excitability

The early studies of cardiac metabolic oscillations showed that they have a profound effect on the excitability and Ca^{2+} handling properties of the cardiac cell. The oscillatory uncoupling of mitochondria depletes cellular ATP levels and drives the activation of ATP-sensitive K^+ (K_{ATP}) channels in the sarcolemma. This will, in turn, produce cyclical changes in the action potential of the cardiomyocyte (Fig. 1A) and this heterogeneity was proposed to be a possible source of ischemia-related arhythmias.

Using the laser flash-induced oscillation, we demonstrated that the action potential duration was tightly coupled to the mitochondrial energetic state. At the onset of $\Delta\Psi_m$ depolarization, the action potential rapidly shortens and the cell quickly becomes inexcitable; this is followed by the parallel recovery of both the metabolic and electrical signals (Fig. 7).[36,70] Stabilizing $\Delta\Psi_m$ by the

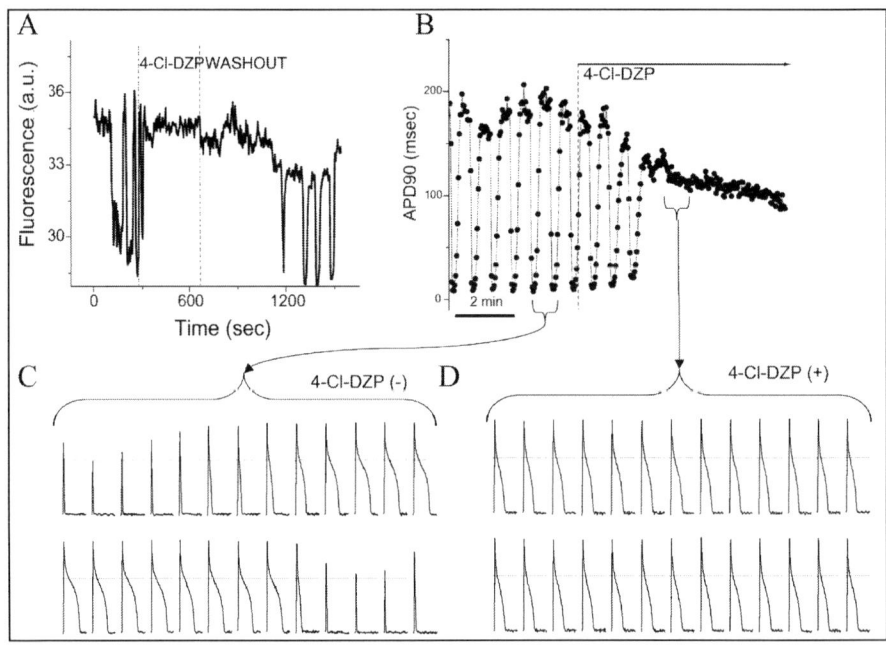

Figure 7. Blockade of mitochondrial oscillations and stabilization of the cellular action potential (AP) by 4'-Cl-DZP. Freshly isolated cardiomyocytes loaded with TMRM (100 nM) at 37°C, where patched and APs were recorded under whole-cell current-clamp conditions on the stage of the microscope. A) This panel shows the reversible effect of acutely added 4'-Cl-DZP (32 μM; between dashed lines) on mitochondrial Δψm oscillations that resume after washout of the MBzR antagonist. B) Mitochondrial oscillations in Δψm and the sarcolemmal action potential duration (APD) were triggered after a highly localized laser flash (3 min before the train of oscillating APDs shown in this panel). APs evoked by brief current injections were recorded during the oscillations. During a synchronized cell-wide depolarization repolarization cycle, the AP shortens in synchrony with fast mitochondrial depolarization.[36] C) During the APD oscillations, the cell becomes inexcitable when Δψm is fully depolarized (remaining upward spikes are from the stimulus only). D) After addition of 64μM 4'-Cl-DZP, a stable AP is restored and Δψm oscillations are suppressed. (Reproduced from Akar, Aon, Tomaselli and O'Rourke (2005) J. Clin. Invest. 115, 3527, with permission of the American Society for Clinical Investigation © 2005).

abovementioned interventions, such as inhibition of the mBzR, not only inhibits the oscillations in mitochondrial variables, but also stabilizes the action potential (Fig. 7). Action potentials were strongly affected only during the synchronized whole-cell mitochondrial oscillations and not when single, or small clusters of, mitochondria were depolarized.

The Mitochondrial Origin of Post-Ischemic Arrhythmias

We have described how the failure of individual mitochondria can scale to involve whole-cell bioenergetics and the integrated function of the cardiac myocyte. Next, we tested if a similar mechanism can occur in the whole heart and contributes to ischemia-related arrhythmias.

After ischemic injury, the early reperfusion phase would be expected to favor mitochondrial criticality since a burst of ROS production and antioxidant depletion are known to occur.[71] Optical mapping studies of isolated perfused guinea-pig hearts subjected to 30 minutes of ischemia demonstrated that persistent ventricular tachycardia and/or fibrillation occurs within minutes of reperfusion (Fig. 8). We used this experimental system to determine if the mBzR

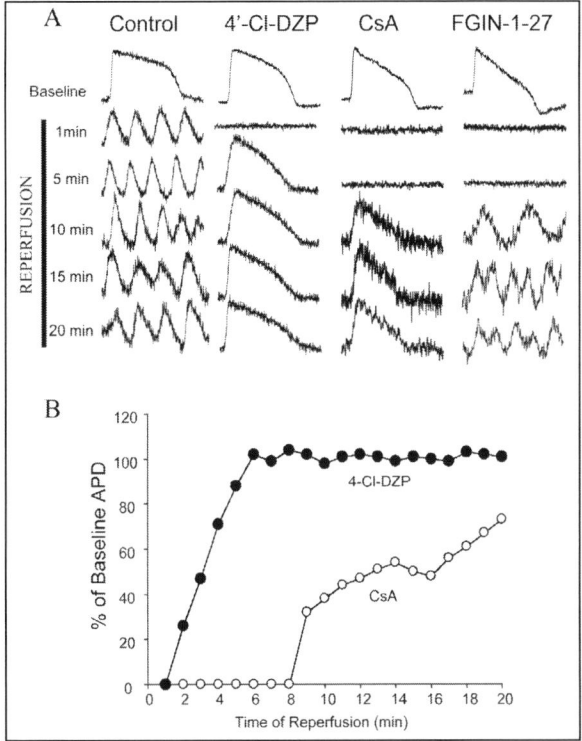

Figure 8. Post-ischemic AP recovery and arrhythmias. A) Representative APs during recovery upon reperfusion in control, 4'-Cl-DZP-, CsA-, and FGIN-1-27-treated hearts. B) Plot of the recovery of APD upon reperfusion normalized to the baseline APD before ischemia in 4'-Cl-DZP- and CsA-treated hearts. (Reproduced from Akar, Aon, Tomaselli and O'Rourke (2005) J. Clin. Invest. 115, 3527, with permission of the American Society for Clinical Investigation © 2005).

antagonist 4'Cl-DZP could prevent post-ischemic arrhythmias, presumably by stabilizing $\Delta\Psi_m$. 4'Cl-DZP had no effect on epicardial action potentials or myocardial conduction velocity in normoxic hearts. Global ischemia induced, within minutes, shortening of the action potential and eventual failure of excitability in untreated controls, but this effect was blunted dose-dependently in hearts perfused with μM concentrations of 4'Cl-DZP.[70] Most dramatically, the tachyarrhythmias upon reperfusion were prevented (Fig. 8). By comparison, CsA, the PTP inhibitor, had no effect on ischemic electrical parameters, and a delayed and incomplete effect on reperfusion arrhythmias (Fig. 8).

The mBzR ligand FGIN-1-27, which enhanced mitochondrial depolarization in single cell studies, shortened the time to inexcitability and conduction block in ischemic hearts, but had no effect in normoxic hearts.

Taken together, the findings supported the idea that loss of $\Delta\Psi_m$ during ischemia and early upon reperfusion, is due to the opening of IMAC, and can be inhibited by mBzR antagonists.[70] This event is coupled with activation of sarcolemmal K_{ATP} channels, creating spatial and perhaps temporal action potential heterogeneity that can be a substrate of ventricular reentry.[36] PTP activation, on the other hand, occurs with some delay after reperfusion.

From these results, we have postulated that the failure of mitochondrial energetics can create "metabolic sinks" in the reperfused myocardium that may constitute sites of functional conduction block. This mechanism is distinct from (but could be occurring in parallel with) blocks caused by the closure of gap junctions between cells, in that the current supporting a wave of depolarization would be annihilated by the metabolic sink; whereas with gap junctional block, an increase in voltage at the wave front could result in propagation via a bypass path (i.e., propagation has a high safety factor ref. 72).

Conclusions

Mitochondria are capable of synchronized oscillations in a number of variables (e.g., volume, $\Delta\Psi_m$, redox, etc.) when studied in suspension or when they are organized as a network in intact cells. In part, this stems from the fact that oxidative phosphorylation is a complex non-linear system which involves ion movements, stored electrochemical gradients, and a semi-permeable membrane barrier to carry out energy transduction. The possibility for charging and discharging the storage element is a common feature of relaxation oscillators in electrical circuits (e.g., a resistor-capacitor circuit) and in biological oscillators such as pacemaker cells in the heart and brain, but the mitochondrial oscillator is unique in terms of its inherent frequency response and amplitude modulation.

A primary ROS-dependent mitochondrial oscillator in intact cardiac cells has been characterized using an integrated experimental and theoretical approach. The mechanism fundamentally determines the cell's response to metabolic stress (whether in a steady polarized or depolarized parametric domain or an oscillatory domain) that scales from the mitochondrion to the whole heart. Moreover, we show that under physiological conditions cardiac mitochondria function as a network of coupled oscillators with a broad range of frequencies. ROS weakly couples mitochondria under normal conditions but becomes a strong coupling messenger when, under oxidative stress, the mitochondrial network attains criticality. Mitochondrial criticality is achieved when a threshold of ROS is overcome and a certain density of mitochondria forms a cluster that spans the whole cell. Under these conditions, the slightest perturbation triggers a depolarization wave throughout the cell. Although locally, mitochondria depolarize in response to a ROS-induced ROS release mechanism, the fact that mitochondria outside the spanning cluster resist depolarization argues against a simple regenerative wave. The mitochondria are also required to be near threshold and belong to a percolation cluster. This requirement means that the spatial organization of mitochondria, which is very different in various cell types, will play a major role in the group dynamics of mitochondrial function. Neighbor-neighbor interaction of mitochondria, and thus functional synchronization, will be most prevalent in closely packed networks and less likely in cells with elongated and widely-spaced mitochondria.

While the focus of this chapter has been on the ROS-dependent mitochondrial oscillator, other mitochondrial oscillatory mechanisms are possible, and may coexist in excitable cells like the cardiomyocyte that contain multiple oscillatory mechanisms. Spontaneous pacemaker firing and oscillations in sarcoplasmic reticulum Ca^{2+} release could also entrain oscillation in mitochondrial function, and a divalent cation-activated intrinsic mitochondrial oscillator may also exist, although it has not been demonstrated in intact cells. Cause and effect is often hard to determine when multiple oscillators are present—this is one reason why the mechanism of oscillatory insulin release from pancreatic β cells has still not been completely resolved, although a clear contribution from glycolysis and Ca^{2+} handling has been proven. Similarly, neonatal cardiac myocytes display alternating periods with and without action potentials, in association with oscillations in $\Delta\Psi_m$. These oscillations were correlated with the intermittent activation of K_{ATP} channels; however, no clear evidence of an intrinsic metabolic oscillator was established.

A connection between the ROS-dependent mitochondrial oscillator and earlier oscillators triggered by enhanced ionic flux across the inner membrane has not been made. Interestingly, in the initial description of oscillations in mitochondrial ionic fluxes by Chance and Yoshioka, these investigators added 1.5-3 mM H_2O_2 and catalase to their mitochondrial suspensions in order to keep a constant supply of oxygen. These conditions could have contributed to oxidative stress in the preparation that could be related to the mitochondrial oscillations observed in living heart cells. Similarly, the role of ROS in divalent-mediated mitochondrial oscillation has not been explored, although the uncoupling effect of Ca^{2+} could, in theory, enhance mitochondrial ROS production according to our view of the relationship between respiration and mitochondrial ROS production at complex III. ROS-independent mitochondrial oscillations have also been described in isolated mitochondria, but this mechanism has not been demonstrated in intact cells.

The evidence that the mitochondria of the cardiac cell behave as a network of oscillators under physiological conditions raises a number of interesting questions to pursue in future investigations. First, while many control systems that are required to respond quickly to changing conditions have been noted to operate close to instability, the emergence of a dominant low-frequency mode associated with pathology in the myocyte begs the question of how close to this instability the network normally operates. Second, the accepted evidence that many signal transduction pathways are ROS-dependent has led us to propose that frequency- and/or amplitude-modulated mitochondrial ROS signals could link the bioenergetic state to acute or long-term (transcriptional) responses in the normal course of energy supply and demand matching in the cell. Mitochondrial ROS bursting during ischemia could also be relevant to the mechanism of ischemic preconditioning or cell injury in the reperfused heart.

Another speculative role for mitochondrial oscillation is the possibility that it serves as a potential intracellular timekeeper. This notion is encouraged by the computational studies that show that the period of the oscillator could be modulated over a broad range of time scales from milliseconds to hours by varying only one parameter. This observation, together with the long-term temporal correlation and power law dependence exhibited by the mitochondrial network could, theoretically, allow a change in one time scale to be felt across the whole frequency range.

References

1. Strogatz SH, Sync. The Emerging Science of Spontaneous Order. New York: Hyperion Books, 2003.
2. Pikovsky A, Rosenblum M, Kurths J. Synchronization: A Universal Concept in Nonlinear Sciences. Vol 29. Cambridge: Cambridge University Press, 2001.
3. van der Pol B, van der Mark J. The heartbeat considered as a relaxation oscillation, and an electrical model of the heart. Phil Mag 1928; 6:763-775.
4. Hess B, Boiteux A. Oscillatory phenomena in biochemistry. Annu Rev Biochem 1971; 40:237-258.
5. Rapp PE. An atlas of cellular oscillators. J Exp Biol 1979; 81:281-306.
6. Berridge MJ, Rapp PE. A comparative survey of the function, mechanism and control of cellular oscillators. J Exp Biol 1979; 81:217-279.
7. Lloyd D, Aon MA, Cortassa S. Why homeodynamics, not homeostasis? Scientific World Journal 2001; 1:133-145.
8. Winfree AT. The prehistory of the Belousov-Zhabotinsky oscillator. J Chem Educ 1984; 61:661-663.
9. Zhabotinsky AM. Periodic course of the oxidation of malonic acid in a solution (Studies on the kinetics of beolusov's reaction). Biofizika 1964; 9:306-311.
10. Duysens LN, Amesz J. Fluorescence spectrophotometry of reduced phosphopyridine nucleotide in intact cells in the near-ultraviolet and visible region. Biochim Biophys Acta 1957; 24(1):19-26.
11. Chance B, Estabrook RW, Ghosh A. Damped sinusoidal oscillations of cytoplasmic reduced pyridine nucleotide in yeast cells. Proc Natl Acad Sci USA 1964; 51:1244-1251.
12. Hommes FA, Schuurmansstekhoven FM. Aperiodic changes of reduced nicotinamide-adenine dinucleotide during anaerobic glycolysis in brewer's yeast. Biochim Biophys Acta 1964; 86:427-428.
13. Chance B, Schoener B, Elsaesser S. Control of the waveform of oscillations of the reduced pyridine nucleotide level in a cell-free extract. Proc Natl Acad Sci USA 1964; 52:337-341.
14. Chance B, Schoener B, Elsaesser S. Metabolic control phenomena involved in damped sinusoidal oscillations of reduced diphosphopyridine nucleotide in a cell-free extract of saccharomyces carlsbergensis. J Biol Chem 1965; 240:3170-3181.
15. Frenkel R. DPNH oscillations in glycolyzing cell free extracts from beef heart. Biochem Biophys Res Commun 1965; 21(5):497-502.
16. Frenkel R. Control of reduced diphosphopyridine nucleotide oscillations in beef heart extracts. II. Oscillations of glycolytic intermediates and adenine nucleotides. Arch Biochem Biophys 1968; 125(1):157-165.
17. Frenkel R. Control of reduced diphosphopyridine nucleotide oscillations in beef heart extracts. I. Effects of modifiers of phosphofructokinase activity. Arch Biochem Biophys 1968; 125(1):151-156.

18. Frenkel R. Control of reduced diphosphopyridine nucleotide oscillations in beef heart extracts. III. Purification and kinetics of beef heart phosphofructokinase. Arch Biochem Biophys 1968; 125(1):166-174.

19. Chance B. Federation of european biochemical societies: Biological and biochemical oscillators. New York: Academic Press, 1973, (proceedings).

20. Lloyd D, Murray DB. The temporal architecture of eukaryotic growth. FEBS Lett 2006; 580(12):2830-2835.

21. Richard P. The rhythm of yeast. FEMS Microbiol Rev 2003; 27(4):547-557.

22. Madsen MF, Dano S, Sorensen PG. On the mechanisms of glycolytic oscillations in yeast. FEBS J 2005; 272(11):2648-2660.

23. Azzi A, Azzone GF. Swelling and shrinkage phenomena in liver mitochondria. II. Low amplitude swelling-shrinkage cycles. Biochim Biophys Acta 1965; 105(2):265-278.

24. Mustafa MG, Utsumi K, Packer L. Damped oscillatory control of mitochondrial respiration and volume. Biochem Biophys Res Commun 1966; 24(3):381-385.

25. Packer L, Utsumi R, Mustafa MG. Oscillatory states of mitochondria. I. Electron and energy transfer pathways. Arch Biochem Biophys 1966; 117(2):381-393.

26. Chance B, Yoshioka T. Sustained oscillations of ionic constituents of mitochondria. Arch Biochem Biophys 1966; 117:451-465.

27. Evtodienko YV. Sustained oscillations of transmembrane Ca2+ fluxes in mitochondria and their possible biological significance. Membr Cell Biol 2000; 14:1-17.

28. Gylkhandanyan AV, Evtodienko YV, Zhabotinsky AM et al. Continuous Sr2+-induced oscillations of the ionic fluxes in mitochondria. FEBS Lett 1976; 66(1):44-47.

29. Maglova LM, Holmuhamedov EL, Zinchenko VP et al. Induction of 2H+/Me2+ exchange in rat-liver mitochondria. Eur J Biochem 1982; 128(1):159-161.

30. Selivanov VA, Ichas F, Holmuhamedov EL et al. A model of mitochondrial Ca(2+)-induced Ca2+ release simulating the Ca2+ oscillations and spikes generated by mitochondria. Biophys Chem 1998; 72(1-2):111-121.

31. Gooch VD, Packer L. Adenine nucleotide control of heart mitochondrial oscillations. Biochim Biophys Acta 1971; 245(1):17-20.

32. Gooch VD, Packer L. Oscillatory systems in mitochondria. Biochim Biophys Acta 1974; 346(3-4):245-260.

33. Gooch VD, Packer L. Oscillatory states of mitochondria: Studies on the oscillatory mechanism of liver and heart mitochondria. Arch Biochem Biophys 1974; 163(2):759-768.

34. O'Rourke B, Ramza BM, Marban E. Oscillations of membrane current and excitability driven by metabolic oscillations in heart cells. Science 1994; 265(5174):962-966.

35. Romashko DN, Marban E, O'Rourke B. Subcellular metabolic transients and mitochondrial redox waves in heart cells. Proc Natl Acad Sci USA 1998; 95(4):1618-1623.

36. Aon MA, Cortassa S, Marban E et al. Synchronized whole cell oscillations in mitochondrial metabolism triggered by a local release of reactive oxygen species in cardiac myocytes. J Biol Chem 2003; 278(45):44735-44744.

37. Kim YV, Kudzina L, Zinchenko VP et al. Chlortetracycline-mediated continuous Ca2+ oscillations in mitochondria of digitonin-treated Tetrahymena pyriformis. Eur J Biochem 1985; 153(3):503-507.

38. Evtodienko Yu V, Teplova V, Khawaja J et al. The Ca(2+)-induced permeability transition pore is involved in Ca(2+)-induced mitochondrial oscillations: A study on permeabilised Ehrlich ascites tumour cells. Cell Calcium 1994; 15(2):143-152.

39. Hajnoczky G, Robb-Gaspers LD, Seitz MB et al. Decoding of cytosolic calcium oscillations in the mitochondria. Cell 1995; 82(3):415-424.

40. Magnus G, Keizer J. Model of beta-cell mitochondrial calcium handling and electrical activity. II. Mitochondrial variables. Am J Physiol 1998; 274(4 Pt 1):C1174-1184.

41. Pedersen MG, Bertram R, Sherman A. Intra- and inter-islet synchronization of metabolically driven insulin secretion. Biophys J 2005; 89(1):107-119.

42. Corkey BE, Tornheim K, Deeney JT et al. Linked oscillations of free Ca2+ and the ATP/ADP ratio in permeabilized RINm5F insulinoma cells supplemented with a glycolyzing cell-free muscle extract. J Biol Chem 1988; 263(9):4254-4258.

43. Lloyd D. Effects of uncoupling of mitochondrial energy conservation on the ultradian clock-driven oscillations in Saccharomyces cerevisiae continuous culture. Mitochondrion 2003; 3(3):139-146.

44. Mironov SL, Richter DW. Oscillations and hypoxic changes of mitochondrial variables in neurons of the brainstem respiratory centre of mice. J Physiol 2001; 533(Pt 1):227-236.

45. Berns MW, Siemens AE, Walter RJ. Mitochondrial fluorescence patterns in rhodamine 6G-stained myocardial cells in vitro: Analysis by real-time computer video microscopy and laser microspot excitation. Cell Biophys 1984; 6(4):263-277.

46. Duchen MR, Leyssens A, Crompton M. Transient mitochondrial depolarizations reflect focal sarcoplasmic reticular calcium release in single rat cardiomyocytes. J Cell Biol 1998; 142(4):975-988.

47. Loew LM, Tuft RA, Carrington W et al. Imaging in five dimensions: Time-dependent membrane potentials in individual mitochondria. Biophys J 1993; 65(6):2396-2407.

48. Buckman JF, Reynolds IJ. Spontaneous changes in mitochondrial membrane potential in cultured neurons. J Neurosci 2001; 21(14):5054-5065.

49. O'Reilly CM, Fogarty KE, Drummond RM et al. Quantitative analysis of spontaneous mitochondrial depolarizations. Biophys J 2003; 85(5):3350-3357.

50. O'Reilly CM, Fogarty KE, Drummond RM et al. Spontaneous mitochondrial depolarizations are independent of SR Ca2+ release. Am J Physiol Cell Physiol 2004; 286(5):C1139-1151.

51. Huser J, Rechenmacher CE, Blatter LA. Imaging the permeability pore transition in single mitochondria. Biophys J 1998; 74(4):2129-2137.

52. Huser J, Blatter LA. Fluctuations in mitochondrial membrane potential caused by repetitive gating of the permeability transition pore. Biochem J 1999; 343(Pt 2):311-317.

53. Vergun O, Votyakova TV, Reynolds IJ. Spontaneous changes in mitochondrial membrane potential in single isolated brain mitochondria. Biophys J 2003; 85(5):3358-3366.

54. Vergun O, Reynolds IJ. Fluctuations in mitochondrial membrane potential in single isolated brain mitochondria: Modulation by adenine nucleotides and Ca2+. Biophys J 2004; 87(5):3585-3593.

55. Ichas F, Jouaville LS, Sidash SS et al. Mitochondrial calcium spiking: A transduction mechanism based on calcium-induced permeability transition involved in cell calcium signalling. FEBS Lett 1994; 348(2):211-215.

56. Zorov DB, Filburn CR, Klotz LO et al. Reactive oxygen species (ROS)-induced ROS release: A new phenomenon accompanying induction of the mitochondrial permeability transition in cardiac myocytes. J Exp Med 2000; 192(7):1001-1014.

57. Zorov DB, Juhaszova M, Sollott SJ. Mitochondrial ROS-induced ROS release: An update and review. Biochim Biophys Acta 2006; 1757(5-6):509-517.

58. O'Rourke B. Pathophysiological and protective roles of mitochondrial ion channels. J Physiol 2000; 529(Pt 1):23-36.

59. O'Rourke B, Ramza BM, Romashko DN et al. Metabolic oscillations in heart cells. Adv Exp Med Biol 1995; 382:165-174.

60. Cortassa S, Aon MA, Winslow RL et al. A mitochondrial oscillator dependent on reactive oxygen species. Biophys J 2004; 87(3):2060-2073.

61. Crompton M, Virji S, Doyle V et al. The mitochondrial permeability transition pore. Biochem Soc Symp 1999; 66:167-179.

62. Duchen MR. Contributions of mitochondria to animal physiology: From homeostatic sensor to calcium signalling and cell death. J Physiol 1999; 516 (Pt 1):1-17.

63. Beavis AD. On the inhibition of the mitochondrial inner membrane anion uniporter by cationic amphiphiles and other drugs. J Biol Chem 1989; 264(3):1508-1515.

64. Beavis AD. Properties of the inner membrane anion channel in intact mitochondria. J Bioenerg Biomembr 1992; 24(1):77-90.

65. Beavis AD, Garlid KD. The mitochondrial inner membrane anion channel: Regulation by divalent cations and protons. J Biol Chem 1987; 262(31):15085-15093.

66. Aon MA, Cortassa S, O'Rourke B. The fundamental organization of cardiac mitochondria as a network of coupled oscillators. Biophys J 2006b; 91(11):4317-4327.

67. Stauffer D, Aharony A. Introduction to Percolation Theory. London: Taylor and Francis, 1994.

68. Feder J. Fractals. New York: Plenum Press, 1988.

69. Aon MA, O'Rourke B, Cortassa S. The fractal architecture of cytoplasmic organization: Scaling, kinetics and emergence in metabolic networks. Mol Cell Biochem 2004b; 256/257:169-184.

70. Akar FG, Aon MA, Tomaselli GF et al. The mitochondrial origin of postischemic arrhythmias. J Clin Invest 2005; 115(12):3527-3535.

71. Bolli R, Marban E. Molecular and cellular mechanisms of myocardial stunning. Physiol Rev 1999; 79(2):609-634.

72. Kleber AG, Rudy Y. Basic mechanisms of cardiac impulse propagation and associated arrhythmias. Physiol Rev 2004; 84(2):431-488.

73. Cortassa S, Aon MA, Marban E et al. An integrated model of cardiac mitochondrial energy metabolism and calcium dynamics. Biophys J 2003; 84(4):2734-2755.

74. O'Rourke B, Cortassa S, Aon MA. Mitochondrial ion channels: Gatekeepers of life and death. Physiology 2005; 20:303-315.

75. Aon MA, Cortassa S, Akar FG et al. Mitochondrial criticality: A new concept at the turning point of life or death. Biochim Biophys Acta 2006; 1762(2):232-240.

76. Aon MA, Cortassa S, O'Rourke B. Percolation and criticality in a mitochondrial network. Proc Natl Acad Sci USA 2004a; 101(13):4447-4452.

CHAPTER 9

Respiratory Oscillations in Yeasts

David Lloyd*

Abstract

Respiratory oscillations in yeasts have been studied in three time domains with periods of (a) about a minute, (b) about 40 min, and (c) about a day. Reactive responses (damped oscillations), rhythms and temperature-compensated clocks have been described for (b) and (c), but a timekeeping clock has not yet been shown for (a). Synchronous populations reveal the time-structure that can only otherwise be studied in single organisms; this is because time-averaging through an asynchronous population conceals its fine structure. Early studies with synchronous cultures made by size selection methods indicated ultradian-clock driven oscillations in respiration, pools of adenylates, total protein, RNA synthesis and many enzyme activities (τ = 40 min in *Schizosaccharomyces pombe*, 30 min in *Candida utilis*), and more recently in self-synchronised continuous cultures of *Saccharomyces cerevisiae* (τ = 48min). Most detailed understanding comes from the latter system, where continuous, noninvasive real-time monitoring (of O_2 uptake, CO_2 production, and NAD(P)H redox state) is combined with frequent discrete time samples (for other redox components, including H_2S, GSH and cytochromes, metabolites, and mRNA levels). A redox switch lies at the heart of this ultradian clock and a plethora of outputs is optimized to a time-base that is genetically-determined and differs in different organisms. It is suggested that the entire temporal landscape of all eukaryotic organisms and the cells of higher plants and animals is constructed on this basis. A time frame for the coordination and coherence of all intracellular processes and the construction and assembly of cellular structures is provided by the ultradian clock. The circadian clock matches these functions to the daily cycle of the external environment.

Introduction

The mitochondrial respiratory chain has a kinetic competence that is defined, not only by its component electron transport steps, but also by the availability of ADP and inorganic phosphate.[1] The principles that underlie respiratory kinetics established by Chance and Williams in a series of papers in the mid-1950s may be used to explain many of the oscillations since observed, both in mitochondria in vitro[2] and in vivo.[3-8] The half-time for the reoxidation of cytochrome a_3 when anaerobic mitochondria are exposed to O_2 is 0.3ms (rat liver mitochondria at 37°C), and the oxidation of flavin takes 200ms. Accompanying ionic changes[2] and energy-conservation reactions in vitro[9] are also measured on time scales of milliseconds or seconds, whereas in vivo they are constrained by complex networks of metabolic interactions and the resulting oscillatory responses are generally much slower.[10,11]

Earlier measurements made on suspensions of mitochondria or bulk samples of organisms from growing cultures have more recently been complemented by in vivo real-time monitoring using minimally-invasive methods (e.g., direct fluorimetric observation of NADH

*David Lloyd—Microbiology (BIOSI 1), School of Biosciences, Cardiff University,
P.O. Box 915, Cardiff CF10 3TL, Wales, UK. Email: lloydd@cf.ac.uk

Cellular Oscillatory Mechanisms, edited by Miguel Maroto and Nicholas A.M. Monk.
©2008 Landes Bioscience and Springer Science+Business Media.

and oxidized flavin,[12] and after administration of suitable fluorophores, mitochondrial inner membrane potential, glutathione and reactive oxygen species[13,14]). Imaging techniques now extend the range of our observations of oscillatory phenomena in living cells to fast[15] and ultra-fast time scales.[15,17]

Mitochondrial respiratory oscillations (τ of the order of minutes) that accompany alkali-cation transport were first described in 1965 in vitro with organelles isolated from pigeon heart or rat liver in four different laboratories.[2] Changes in optical transmittance due to volume changes, H^+, K^+, respiration rate and morphology were monitored,[18] and it was demonstrated that fluxes of ATP and ADP may be an important synchronizing as well as a controlling factor of energy flows in this system. An artificially-synchronized system (using ATP) could be modulated by the K^+ ionophore, valinomycin.[19] Oligomycin or atractylate addition abolished both the natural and artificially-induced synchrony. Similar experiments have not been performed using isolated yeast mitochondria, but the data obtained with animal mitochondria provides important lessons for our understanding of in vivo measurements in yeasts.

Minute-Long Oscillations in *S. cerevisiae*

In self-synchronized continuous cultures of *S. cerevisiae*, in addition to the circa 40min ultradian clock-driven respiratory cycles, another oscillatory phenomenon is observed (M. Roussel and D. Lloyd, unpublished experiments). Although evident in the traditional monitoring procedure using an oxygen eletrode,[20-22] the more sensitive and faster-responding membrane-inlet mass spectrometer probe[23-25] provides a better means of continuous readout. The amplitude is usually only less than one tenth that of the *circa* 40 min clock output and the period is *circa* 3min. Unpublished experiments (M. Roussel and D.Lloyd) indicate concomitant oscillations in CO_2 output and a complex relationship with the ultradian clock-driven rhythm, as well as the enveloping cell cycle-division cycle-associated respiratory oscillations.

When this strain of yeast is examined by 2-photon laser excitation after loading with the fluorophores, tetramethylrhodamine ethyl ester (a voltage-sensitive dye that accumulates in mitochondria, due to the mitochondrial inner membrane potential) and dichlorodihydrofluorescein (for reactive oxygen species, especially H_2O_2),[13,14] oscillations with periods of about a minute are again evident. In this case, the organisms were continuously perfused in phosphate-buffered saline at pH 7.4, containing 5mM glucose, on the surface of poly-*L*-lysine coated glass (as compared with continuously-stirred growing suspensions in the continuous culture). The mechanisms involved in the generation of these oscillations have not been further investigated, but may well involve the H^+, K^+ and volume changes previously described for animal mitochondria in vitro.[2,18,19]

Ultradian (τ 30-50min) Oscillations in Synchronous Cultures of Yeasts

Saccharomyces cerevisiae

Oscillations of respiratory activity with one maximum occurring per cell-cycle have been observed in *S. cerevisiae* in synchronous cultures prepared by a size-selection method, irrespective of whether growth was in a defined medium[26,27] or in a complex medium.[28,29] Oscillations observed in respiratory activity in glucose-grown cultures were not evident when maltose was the carbon source.[30] Small perturbations, due to the drop-wise addition of nutrients or alkali, in continuous cultures, give rise to synchrony of growth and division, as indicated by periodicity of the budding cycle. In such cultures, large amplitude excursions of dissolved O_2, CO_2 production and heat evolution were observed.[31-35] The redox state of these cultures, as shown by direct monitoring of NADH fluorescence[34] also showed cell cycle related oscillations.

Schizosaccharomyces pombe

Single stepwise increases in oxygen uptake rate per ml of culture were observed during the cell-cycle of *Schizosaccharomyces pombe* synchronized by a nutritional induction method in a complex growth medium;[36] these authors claimed to find a doubling of mitochondrial numbers per cell coinciding with the abrupt increases in respiration rate. However the difficulties of estimation of mitochondrial numbers in sectioned organisms necessitate a more thorough investigation before this claim is confirmed, and it seems unlikely that respiration rate is proportional to mitochondrial numbers rather than mass.[37] A more complex progress curve for oxygen uptake was obtained in this species when grown synchronously in a defined medium (containing 1% glucose) after a density-gradient centrifugation size selection procedure.[4] In this case, both total cell protein and respiration increase exponentially overall so as to double during the cell-cycle, but an oscillation in oxygen uptake also occurred so as to produce two maxima per cycle (Fig. 1). The first maximum was observed during the phase of cell elongation prior to cell division and the second maximum coincided with the doubling in cell numbers. A doubling of the respiratory rate of samples withdrawn from the culture at a respiratory maximum was produced when 16 μM-carbonyl cyanide m-chlorophenyl-hydrazone (CCCP, an agent that removes the linkage of energy conservation to electron transport) was added. Organisms taken at the minima showed a less marked response to this uncoupler. Heat production of the culture increased uniformly through the cell-cycle. Addition of concentrations of antimycin A or CN^- sufficient to give about 50% inhibition produced no attenuation of the respiratory oscillation, and on the basis of these results[4] it was concluded that the respiration of the synchronous culture has two components. One of these increases exponentially at all times in the cycle, cannot be easily uncoupled and is preferentially blocked by inhibitors of electron transport acting at phosphorylation Sites II or III. The second component consists of easily-uncoupled electron transport chains which are only inhibited by high concentrations of antimycin A or CN^-. The activity of this component oscillates with a periodicity equal to 0.5 of a cell cycle, presumably due to the periodic expression of activity of a rate-limiting entity.

When glucose is replaced by 1% glycerol as the carbon source, oxygen uptake rates show two steps per cycle with timings of the abrupt increases being similar to those found in glucose-grown cells[38]: this suggests that respiratory oscillations observed with glucose arise from interactions between the respiratory system and glycolysis.

Periodic increases in total amounts of several mitochondrial enzymes were observed in glucose-repressed *Schiz. Pombe*.[34] In this case "peak" patterns may correspond to the oscillatory respiration observed in these cultures.

In a continuous culture of *Schiz. pombe* growing in the presence of 1% glucose the time course of synthesis of cytochromes $a + a_3$ is similar to that of b_{563} (b_t) (Fig. 2); both cytochromes reach two maxima per cell-cycle.[40] These cytochromes (the synthesis of which are partially dependent on the mitochondrial protein synthesis system), show a completely different pattern of development from cytochromes c_{548}, b_{554} and b_{540}, all of which increase linearly over the first part of the cycle, then plateau off. Thus the ratio of individual cytochrome components of the inner mitochondrial membrane varies considerably throughout the cell-cycle. Comparison of the spectroscopically-detectable cytochromes $a + a_3$ with the cytochrome c oxidase activities of extracts reveals that the increase in glucose-reducible a-type cytochrome over the first third of the cell-cycle does not result in a detectable increase in enzyme activity. The trough of enzyme activity represents a real disappearance in spectrophotometrically-detectable haemoprotein, and the subsequent maximum in the haemprotein is also reflected in cytochrome c oxidase activity. The control mechanisms involved in this complex pattern of changes remains to be elucidated. Variation in the ratio cytochrome a_3: cytochrome a over the range 0.4-1.3 was observed during the cell-cycle indicating that the synthesis of the two components of the cytochrome c oxidase complex do not occur together. Cytochrome $a + a_3$ shows a single step per cell-cycle, the other three cytochromes (2 b-type and 1 c-type) show a double step

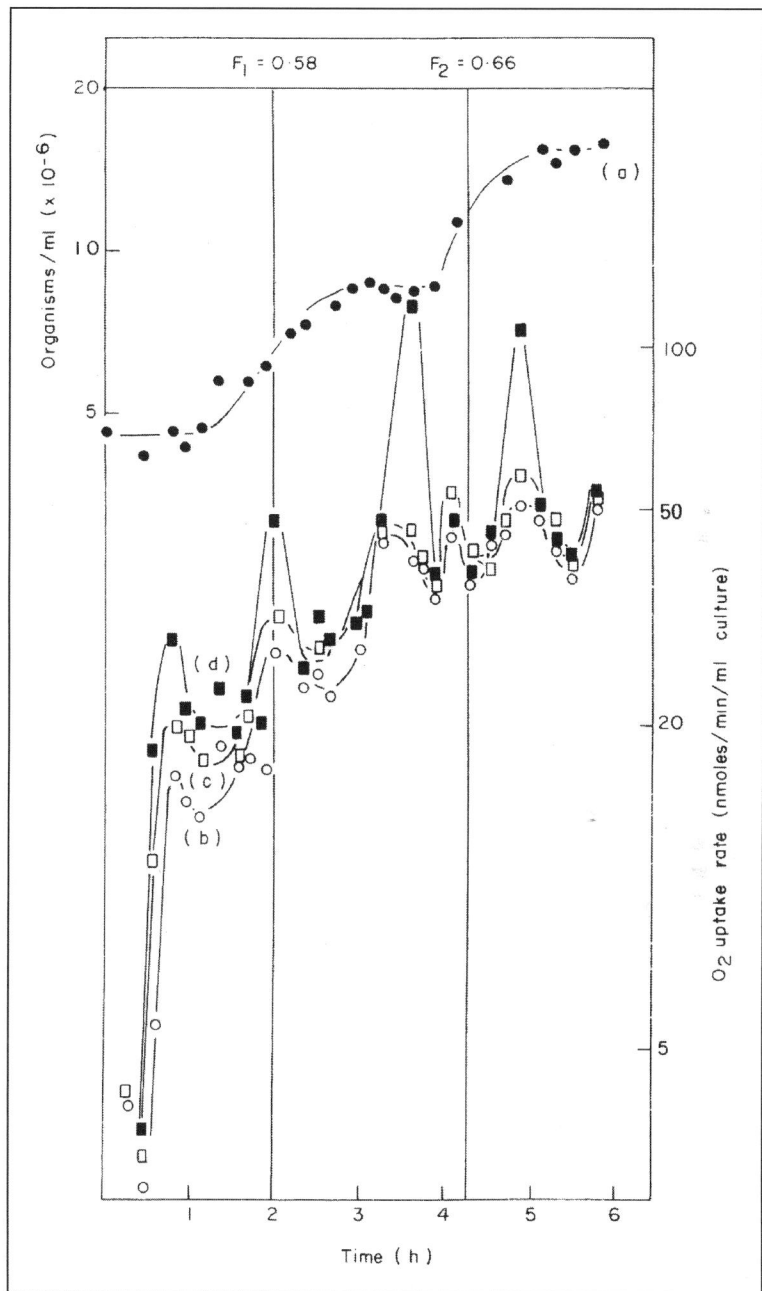

Figure 1. Oxygen uptake of yeast suspensions from a synchronous culture of glucose-grown *Schizosaccharomyces pombe* and the effect of CCCP. F_1 and F_2 denote synchrony indices, [130] of the first and second doublings in cell numbers (a) respectively (mid-point indicated by a vertical line). Oxygen uptake measurements on culture samples removed at frequent intervals from a synchronous culture were made in the absence (b) or the presence of 8.1 μM-CCCP (c) or 16.2 μM-CCCP (d). (Reproduced with permission from ref. 4.)

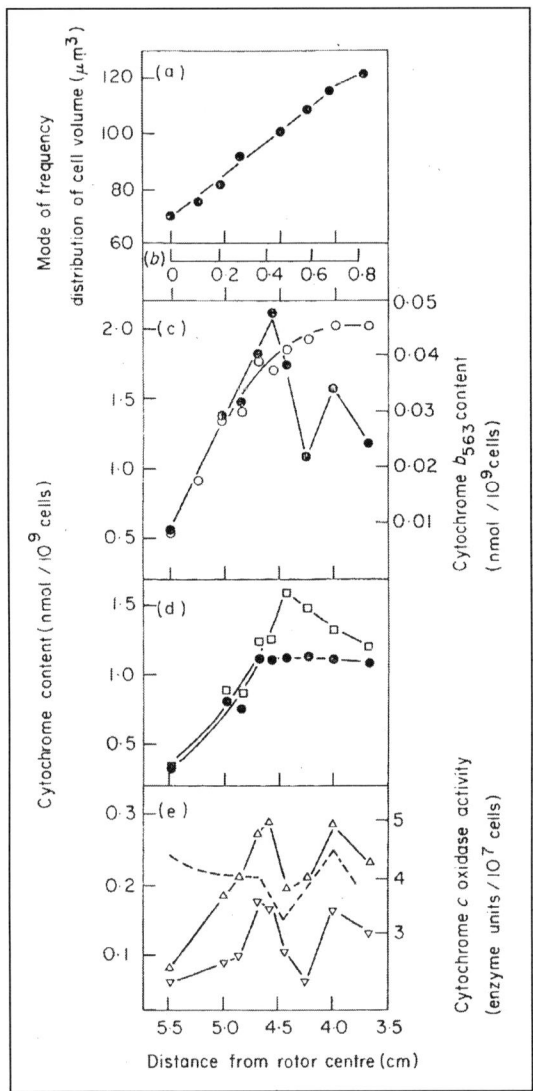

Figure 2. Cellular contents of cytochromes after analysis of the cell-cycle by isopycnic zonal centrifugation on a dextran gradient of cells from a glucose-repressed exponentially-growing culture of *Schizosaccharomyces pombe*. 30 ml of cell suspension (containing 15.8 g wet wt cells) was loaded on the dextran gradients in a Beckman Ti-14(B29) zonal rotor. Centrifugation was at 35,000 rev/min for 50 min (2×10^6 g min at the sample zone: $\int \omega^2$ dt = 4.53×10^{10} rad^2 s^{-1}. Difference spectra (reduced-oxidized) of intact cells were recorded in successive fractions removed from the rotor; reduction was in the presence of 1% glucose, oxidation was in the presence of 0.1% H_2O_2. Spectra were recorded in a path length of 2 mm with a spectral bandwidth 2 nm, at 77K on cell suspensions at 3×10^9 cells/ml. a) Modes of frequency distribution of cell volumes in successive fractions removed from the rotor. b) Resolved portion of the cell-cycle, normalized with respect to a cell volume of 115 μm^3 at 0.67 of a cell cycle. (c) c_{548} (-O-) and b_{563} (-●-). (d) b_{554}-□-) and b_{560} (-●-) (e) $a + a_3$ (measured at 445-458 nm(-Δ-) and at 600-630 nm (-∇-) respectively, together with cytochrome *c* oxidase activity plotted as a function of the cell-cycle, (---) as determined in a separate experiment. (Reproduced with permission from ref. 40.)

pattern. Mitochondrial ATPase in cell-free extracts prepared at 15 min intervals through more than two cell-division cycles also showed the 40 min oscillation.[10] Levels of NADH and flavin fluorescence were also oscillatory.[1] Burgeoning understanding of the control mechanisms that govern cell cycle progression in this organism have led to further studies. That these 'epigenetic oscillations' in energy-yielding components and functions represent the outputs of an ultradian clock has been confirmed.[42,43] In these experiments, the septum index (percentage of cells in the final stage of the cell division cycle, CDC) was assessed by examination of 10^3 organisms microscopically at 10 min intervals.[44] The ultradian rhythm of septation becomes evident when organisms are transferred to glucose-containing media after slow growth in LD 12, 12 (with xylulose) at 30°C. Expression of the rhythm in the population does not occur if the organisms have not been synchronized with respect to their circadian cycle. Another more convenient method relies on at least three cycles of temperature changes (0.25 h, 0.5 h at 27°C, 33°C or 0.5 h, 0.25 h at 33°, 27°C). These conditions of temperature are well within the normal range for growth, and are thus unlikely to stress the organism. Single, more extreme chilling or heat-shock treatments were ineffective. However, a broad range of entrainment (between 24min and 70 min) was demonstrated. Unlike circadian rhythmicity in this organism (see below), light-dark cycles could not entrain, even after more than 20 cycles at high light intensities (up to 12000 _Einsteins m^{-2}s^{-1}). The free-running period of the rhythm was within the range 40-44 min between 26°C and 34°C, and its persistence for more than 26 cycles with little damping suggests intercellular communication between cells of the population. Different strains of *Schiz. pombe* show slightly different ultradian clock periods: e.g., WT Cardiff, 46 min; WT Tübingen 40-44 min; WT EMBL, 35 min.[45] Different growth media or different conditions (e.g., aerobiosis or anaerobiosis) do not measurably affect the clock period.[42]

A manometric method was used to reexamine gas exchange in *Schiz. pombe* (F. Kippert, unpublished data). Periods of 42 min (for W.T. Tübingen) were again found for O_2 uptake as well as for CO_2 production in respiring cultures (and also for fermentative CO_2 evolution). Good temperature compensation was demonstrated. When the CDC was blocked with hydroxyurea, the oscillations persisted. Acidification of the culture medium measured with bromophenol blue also showed a 42 min periodicity. These data suggest that the ultradian clock has several outputs in rapidly growing organisms, just as does the circadian clock under conditions where growth is slow. Carbon dioxide oscillations reported by Novak and Mitchison[46,47] may also represent ultradian clock outputs, although the necessary criteria were not tested.

Investigations of CDC control in *Schiz. pombe* were initiated. As well as the rhythm of septation, DNA synthesis shows a clear 42 min rhythm, as does the cdc^{2+} protein kinase.[45] Using temperature-sensitive mutants, and a method of temperature cycling appropriate to these organisms, it was possible to show separate ultradian controls over S phase and mitosis. The wee 1 protein kinase is implicated as a site of interaction of the ultradian clock with the CDC control circuitry. Evidently the variety of cdc mutants available leads to opportunities for further study. One of the few chemical agents generally affecting period length of the circadian rhythms is Li$^+$.[48,49] Similar effects are seen with ultradian clock-controlled outputs in phosphoinositol-limited *Schiz. pombe* where 1 mM LiCl increased period length from 42 min to 1 h. One site of action of Li$^+$ is on the inositol cycle, phosphoinositol monophosphatase is especially sensitive. Monoamine oxidase (type A) inhibitors also perturb the ultradian clock. These and other experiments have implicated the participation of Ca^{2+} and second messengers in ultradian clock function in *Schiz. pombe*. More recently, mitogen-activated protein kinase and cAMP/protein kinase A have been investigated and found to be essential to the functioning of the ultradian clock in this yeast.[50]

The respiration rates of cultures of *Schiz. pombe* synchronized by the addition and subsequent removal of 2 mM-2'deoxyadenosine (an inhibitor of DNA synthesis) also show an oscillatory pattern.[51] Oscillatory respiration ($\tau \cong 40$ min) was observed 1.5 h before the removal of the inhibitor and continued through the subsequent period of synchronous growth (Fig. 3). However, three maxima were found during this period and, in contrast with the findings from synchronous cultures

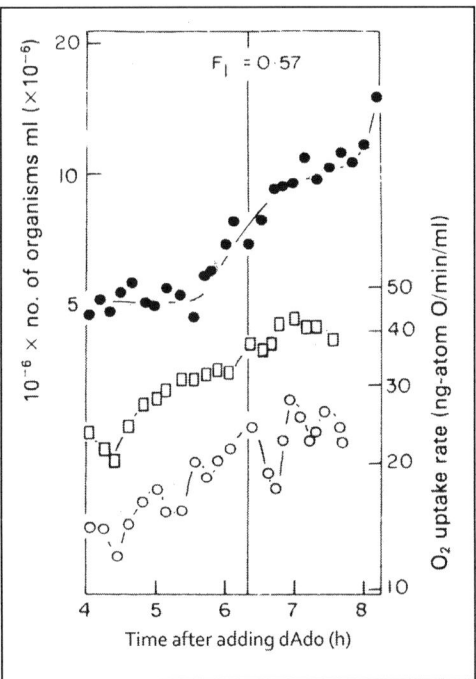

Figure 3. Effect of CCCP on oxygen uptake in cell suspensions from a 2-[1] deoxyadenosine-synchronized culture of *Schiz. pombe*. Deoxyadenosine was added to an exponential culture at zero time and, after 4h incubation, removed by centrifugation; cells were resuspended in fresh medium lacking the inhibitor. F_1 is the synchrony index of the first synchronous doubling (mid-point indicated by vertical line) in cell numbers (●). Oxygen uptake measurements on culture samples removed at approximately 10 min intervals were made in the absence (○) or in the presence of 9.8μM-CCCP (□). (Reproduced with permission from ref. 51.)

prepared by selection, respiration was preferentially stimulated by CCCP at minima rather than maxima; heat dissipation increased continuously either in the presence or absence of this uncoupler. Thus the underlying mechanisms responsible for the expression of respiratory activity in this organism may be quite different in selection- and induction-synchronized cultures. Adenine nucleotide pools showed oscillations in these cultures (Fig. 4).

Candida utilis

Synchronous cultures of the budding yeast, *C. utilis*, prepared by continuous flow size selection, showed respiratory oscillations when the carbon source was either glucose (Fig. 5) acetate or glycerol.[8] Whereas the periodicity of the oscillations (about one-third of the cell cycle time i.e., 30 min) was unaltered by the nature of the carbon source, respiratory maxima and minima showed different uncoupler and inhibitor sensitivities when grown on different substrates. When either acetate or glycerol was the carbon source, the inhibitory effects of CN^- (Fig. 6) and DCCD [an inhibitor of ATP synthase[53]] were greater at respiratory maxima, while maximal uncoupling of respiration by CCCP was achieved at respiratory minima. When cells were grown synchronously in the presence of glucose, the effects of these compounds were different (Table 1). Heat evolution in these cultures increased smoothly. The respiratory oscillations observed in acetate and glycerol-grown synchronous cultures can therefore be explained as

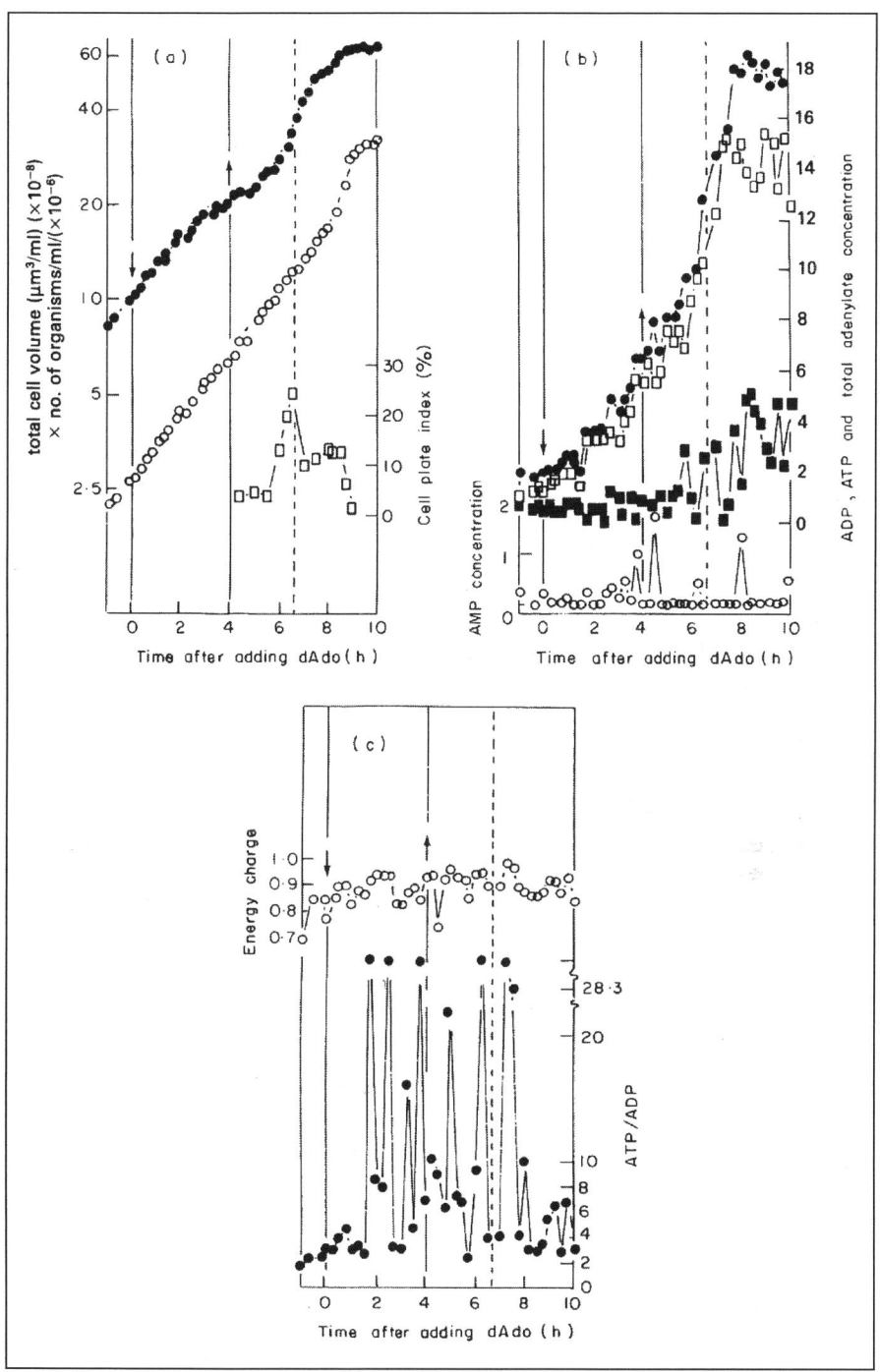

Figure 4. Please see figure legend on following page.

Figure 4, viewed on previous page. Changes in individual adenine nucleotide pools, total adenylates, energy charge and the ATP/ADP ratio in deoxyadenosine-synchronized cultures of *Schiz. pombe.* Culture samples were rapidly mixed and extracted with trichloroacetic acid; adenylates were assayed by the intensity of emission of bioluminescence on reaction with firefly luciferase. a) Cell numbers (●), total cell volume (O) and cell plate index (□); b) Total adenylates (●) and the individual pool sizes of ATP (□), ADP (■) and AMP (O); all expressed as nmol (ml culture)$^{-1}$. c) Energy charge (O) and ATP/ADP ratio (●).Deoxyadenosine was added at the first arrow (and solid vertical line) and removed by centrifugation and resuspension in fresh medium at the second arrow (and solid vertical line). The vertical broken line indicates the mid-point of the first synchronous doubling in yeast numbers. (Reproduced with permission from ref. 52.)

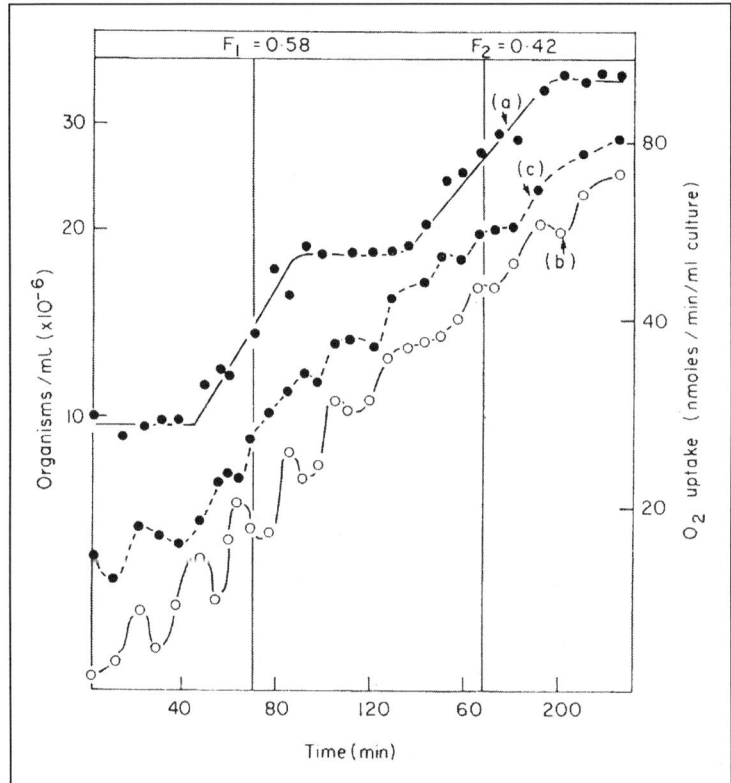

Figure 5. Oxygen-uptake of yeast suspension from a synchronous culture of *Candida utilis* growing in the presence of 1% glucose and the effect of CCCP. F_1 and F_2 denote the synchrony indices of the first and second doubling in cell numbers (a) respectively. O_2-uptake measurements on culture samples removed at frequent intervals from a synchronous culture were made in the absence (b), or the presence of 1.12 μM-CCCP (c). (Experiment of R.K. Poole.)

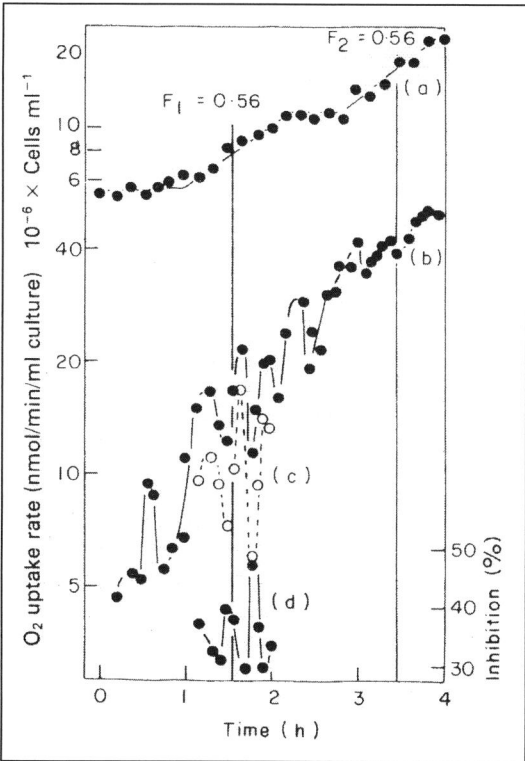

Figure 6. Effects of cyanide on respiratory oscillations in a synchronously dividing culture of *C. utilis* with glucose as carbon source. The synchronous culture initially contained 10% of the original population of the exponentially growing culture and was concentrated fourfold by centrifugation at 200 *g* for 2 min followed by resuspension in conditioned growth medium. At intervals, samples were withdrawn from the culture and rates of respiration were determined in the presence or absence of KCN. (a) Cell numbers; (b) respiration rate in the absence of KCN; (c) respiration rate in the presence of 10μM-KCN: (d) inhibition of respiration (%) resulting from addition of KCN. (Reproduced with permission from ref. 8.)

Table 1. Cell cycle times and the effects of KCN, DCCD and CCCP on the respiration of synchronous cultures of Candida utilis

| Carbon Source | Cell Cycle Time (min) | | Effect of | | |
	First Cycle	Second Cycle	KCN	DCCD	CCCP
Glucose	94.6 ± 17.4(10)	102.8 ± 12.1(9)	–	–	–
Acetate	110.8 ± 16.4(12)	118.1 ± 12.1(11)	+	+	–
Glycerol	91.4 ± 11.3(9)	98.2 ± 9.5(7)	+	+	–

Cell cycle times (mean values ± standard deviations, for the number of experiments shown in parentheses) were measured from the time of selection to the first mid-point of increase in cell numbers (first cycle), and from the first to second mid-points of increases in cell numbers (second cycle). + indicates maximum effect at respiratory maxima; – indicates maximum effect at respiratory minima. (Reproduced with permission from ref. 8.)

reflecting in vivo mitochondrial respiratory control.[1] It was suggested that the oscillations in glucose-grown cells reflect a more complicated control mechanism, in that secondary interactions between the products of mitochondrial energy conservation and the initial reactions of glucose catabolism via feedback loops and allosteric control sites are also involved.

Variations in the participation of the Embden-Meyerhof-Parnas pathway and hexose monophosphate pathway in glucose metabolism were reported following radiorespirometric measurements of phased cultures of *C. utilis*;[54] O_2 consumption and adenylate pools show oscillatory changes during the cell cycle when cells growing with glycerol were limited by nitrogen sources or by iron.

Saccharomyces cerevisiae: Self Synchronized Continuous Culture

Another respiratory ultradian rhythm, apparently different from others previously identified occurs in continuous cultures of *S. cerevisiae*. The phenomenon can be demonstrated with glucose, acetaldehyde or ethanol as major carbon source;[55,56] therefore they are not glycolytic oscillations. With ethanol, continuous monitoring of NADH indicates an oscillation of NADH (Fig. 7), with a complex waveform, and with the predominant period of 45 min identical with that in dissolved O_2.[57] Intracellular GSH also oscillates with the same period as dissolved oxygen. These respiratory oscillations are extremely sensitive to perturbation by pulse addition of Na nitroprusside, and this effect appears to be specifically mediated by nitrosonium ions (NO^+), as NO- (gas) or NO-donors are not effective.[58] Oscillations gradually recover after the

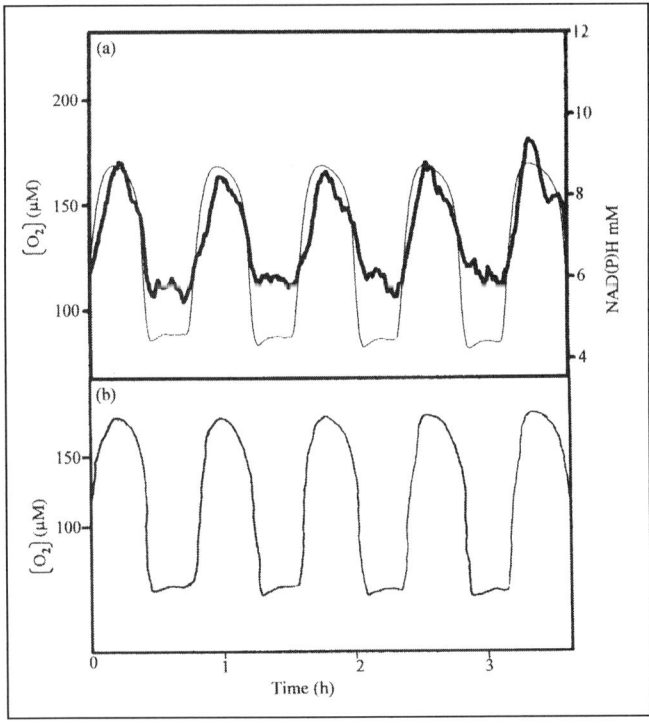

Figure 7. Dissolved O_2 and reduced nicotinamide nucleotide fluorescence in a continuous culture of *S. cerevisiae*. a) Simultaneous O_2 electrode and fluorimetric(heavy line) monitoring (366 → 450 nm) in the same culture: fluorescence emission was calibrated by nicotinamide nucleotide extraction from the culture. b) Control cultures (no UV irradiation). (Reproduced with permission from ref. 62.)

perturbation and the time for recovery is concentration dependent. Preferred target sites are probably either thiols or protein metal centres. GSH itself also produces a marked effect on the respiratory oscillations[59] leading to an interruption of oscillatory behaviour due to respiratory inhibition. In these continuous cultures, growth (the mean cell cycle time) is controlled by the dilution rate with inflowing growth medium,[20,55] but the respiratory oscillation shows timekeeping characteristics,[21,60] in that step-wise changes of temperature reveal temperature-compensated periodicity. The nicotinamide nucleotide[61] and glutathione pools[59] oscillate with distinct phase-relationships with the respiratory cycles, as do mitochondrial energy states.[62,63] Conserved signalling pathways are implicated as indicated by the period-lengthening effects of Li^+ [64] and phase shifting by H_2S which acts as the population synchronizer.[65] Cell-cell communication involves acetaldehyde as an extremely mobile (highly diffusible) but evanescent (oxidizable) secreted metabolite.[66] Possibly other small molecules with similar characteristics are also implicated.

Genome-wide expression levels revealed the pervasive nature of the 40 min timeframe,[67] where the entire transcriptome showed a low amplitude oscillation, with 27% of these transcripts showing a high oscillation strength. Transcripts were either maximally expressed in the oxidative (high respiration; ~10% of all transcripts) or the reductive (low respiration; ~90% of all transcripts) states of the cycle. Therefore, gene expression shows two blocks of redox superclusters that extend beyond central metabolism and mitochondrial energetics to other highly-conserved cellular processes (peroxisome functions and regulators of protein, RNA and DNA synthesis, repair and turnover). Of the core transcripts, 35% have a significant sequence homology to higher eukaryotes; this suggests that what we observe is a basic universal necessity to provide temporal coherence of all higher living systems. At its core is the oscillatory intracellular redox state, but the entire intracellular network of biochemical reactions is entrained to its fundamental rhythm.

Mitochondrial Respiratory Dynamics in Vivo During Growth

The respiratory oscillations in yeast growing in continuous culture represent a high-amplitude variation in the structure and function of the organelles.[62,63] The mechanism had been previously elucidated in the cell-division synchronized cultures of the soil amoeba, *Acanthamoeba castellanii*, where measurements of adenine nucleotide pools clearly indicated a process of in vivo mitochondrial respiratory control (i.e., restriction of respiratory chain activity by the availability of ADP, which in turn depends on biosynthetic ATP utilization rates.[71] This research led to the suggestion that the control of mitochondrial respiratory rates lies in an "epigenetic" control circuit with a slow (τ = 69 min for *A. castellanii*) dynamic. Thus the mitochondria dance to a "slow drum beat" played elsewhere.[11] The yeast system obeys similar rules, but in this case the ultradian period is about 40min, again the observed cycles are dictated by the slower time-scales of the energy-requiring processes by biosynthesis, so that the changing levels of dissolved O_2 we observe in cultures of the growing cells are a consequence of the ultradian clock-driven cycles of energy demand.[62] Inner mitochondrial membranes show structural changes (Fig. 8) typical of alternating states of ADP-driven energization and "resting" phases, as well as mitochondrial membrane potential and redox changes of respiratory chain components (e.g., NADH).[61] Addition of compounds that uncouple energy conservation from electron transport (protonophores such as S_{13} or CCCP) to the continuous culture confirms that resetting of the respiratory oscillations at low concentrations occurs. At higher concentrations these treatments synchronize cell-division events.[68] At even higher protonophore concentrations, cell cycle delay becomes evident. These data confirm that control of mitochondrial activities in situ does not reside primarily in the mitochondria themselves, as the cycles of mitochondrial energization (τ circa 40 min) are at least two orders of magnitude slower than for isolated organelles (τ typically measured in sec, (Fig. 8). The mitochondria in the cell are enslaved by slower processes. On a still longer time scale, cell division cycle timekeeping depends on the functioning of the ultradian clock.

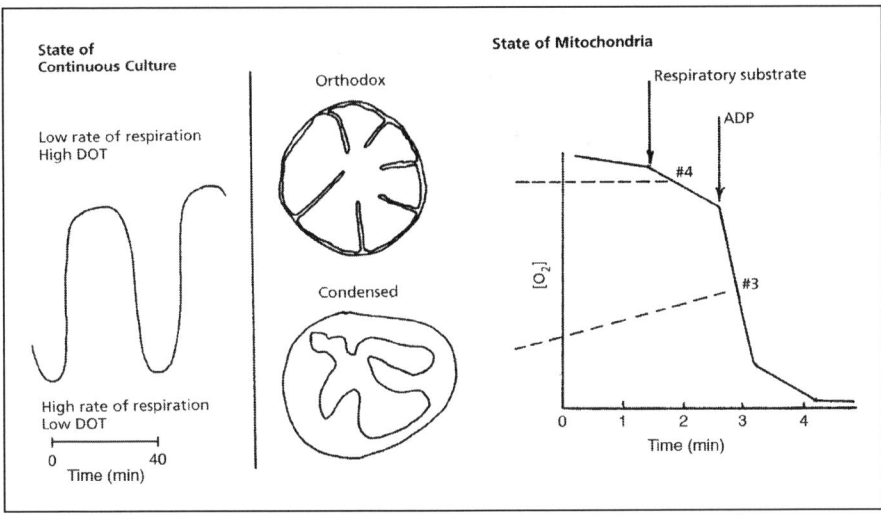

Figure 8. Respiratory oscillations in a continuous culture of *S. cerevisiae*: maxima and minima corresponds to extremes of changes in mitochondrial structure that accompany altered metabolic status during energy conservation in vitro. DOT, dissolved oxygen tension in the culture medium; #3 mitochondrial energized state, #4 resting state. The 40 min cycle in vivo is slower than mitonchondrial transitions in vitro. (Reproduced with permission from ref. 63.)

Although cytochrome *c* oxidase, the terminal mitochondrial electron acceptor, is responsible for the efficient and safe 4 electron reduction of O_2 to H_2O, a minor product is H_2O_2, accounting for about 0.1% of total O_2 consumption in mitochondria.[69,70] Two sites for "electron leakage" along the respiratory chain have been highlighted. These are at Sites I and III, and are assigned to the transient exposure of autoxidizable FeS cluster[71] and semi-ubiquinone[72] to intracellular O_2. Whereas the former source of ROS yields predominantly intramitochondrial radicals, the latter produces ROS both there and in the extramirochondrial cytosol about equally.[73] Other sites include the reduced nicotinamide nucleotide-driven plasma membrane and endoplasmic reticulum electron transport chains, peroxisomes and by cytochrome P450.[74] Reactions of ROS include their own interconversions, reaction with NO to form the highly reactive peroxynitrite and the peroxidation of membrane lipids, both low mol. wt. and protein thiols, and nucleic acids.[75]

Oxidative Stress and Signalling by ROS

Further consequences result from the temporal organization of mitochondrial energy generation. Levels of reactive O_2 species (O_2^-, H_2O_2, HO and $^1O_2$) change cyclically on a 40min time-base, as the ultradian coordination unfolds. This occurs as a result of the inherently "leaky" electron transport reactions of the respiratory chain.[69] However, in higher eukaryotes, animals and plants, ROS have diverse signalling roles, where they convey pivotal informational transfer in mitochondrial synchrony (e.g., in cardiomyocytes).[76] They also induce or suppress gene expression, activate signalling cascades and induce apoptosis.[77]

In yeast, we have integrated the observations of ultradian cycles of mitochondrial respiration, production of ROS and the hypothesis of a finite lifetime of the organism being determined by a definite number of the circa- 40 min periods (Fig. 9).[78] Apoptosis has been observed in yeasts[79,80] as has ultradian cycling of sensitivity to H_2O_2.[82] The pervasive and all-inclusive characteristic of the circa 40 min ultradian clock is further revealed by monitoring the DNA content of cells by flow cytometry after staining with propidium iodide. Within the

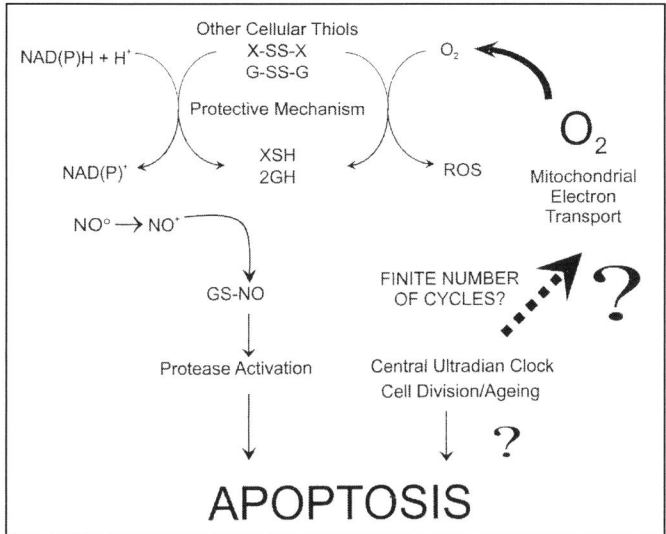

Figure 9. The redox switch, central to the operation of the ultradian ($\tau \approx 40$ min) clock in yeast is closely coupled to mitochondrial electron transport, a major source of reactive oxygen species (ROS). Apoptosis and cell senescence (aging) may be determined by the number of ultradian respiratory cycles experienced. (Reproduced with permission from ref. 78.)

time frame of the 40 min cycle, a 10-15 min period is conducive to DNA synthesis and replication; this window opens during the reductive phase of the clock cycle.[67] About 8% of the total population undergo this transition in each round of the respiratory oscillation. Thus, respiration is tightly coupled to the nuclear DNA synthesis cycle; furthermore a major burst of RNA-centred biosynthetic activity occurs at this stage and it is regulated by transcriptional regulation of a cohort of genes that also include the sulphur regulation transcriptional complex (Met-4-Cbf1-Met28-Met31-Met23-Met30).[22,83] It is important for the separation of incompatible reactions that biochemical reactions sensitive to reactive oxygen species occur during this time when oxygen uptake rates are minimal, and H_2S and GSH levels are highest.

Circadian Oscillations in Yeasts

The first reports that yeast is sensitive to blue light and that the cell-division cycle of a yeast could be entrained by LD cycles opened up a new field of research.[84,85] As in other lower eukaryotes, mitochondrial cytochromes were implicated as being involved in the photoentrainment pathway,[84] and more detailed studies of well-characterized mitochondrial and cytoplasmic cytochrome-deficient mutants[86] confirmed this for *S. cerevisiae*. Photochemical action spectra for the inhibition of growth by visible light gave a maximum at 408 nm in the Soret region of the cytochrome absorption spectrum. Resistance to this blue-light effect was greatest in strains where all three types of cytochrome (*b,c* and *a*) had been deleted; these results were in accord with previously reported haem chromophoremediated photodynamic effects.

At 12°C where the generation time was about 31 h, cultures of *S. cerevisiae* could be entrained to LD 10, 14 cycles; about 50% of the organisms produced buds in each cycle, and this process began at or just before the dark phases.[87] Similar results were obtained in LD 12, 12 or LD 14, 10 cycles, and free-runs in complete darkness after these entrainment regimens gave oscillations with a period of 26-28 h. Persistence for as long as 7-8 days in constant dark was observed. Uptake of [^{14}C]-histidine or lysine was used to measure transport rates through the plasma membrane; again, free-running circadian rhythms were observed under constant darkness, sometimes with a bimodal waveform (peaks at subjective dawn, shoulders at subjective dusk).

In a mutant (lacking cytochromes aa_3, b and c), attempts to entrain nutrient uptake to a LD 14, 10 cycle were ineffectual.[89]

Schiz. pombe exhibits cell cycle-dependent variation in sensitivity to 15 min heat shocks (49°C) and (as for S-phase) shifting forward of heat sensitivity could be achieved by treatment with 0.2% 2-phenylethanol.[89-90] Cultures kept at 20°C or 30°C were exposed to 55°C temperatures and colony formation on plates was assessed. The circadian rhythm of survival presumably represents an evolutionary adaptation to daily temperature cycle, persistent in constant darkness ($\tau = 27$ h), and shows temperature compensation.[91] A circadian cycle of cell division of *Schiz. pombe* can be monitored by changes in the septation index in cultures maintained at low temperature. This can be synchronized either by temperature or LD cycle.[92] Growth of these cultures is light-sensitive. Slowly metabolized-sugars (giving generation times longer than 1 day, e.g., mannose for *Schiz. pombe*, trehalose for *S. cerevisiae*) are suitable for circadian experiments at higher temperatures. Rhythmic acidification of the culture media also occurs (F. Kippert, personal communication). Experiments with cytochrome-deficient strains of *Schiz. pombe* suggest that mitochondrial cytochrome b is necessary for photoentrainment; a 'blind' mutant can still be synchronized by temperature cycles.[92]

Other Oscillations

As well as the three types of oscillatory behaviour described above, other reports have indicated periodic phenomena in yeasts. For example, a burgeoning literature describes in minute detail the mechanism of glycolytic oscillations, without any clear evidence for unique functions;[93] these can be modulated by mitochondrial functions (e.g., inhibition of mitochondrial activities in *S. cerevisiae* affect glycolytic periodicities[94]). Also, acetaldehyde, a secondary product of glycolysis, is a key effector of the respiratory oscillations that can phase shift[66] the metronomic time-keeping of the ultradian clock[22] and occupies a central role in the redox switch core of the 40 min oscillator.[83]

Metabolic oscillations involving pulsatile NH_4^+ release have been implicated in the production of organized growth in colonies,[95] although other possible effectors have not been excluded from participation.[96]

Cell-cell signalling between individual yeasts can now be observed microscopically.[15] Yeast should perhaps not be regarded as a unicellular organism, as many facets of its behaviour in the laboratory[97] indicate cooperative activity between individuals that reflect its natural existence as a biofilm (e.g., on the surfaces of grapes), or in flocs, aggregates or colonies.

Electrically-observed sustained oscillations (periods in the range 3-9 min) in growing yeast cultures[98] have been attributed to glycolytic oscillations, but this claim has to be further substantiated. It seems more likely that AC impedance is a function of plasma membrane electrochemical potential,[99] a property used to control continuous yeast culture growth and often resulting in periodic or chaotic outputs.

Functions of Oscillations

A range of functions have been designated for oscillatory performance in living systems (Table 2). Separation of incompatible processes (e.g., oxidative vs. reductive) lies at the redox switching core[22,61,83] of the *circa* 40 min oscillator, and perhaps still echoes the ancestral conflict between the archaeal host and its newly-acquired proteobacterial endosybiont[83,100] in a SO_4^{2-}-rich primordial environment. The respiratory organelle is in some senses still partially enslaved,[11,62,63,101] and even today dances to a slower tune that has evolved to ensure cohesion of the massively-interconnected cellular network.[22,83,102] On this timescale, the massive parallel-processing integrally required for the function of the network requires a strict time frame for convergence. The recent data from the self-synchronised (spontaneously-organized) continuous culture of *S. cerevisiae* clarifies all the earlier observations on synchronous cultures of yeasts and also provides a more amenable system for further studies by powerful new technologies for continuous noninvasive investigations. The coherence of the intracellular machine requires strict autodynamic performance that encompasses metabolic, transcriptional, translational and cell division cycle events.

Table 2. *Functions of oscillations/rhythms/clocks*

---

1. Increased energy efficiency? e.g., in glycolysis
2. Signalling e.g., Ca^{2+} oscillator, $O_2^{-\bullet}$ Amplitude modulation, or frequency modulation
3. Spatial organization e.g., in segmentation, the somite "clock"
4. Temporal organization
   a. Matching intracellular/interorganism events with the environmental cycles e.g., circadian rhythms, seasonal rhythm.
   b. Separating incompatible processes e.g., photosynthesis producing oxygen vs. nitrogen fixation
   c. Coordinating events in different compartments of the cell or of the organism e.g., mitochondrion/nucleus - cyosol
5. Entrainment by
   a. Phase
   b. Frequency
6. Prediction (e.g., dawn or dusk by circadian rhythms)
7. Responsiveness
8. Biological "fitness"

The more rapid events reflected in the minute time domain respiratory oscillations is likely to result from ion transport across mitochondrial membranes during energy yielding processes.[8,19] They probably also indicate inter-compartment signalling functions (e.g., by Ca^{2+} and reactive oxygen species).[77,105,104]

Circadian rhythmicity, a higher-order output of the autodynamic cellular network, has evolved to match the activities of the organism to the environment cycles that result from the daily rotation of the earth. The optimization of network functions within this 24 h time-frame gives increased biological "fitness" arising from anticipatory advantages.[105] There has been a general underestimation of the temporal complexity and extreme dynamicity of living processes (e.g., the rapid dynamics of protein turnover has become appreciated only in the past decade). Attempts to study the "circadian clock" and its control without due consideration of the whirlpool of cellular dynamics proceeding on rapid time scales,[106] is unlikely to yield a comprehensive understanding.[107,108]

Models that incorporate interlinked feedback and feedforward controlled circuits as demanded by the ever-growing family of "canonical" circadian clock genes become necessarily more intricate with increasing mathematical complexity, [109] even if techniques for dimensional reduction are available.[110] Where more than two state variables are involved, then perhaps quasiperiodic or chaotic dynamics may provide appropriate models.[111] Chaos occurs in complex open nonlinear systems, including biological ones, and there are strong indications that, as well as in population dynamics and in epidemics, some normal physiological states (e.g., of brain and heart) may be described as chaotic.

Chaotic operation has been experimentally demonstrated in continuous cultures of *S. cerevisiae* under several different conditions:

1. Under "permittistatical" control (i.e., using output from an AC impedence measuring device to control the growth medium supply rate.[99]
2. Addition of the monoamine oxidase A-type inhibitor, phenelzine, to a pH-controlled culture leads to a period-doubling, often the first step towards chaos.[64] Further work confirms this and investigates the transcriptional controls involved (C.M. Li and R.R.Klevecz, unpublished data).
3. Stepwise decreases in culture pH reveals a progressive increase in complexity of trajectories and the eventual uncovering of a strange attractor.[112]
4. In a long-term experiment months continuous culture 40,000 data points collected using an immersed direct inlet mass spectrometer probe to measure dissolved O2, CO2, and H2S (Fig. 10) reveal a chaotic attractor (M. Roussel and D. Lloyd, unpublished).

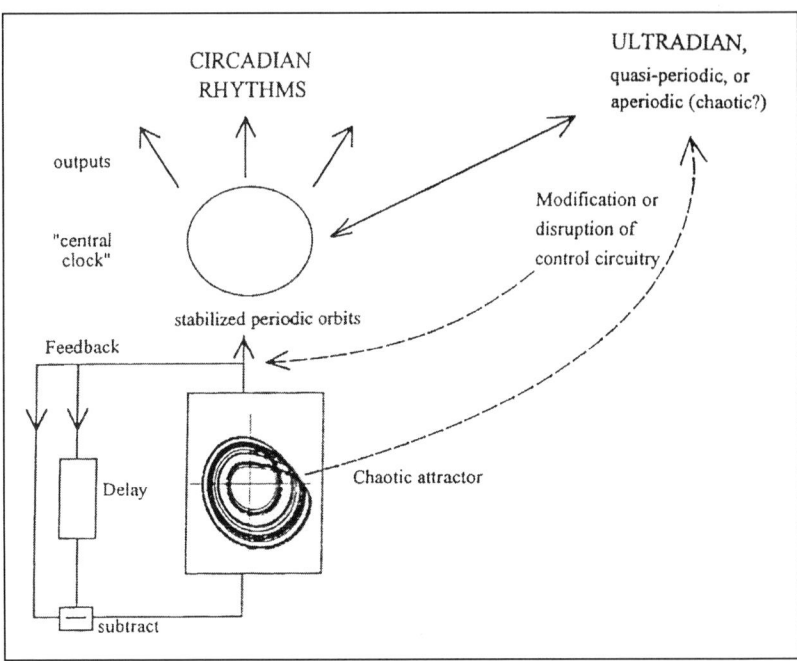

Figure 10. A controlled chaotic attractor requires three state variables and feedback with delay. Multi-frequency outputs can be selected by modification arhythmia of control. Loss of control (e.g., by mutation or exposure to intense continuous light) gives a rhythmia or high-frequency outputs. (Reproduced with permission from ref. 125.)

Even a very simple model of the circadian system shows chaotic dynamics.[113] In most situations chaos is regarded as a nuisance since the onset of chaotic operation sets a limit to the range of useful operation. Why then have some living systems incorporated chaotic function? Explanations have invoked unpredictability as advantageous in the search for novelty in form and function.

An answer to the question "what is the use of chaos" became much easier when Ott, Grebogi and Yorke pointed out that the exploitation of chaos becomes possible when it can be controlled.[114] A typical chaotic attractor has an infinite number of orbits embedded within it. A general method was proposed whereby it is possible to choose a low period unstable orbit which improves system performance and into apply small time-dependent perturbations in order to stabilize that orbit. This technique has since been shown to work for mechanical, electronic, and chemical systems.[115] In view of the generality of the principles, it would be most surprising if the advantages of controlled chaos had not been made available during the evolution of living organisms.[116] These benefits are not inconsiderable; instead of a fixed period limit cycle, the controlled chaotic attractor provides a single multi-oscillator capable of tuneable outputs of variable frequencies. Such a system can switch rapidly from one state to another, thereby providing multiple use a single system configuration. It can be shown that a controlled chaotic attractor can quickly and easily be tuned to optimal system performance, and is robust to external noise. Controlled chaos can lead to system diversity and to the development of increased complexity.

Several methods are now recognised ain physical systems for the control of chaos,[117] none of these require novel control elements in terms of previously recognised principles of metabolic control (feedback inhibition, feed forward activation, and time delay). The continuous control of chaos by self-controlling feedback, developed in numerical simulations for electronic

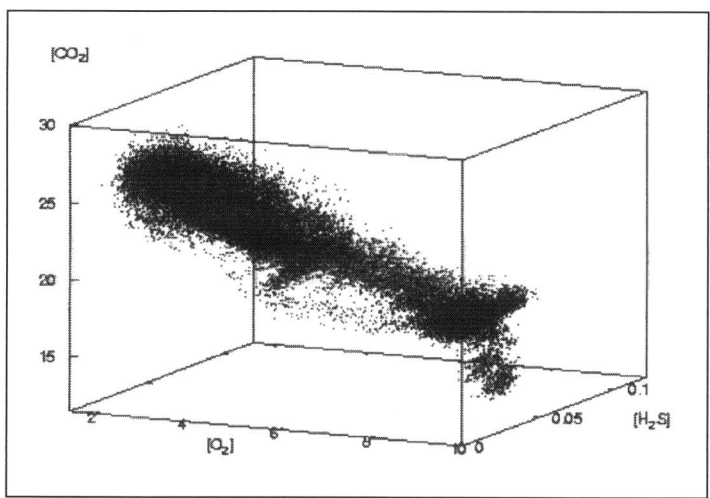

Figure 11. Membrane inlet mass spectrometer signals for dissolved O_2, CO_2 and H_2S (m/z = 32, 44 and 34 relative to Argon at m/z = 44) in a continuous culture of *S.cerevisiae*. The 40,000 data points form a chaotic attractor with a leading Lyapunov exponent of $0.752 \pm 0.004 h^{-1}$ (95% confidence). Unpublished experiments of M. Roussel and D. Lloyd.

circuit design (A.Tamecevicius, personal communication), provides an excellent example (Fig. 11) of the simplicity and in principle the applicability of these methods to metabolic and transcriptional circuitry.[118]

I propose that in its optimised states, the controlled chaotic cellular attractor provides the stabilised orbits of the biological clocks that we recognise as necessary time-bases in the circadian, ultradian and minute-long domains. Domination of output by the circadian system can be overcome experimentally (e.g., in *Drosophila*,[119] or in rats reared continuously in bright light, in *Lingulodinium (Gonyaulax polyedra)* at low temperature, in per0 mutants of *Drosophila* or Neurospora or in optic-tract sectioned insects. Less drastic interference(e.g., in *Drosophila* in the presence of D_2O or in some other *per* mutants)[120,121] may give arrhythmic quasiperiodic or short period (ultradian) operation has been reported for lower eukaryotes as well as for humans (see examples ref. 122)

The hypothesis that a controlled chaotic attractor may provide the central oscillator responsible for the generation of circadian and ultradian rhythms[123-125] may be tested by seeking chaotic dynamics in those systems where controls have been disrupted.

A controlled chaotic attractor (Fig. 11) may be used to model this multilayered complexity, where coherent operation requires the interweaving and intertwining of processes on many timescales from the extremely rapid (ns) protein side-chain movements to the *circa* 40 min ultradian clock time base and circadian and annually-controlled events of life processes. Metazoan and plant evolution has interactions between cells as a key step, and the generation of oscillatory signalling has its earliest beginnings in the lower organisms.

Thus in zebrafish, the 'segmentation clock' that functions in vertebrate embryos to organize key stages in development involves coupled oscillators facilitating synchronised oscillation and collective behaviour of neighbouring cells. The robust nature of these complex processes and the minimization of external noise is an excellent example of the essential nature of oscillatory biological systems.[127]

In cell lines derived from mammalian sources the characteristics can now be detected, studied and related to early evolutionary beginnings. In the case of hepaticytes cell-cell synchronization involves gangliosides and/or catecholamines.[128,129]

Even in yeast, synchronization of cell monolayers perfused with glucose and O_2 occurs by a process of self-organisation spontaneously, and redox oscillations initiated in individual mitochondria spread through each cell and then across the whole field of cells under observation.[15]

References

1. Chance B, Williams GR. The respiratory chain and oxidative phosphorylation. Adv Enzymol 1956; 17:65-134.
2. Gooch VD, Packer L. Oscillatory systems in mitochondria. Biochim Biophys Acta 1974; 346:245-260.
3. Mochan E, Pye EK. Respiratory oscillations in adapting yeast cultures. Nat New Biol 1973; 242(119):177-179.
4. Poole RK, Lloyd D, Kemp RB. Respiratory oscillations and heat evolution in synchronously-dividing cultures of the fission yeast Schizosaccharomyces pombe 972h. J Gen Microbiol 1973; 77:209-220.
5. Edwards C, Statham M, Lloyd D. Establishment by large-scale synchronous cultures of the trypanosomatid, Crithidia fasciculata by cell-size election: Changes in respiration and adenylate charge through the cell cycle. J Gen Microbiol 1975; 88:149-152.
6. Lloyd D, Phillips SA, Statham M. Oscillations of respiration adenine nucleotide levels and heat evolution in synchronous cultures of Tetrahymena pyriformis prepared by continuous flow selection. J Gen Microbiol 1978; 106:19-26.
7. Edwards SW, Lloyd D. Oscillations of respiration and adenine nucleotides in synchronous cultures of Acanthamoeba castellanii: Mitochondrial respiratory control in vivo. J Gen Microbiol 1978; 108:197-204.
8. Kader J, Lloyd D. Respiratory oscillations and heat evolution in synchronous cultures of Candida utilis. J Gen Microbiol 1979; 114:455-461.
9. Mitchell PD. Foundations of vectorial metabolism and osmochemistry. Biosci Reports 2004; 24:386-435.
10. Lloyd D, Edwards SW. Mitochondrial adenosine triphosphatase of the fission yeast, Schizosaccharomyces pombe 972⁻: Changes in activity and oligomycin sensitivity during the cell cycle of catabolite-repressed and de-repressed cells. Biochem J 1977; 162:39-46.
11. Lloyd D, Edwards SW. Epigenetic oscillations during the cell cycles of lower eukaryotes are coupled to a clock: Life's slow dance to the music of time. In: Edmunds Jr LN, ed. Cell Cycle Clocks. New York: Plenum Press, 1984:107-145.
12. Chance B, Legallais V, Sorge J et al. A versatile time-sharing multichannel spectrophotometer, reflectometer and fluorometer. Anal Biochem 1975; 66:498-514.
13. Aon MA, Cortassa S, Marbán E et al. Synchronized whole-cell oscillations in mitochondrial metabolism triggered by a local release of reactive oxygen species in cardiac myocytes. J Biol Chem 2003; 278:44735-44744.
14. Lemar KM, Passa O, Aon MA et al. Allyl alcohol and garlic (Allium sativium) extract produce oxidative stress in Candida albicans. Microbiology 2005; 151:3257-3265.
15. Lloyd D, Lemar KM, Murray DB et al. Yeast respiratory oscillations monitored in continuous cultures and evaluated by 2-photon laser microscopy. VIII Congreso de la Sociedad Ibérica de Cytometria 2003; 59.
16. Digman MA, Brown CM, Sengupta P et al. Measuring fast dynamics in solutions and cells with a laser scanning microscope. Biophys J 2005; 89:1317-1327.
17. Wiseman PW, Brown CM, Webb et al. Spatial mapping of integrin interactions and dynamics during the cell migration by image correlation microscopy. J Cell Sci 2004; 117:5521-5524.
18. Gooch VD, Packer L. Adenine nucleotide control of heart mitochondrial oscillations. Biochim Biophys Acta 1971; 245:17-20.
19. Boiteux A, Degn H. Oscillating respiration in mitochondria. Hoppe Seylers Z Physiol Chem 1972; 353:696-701.
20. Satroutdinov AD, Kuriyama H, Kobayashi H. Oscillatory metabolism of Saccharomyces cerevisiae in continuous culture. FEMS Microbiol Lett 1992; 77:261-267.
21. Murray DB, Roller S, Kuriyama H et al. Clock control of ultradian respiratory oscillation found during yeast continuous culture. J Bacteriol 2001; 183:7253-7259.
22. Lloyd D, Murray DB. Ultradian clock: Metronome for intracellular orchestration. Trends Biochem Sci 2005; 30:373-377.
23. Lloyd D, Bohátka S, Szilagy J. Quadrupole mass spectrometry in the monitoring and control of fermentations. Biosensors 1985; 1:179-212.
24. Degn H, Cox RP, Lloyd D. Membrane inlet mass spectrometry: Applications to direct measurement of biological gaseous exchange. Meth Biochem Anal. 1985:31:165-194.
25. Lloyd D, Thomas KL, Cowie G et al. Direct interface of chemistry to microbiological systems: Membrane inlet mass spectrometry. J Microb Meth 2002; 50:175-188.

26. Kuenzi MT, Fiechter M. Changes in carbohydrate composition and trehalase activity during the budding cycle of yeast. Arch Mikrobiol 1969; 64:396-407.

27. Nosoh Y, Takamiya A. Synchronization of budding cycle in yeast cells and effect of carbon monoxide and nitrogen-deficiency on the synchrony. Plant and Cell Physiol 1962; 3:53-56.

28. von Meyenburg HK. Energetics of the budding cycle of yeast growth. Arch Microbiol 1969; 66:289-303.

29. Wiemken A, Matile P, Moore H. Vacuolar dynamics in synchronously budding yeast. Arch Microbiol 1970; 70:89-103.

30. Dharmalignam K, Jayaraman J. Mitochondriogenesis in synchronous culture of yeast. Oscillatory pattern of respiration. Arch Biochem Biophys 1973; 157:197-202.

31. Parulekar SJ, Semiones GB, Rolf MJ et al. Induction and elimination of oscillations in continuous cultures of yeast (Saccharomyes cerevisiae). Biotech Bioeng 1986; 28:700-710.

32. Strässle C, Sonnleitner B, Fiechter A. A predictive model for the spontaneous synchronization of yeast (Saccharomyes cerevisiae) grown in continuous culture. J Biotech 1988; 7:299-318.

33. Martegani E, Porro D, Ranzi BM et al. Involvement of a cell size control mechanism in the induction and maintenance of oscillations in continuous cultures of budding yeast. Biotech Bioeng 1990; 36:453-459.

34. Münch T, Sonnleitner B, Fiechter AS. New insights into the synchronization mechanism with forced synchronous cultures of Saccharomyces cerevisiae. J Biotech 1992; 24:299-314.

35. Auberson LCM, Kanbier T, von Stockar. Monitoring yeast cultures by calorimetry. J Biotech 1993; 29:205-215.

36. Osumi M, Sando N. Division of yeast mitochondria in synchronous culture. J Elect Micros 1969; 18:47-56.

37. Lloyd D, Poole RK, Edwards SE. The Cell Division Cycle: Temporal Organization and Control of Cellular Growth and Reproduction. London: Academic Press, 1984.

38. Poole RK, Lloyd D. Changes in respiratory activities during the cell-cycle of the fission yeast Schizosaccharomyces pombe 972h⁻ growing in the presence of glycerol. Biochem J 1974; 144:141-148.

39. Poole RK, Lloyd D. Changes in enzyme activities in synchronously dividing cultures of the fission yeast Schizosaccharomyces pombe 972h⁻. Biochem J 1973; 136:195-207.

40. Poole RK, Lloyd D, Chance B. Development of cytochromes of Schizosaccharomyces pombe during the cell cycle. Biochem J 1974; 138:201-210.

41. Bashford CL, Chance B, Lloyd D et al. Oscillations of redox states in synchronously dividing cultures of Acanthamoeba castellanii and Schizosaccharomyces pombe. Biophys J 1980; 29:1-12.

42. Kippert F, Lloyd D. The ultradian clock of Schizosaccharmomyces pombe: Environmental stability, but genetic variability. J Interdisc Cycle Res 1991; 22:138-139.

43. Kippert F, Lloyd D. A temperature-compensated clock ticks in Schizosaccharomyces pombe. Microbiology 1995; 141:883-890.

44. Kippert F, Lloyd D. The fluorochrome aniline blue, specifically stains the septum of both live and fixed Schizosaccharomyces pombe. FEMS Microbiol Lett 1995; 132:215-219.

45. Kippert F. The ultradian clock and the cell cycle in Schizosaccharomyces pombe. M. Phil Thesis; Cardiff: University of Wales, 1992.

46. Novak B, Mitchison JM. CO₂ production in cell-free extracts of yeast detects cell cycle changes. J Cell Sci 1986; 86:191-206.

47. Mitchison JM, Creanor J, Novak B. Coordination of growth and division during the cell cycle of the fission yeast. Coldspring Harbor Symp Quant Biol 1991; 56:557-565.

48. Johnsson A, Engelmann W, Pflug B et al. Period lengthening of human circadian rhythms by lithium carbonate, a prophylactic for depressive disorders. Int J Chronobiol 1983; 8:129-147.

49. Klemfuss H. Rhythms and the pharmacology of lithium. Pharmacol Ther 1992; 56:53-78.

50. Kippert F. Cellular signalling and the complexity of biological timing: Insights from the ultradian clock of Schizosaccharomyces pombe. Philos Trans Soc Lond B Biol Sci 2001; 356:1725-1733.

51. Poole RK. Development of respiratory activity during the cell cycle of Schizosaccharomyces pombe 972h⁻: Respiratory oscillations and heat dissipation in cultures synchronized with 2'-deoxyadenosine. J Gen Microbiol 1977; 103:19-27.

52. Poole RK, Salmon I. The pool sizes of adenine nucleotides in exponentially growing stationary phase and 2'-deoxyadenosine-synchronized cultures of Schizosaccharomyces pombe 972h⁻¹. J Gen Microbiol 1978; 106:153-164.

53. Kovac L. Oligomycin-like inhibition of yeast respiration by N,N¹-dicyclohexylcarbodiimide and the nature of energy coupling in intact yeast cells. Biochim Biophys Acta 1970; 205:520-523.

54. Thomas KC, Dawson PSS. Variations in the adenylate energy charge during phased growth (cell cycle) of Candida utilis under energy excess and energy-limiting growth conditions. J Bacteriol 1977; 132:36-43.

55. Keulers M, Satroutdinov AD, Suzuki T et al. Synchronization affector of autonomous short-period sustained oscillation of Saccharomyces cerevisiae. Yeast 1996; 12:673-682.

56. Keulers M, Satroutdinov AD, Kuriyama H. Oscillations in ethanol-grown Saccharomyces cerevisiae. FEMS Microbiol Lett 1996; 142:253-258.

57. Murray DB, Engelen FAA, Keulers M et al. NO$^+$, but not NO, inhibits respiratory oscillations in ethanol-grown chemostat cultures of Saccharomyces cerevisiae. FEBS Lett 1998; 431:297-299.

58. Lloyd D, Murray DB, Engelen FAA et al. NO$^+$, but not NO, inhibits respiratory oscillations in ethanol-grown chemostat cultures of Saccharomyces cerevisiae. Biochem Soc Trans 1998; 26:S339.

59. Murray DB, Engelen FAA, Lloyd D et al. Involvement of glutathione in the regulation of respiratory oscillation during a h of continuous culture of Saccharomyces cerevisiae. Microbiology 1999; 145:2739-2745.

60. Lloyd D, Edwards SW, Fry JC. Temperature-compensated oscillations in respiration and cellular protein content in synchronous cultures of Acanthamoeba castellanii. Proc Natl Acad Sci USA 1982; 70:3786-3788.

61. Lloyd D, Murray DB. Redox cycling of intracellular thiols: State variables for ultradian, cell division cycle and circadian cycles. In: Vanden Driessche T, Guisset JL, DeVries GP, eds. Redox Behaviour of Circadian Systems. Kluwer: Amsterdam, 2000:85-94.

62. Lloyd D, Salgado ELJ, Turner MP et al. Respiratory oscillations in yeast: Clock-driven mitochondrial cycles of energization. FEBS Lett 2002; 519:41-44.

63. Lloyd D, Salgado ELJ, Turner MP et al. Cycles of mitochondrial energization driven by the ultradian clock in a continuous culture of Saccharomyces cerevisiae. Microbiology 2002; 148:3715-3724.

64. Salgado LEJ, Murray DB, Lloyd D. Some antidepressant agents (Li$^+$, monoamine oxidase type A inhibitors) perturb the ultradian clock in Saccharomyces cerevisiae. Biol Rhythm Res 2002; 33:351-361.

65. Sohn HY, Murray DB, Kuriyama H. Ultradian oscillation of Saccharomyces cerevisiae: H$_2$S mediates population synchrony. Yeast 2000; 16:1185-1190.

66. Murray DB, Klevecz RR, Lloyd D. Generation and maintenance of synchrony in Saccharomyces cerevisiae in continuous culture. Exp Cell Res 2003; 287:10-15.

67. Klevecz RR, Bolen J, Forrest G et al. A genome wide oscillation in transcription gates DNA replication and cell cycle. Proc Nat Acad Sci USA 2004; 101:1200-1205.

67b. Klevecz RR, Dynamic architecture of the yeast all cycle uncovered by wavelet decomposition of expression microarray data. Funct Integr Genomics 2000; 1:186-192.

67c. Klevecz RR, Dowse HB. Tuning in the transcriptome: Basins of attraction in the yeast cell cycle. Cell Proliferation 2000; 33:209-218.

67d. Klevecz RR, Murray DB. Genome wide oscillations in expression. Wavelet analysis of time series data from yeast expression arrays. Mol Biol Rep 2001; 28:73-82, (uncovers the dynamic architecture of the phenotype).

67e. Moloshok TD, Klevecz RR, Grant JD et al. Application of Baysian decomposition for analysing microarray data. Bioinformatics 2002; 18:566-575.

68. Lloyd D. Effects of uncoupling of mitochondrial energy conservation on the ultradian clock-driven oscillations in Saccharomyces cerevisiae continuous culture. Mitochondrion 2003; 3:139-146.

69. Boveris A, Chance B. The mitochondrial generation of hydrogen peroxide. General properties and effect of hyperbaric oxygen. Biochem J 1973; 134:707-716.

70. Hansford RG, Hogue, Mildaziene V. Dependence of H$_2$O$_2$ formation by rat heart mitochondria on substrate availability and donor age. J Bioeng Biomemb 1997; 29:89-95.

71. Cadenas E, Boveris A, Ragan CI et al. Production of superoxide radicals and H$_2$O$_2$ by NADH ubiquinone reductase and ubiquinone cytochrome c reduction from beef heart mitochondria. Arch Biochem Biophys 1977; 180:248-257.

72. Ksenzenko M, Konstantiov AA, Khomotov GB et al. Effect of electron transport inhibitors on superoxide generation in the cytochrome bc$_1$ site of the mitochondrial respiratory chain. FEBS Lett 1983; 155:19-23.

73. Aon MA, Cortassa S, Marbán E et al. Cell oscillations in mitochondrial metabolism triggered by a local release of reactive oxygen species in cardiac myocytes. J Biol Chem 2003; 278:44735-44744.

74. Jezek P, Hlavatá L. Mitochondria in homeostasis of reactive oxygen species. Int J Biochem Cell Biol 2005; 37:2478-2503.

75. Packer MA, Porteous CM, Murphy MP. Superoxide formation in the presence of nitric acid forms peroxynitrite. Biochem Mol Biol Int 1996; 40:527-534.

76. Aon MA, Cortassa S, Akar FG et al. Mitochondrial criticality: A new concept at the turning point of life or death. Biochim Biophys Acta 2006; 1762:232-240.
77. Hancock JT, Desikan R, Neill SJ. Role of reactive oxygen species in cell signalling pathways. Biochem Soc Trans 2001; 29:345-350.
78. Lloyd D, Lemar KM, Salgado LE et al. Respiratory oscillations in yeast: Mitochondrial reactive oxygen species, apoptosis and time, a hypothesis. FEMS Yeast Res 2003; 3:333-339.
79. Madeo F, Frölich E, Frölich KU. A yeast mutant showing diagnostic markers of early and late apoptosis. J Cell Biol 1997; 139:729-734.
80. Lemar KM, Müller CT, Plummer S et al. Cell death mechanisms in the human opportunistic pathogen, Candida albicans. J Eukaryot Microbiol 2003; 50:(Suppl):685-686.
81. Silva RD, Sotoca R, Johansson B et al. Hyperosmotic stress induces metacaspase- and mitochondria-dependent apotosis in Saccharomyces cerevisiae. Mol Microbiol 2005; 58:824-834.
82. Wang J, Lui W, Uno T et al. Cellular stress responses oscillation of energy metabolism in the yeast, Saccharomyces serevisiae. FEMS Microbiol Lett 2000; 189:9-13.
83. Lloyd D, Murray DB. The temporal architecture of eukaryotic growth. FEBS Lett 2006; 580:2830-2835.
84. Ninnemann H, Butler WL, Epel BL. Inhibition of respiration in yeast by light. Biochim Biophys Acta 1970; 205:499-506.
85. Wille Jr JJ. Light entrained circadian oscillations of growth rate in the yeast Candida utilis. In: Scheving LE, Halberg F, Pauly JE, eds. Chronobiology. Tokyo: Igaku Shoin, 1974:72-77.
86. Ulaszewski S, Mamouneas T, Shen SK et al. Light effects in yeast: Evidence for participation of cytochromes in photoinhibition of growth and transport in Saccharomyces cerevisiae cultured at low temperatures. J Bact 1979; 138:523-529.
87. Edmunds Jr LN. Light effects in yeast: Persisting oscillations in all division activity and amino acid transport in cultures of Saccharomyces cerevisiae entrained by light-dark cycles. Photochem Photobiol 1979; 30:595-601.
88. Bullock JG, Coakley WT. Effect of heat on the viability of Schizosaccharomyces pombe 972h⁻ growing in synchronous cultures. Expl Cell Res 1976; 103:447-447.
89. Bullock JG, Coakley WT. Investigation into the mechanisms and repair of heat damage to Schizosaccharomyces pombe growing in synchronous cultures. J Therm Biol 1978; 3:159-162.
90. Bullock JG, Coakley WT. The cell cycle thermal-inactivation sensitive stage of Schizosaccharomyces pombe is independent of 2-phenylethanol-induced changes in S phase location. Expl Cell Res 1979; 121:441-444.
91. Kippert F. Circadian control of heat tolerance in stationary phase cultures of Schizosaccharomyces pombe. Arch Microbiol 1989; 155:177-170.
92. Kippert F, Engelman W, Ninnemann H. "Blind" cytochrome b mutant of yeast can still be entrained to 24h temperature cycles. J Interdisc Cycle Res 1991; 22:137-138.
93. Lloyd D, Stupfel M. The occurrence and functions of ultradian rhythms. Biol Rev 1991; 61:275-299.
94. Aon MA, Cortassa S, Westerhoff HV et al. Dynamic regulation of yeast glycolytic oscillations by mitochondrial functions. J Cell Sci 1991; 99:325-334.
95. Palkova Z, Devaux F, Icicova M et al. Ammonia pulses and metabolic oscillations guide yeast colony development. Mol Biol Cell 2002; 13:3901-3914.
96. Murray DB. On the temporal organisation of Saccharomyces cerevisiae. Curr Genomics 2004; 5:65-671.
97. Dickinson JR. Are yeasts free-living unicellular eukaryotes? J Appl Microbiol 2005; 41:445-447.
98. Male T, Feder J, Giaever GN et al. Oscillations in yeast observed electrically. Biol Rhythm Res 1999; 370.
99. Davey HM, Davey CM, Woodward AM et al. Oscillatory stochastic and chaotic growth fluctuations in permittistatically controlled yeast cultures. BioSystems 1996; 39:43-61.
100. Searcy DG. Metabolic integration during the evolutionary origin of mitochondria. Cell Res 2003; 13:229-238.
101. Lloyd D, Edwards SW. Temperature-compensated ultradian rhythms in lower eukaryotes: Timers for cell cycle and circadian events. Prog Clin Biol Res 1987; 227A:131-151.
102. Lloyd D. Systems dynamics of biology. J Appl Biomed 2005; 3:1-12.
103. Dewitt HS, Laffafian I, Hallett MB. Phagosomal oxidative activity during β2 integrin (CR³)-mediated phagocytosis by neutrophils is triggered by a nonrestricted Ca^{2+} signal: Ca^{2+} controls time not space. J Cell Sci 2003; 116:2857-2865.
104. O'Rourke B, Cortassa S, Aon MA. Mitochondrial ion channels: Gatekeepers of life and death. Physiol 2005; 20:203-215.
105. Lloyd D. Circadian and ultradian clock-controlled rhythms in unicellular microorganisms. Adv Microb Physiol. 1997:39:291-338.

106. Lloyd D, Gilbert DA. Temporal organization of the cell division cycle of eukaryote microbes. Symp Soc Gen Microbiol 1998; 56:251-278.
107. Schibler U, Naef F. Cellular oscillators: Rhythmic gene expression and metabolism. Curr Opin Cell Biol 2005; 17:223-229.
108. Gillette MU, Sejnowski TJ. Biological clocks coordinately keep life on time. Science 2005; 309:1196-1198.
109. Forger DB, Peskin CS. Model based conjectures on mammalian clock controversies. J Theor Biol 2004:203:533-539.
110. Indic P, Gurdziel K, Kronauer RE et al. Development of a two-dimensional manifold to represent high dimension mathematical models of the intracellular mammalian circadian clock. J Biol Rhythm 2006; 21:222-232.
111. Lloyd AL, Lloyd D. Chaos: Its significance and detection in biology. Biol Rhythm Res 1995; 26:233-252.
112. Murray DB, Lloyd D. A tuneable attractor underlies yeast respiratory dynamics. Biosystems 2006, (in press).
113. De Doede J, Olofson E, Rietveld WJ. A mathematical model of the circadian system with a delayed feedback loop. J Interdisc Cycle Res 1992; 23:142-144.
114. Ott E, Grebogi C, Yorke JA. Controlling chaos. Phys Rev Lett 1990; 64:1196-1199.
115. In: Ott E, Sauer T, Yorke JA, eds. Coping with Chaos: Analysis of Chaotic Data and The Exploitation of Chaotic Systems. New York: John Wiley and Sons Inc., 1994.
116. Lloyd AL, Lloyd D. Hypothesis: The central oscillator of the circadian clock is a controlled chaotic attractor. BioSystems 1993; 29:77-85.
117. Shinbrot T, Grebogi C, Ott E et al. Using small perturbations to control chaos. Nature 1993; 363:411-417.
118. Pyragas K. Continuous control of chaos by self-controlling feedback. Phys Lett A 1993; 170:421-428.
119. Dowse HB, Ringo JM. Further evidence that the circadian clock in Drosophila is a population of coupled ultradian oscillators. J Biol Rhythm 1987; 2:65-76.
120. Dowse H, Ringo J. Do ultradian oscillators underlie the circadian clock in Drosophila? In: Lloyd D, Rossi E, eds. Ultradian Rhythms in Life Processes. London: Springer-Verlag, 1992:105-117.
121. Power JM, Ringo JM, Dowse HB. The effects of period mutations and light on the activity rhythms of Drosophila melanogaster. J Biol Rhythm 1995; 10:267-280.
122. In: Lloyd D, Rossi EL, eds. Ultradian Rhythms in Life Processes. An Inquiry into Fundamental Principles of Chronobiology and Psychobiology. London: Springer-Verlag, 1992.
123. Lloyd D. A controlled chaotic attractor controls life. In: Gnaiger E, Gellerich F, Wyss M, eds. What Is Controlling Life 250 Years After Erwin Schrödinger's What is Life. Innsbruck: Innsbruck University Press, 1994.
124. Lloyd D, Lloyd AL. Hypothesis. A controlled chaotic attractor constitutes the central oscillator of the circadian clock. Bull Group d' Etudes des Rhythmes Biologiques 1994; 26:188-192.
125. Lloyd D, Lloyd AL. A controlled chaotic attractor could provide a tuneable oscillator for circadian clocks. Biol Rhythm Res 1994; 25:35-40.
126. Klevecz RR. A precise circadian clock from chaotic cell cycle oscillations. In: Lloyd D, Rossi EL, eds. Ultradian Rhythms in Life Processes. London: Springer Verlag, 1992.
127. Horikawa K, Ishimatsu K, Yoshimoto E et al. Noise-resistant and synchronized oscillation of the segmentation clock. Nature 2006; 441:719-723.
128. Brodsky VY. Direct cell-cell communication; a new approach derived from recent data on the nature and self-organisation of ultradian (circahoralian) intracellular rhythms. Biol Rev 2006; 81:143-162.
129. Brodsky VY, Zvezdina ND, Fateeva VI et al. Involvement of protein kinases in self-organization of the rhythm of protein synthesis by cell-cell communication. Cell Biol Int 2007;31(1):65-73.
130. Blumenthal LK, Zahler SA. Index for measurement of synchronization of populations. Science 1962; 135:724-726.

Stochastic Phase Oscillator Models for Circadian Clocks

Jacques Rougemont and Felix Naef*

Background

Circadian Rhythms

Periodic environments like we experience on the surface of planet earth lead living organisms to evolve molecular anticipation devices known a circadian clocks. The word circadian refers to the period of these oscillations which last about (circa) one day (dies). A frequently felt manifestation of this oscillator is experienced by travelers crossing timezones, when the local external cues are suddenly set out of phase with respect to our internal timing, resulting in a discomfort called jetlag. Although we might be less conscious about them, the circadian pacemaker also regulates a number of our basic daily physiological functions such as hourly changes in our body temperature or heart beat rate. Such clocks are found throughout the tree of life, in bacteria, plants, insects, funghi, vertebrates and mammals. Since the 1970s,[1] genetics and molecular biology has begun to disentangle the molecular circuitries by which cell-autonomous oscillations can be maintained, and how external light or temperature entrainment cues are relayed to this pacemaker. The three defining characteristics of these oscillators is that (i) rhythms persists in constant conditions (after external cues have been removed); (ii) phases can be reset by light, temperature or hormone pulses; (iii) the period of oscillation is temperature compensated in a physiological range. A commonality across the many species whose oscillators were studied is the recurrence of negative feedback circuits among the core clock genes.[2] Several species including Arabidopsis Thaliana, Drosophila melanogaster and mouse, use interlocked feedback loops, with up to three loops in Arabidopsis.[3,4] The resulting redundancy is thought to provide not only robustness,[5] but also the necessary flexibility to allow accurate timekeeping despite seasonal changes in photoperiod duration[3] or temperature variations. Interesting recent findings in cyanobacteria have shown that the circadian oscillator in the complete photo-autotroph *Synechococcus Elongatus* can tick independent of transcription and translation,[6,7] (reviewed in ref. 8), and that it is instead driven by a phosphorylation cycle. The possibility of a phosphorylation cycle has also been hypothesized in higher organisms[9] but remains to be validated experimentally.

In higher organisms timing is organized in a hierarchical manner with central and peripheral clocks. In mammals, the central clock consists of two nuclei of about 10,000 neurons (true) called the suprachiasmatic nuclei (SCN), which receives direct input about external light cues via the retinohypothalamic tract from the retina. Peripheral clocks are ticking in most of

*Corresponding Author: Felix Naef—Swiss Institute of Experimental Cancer Research (ISREC), Ecole Polytechnique Fédérale de Lausanne (EPFL), CH-1015 Lausanne, Switzerland. Email: felix.naef@isrec.ch

Cellular Oscillatory Mechanisms, edited by Miguel Maroto and Nicholas A.M. Monk. ©2008 Landes Bioscience and Springer Science+Business Media.

our organs, including liver, kidney, lung.[10] These are coordinated, or driven, by the SCN via humoral signals under normal conditions, but their phase can be shifted by local cues such as feeding in rodents.[11] Studying how the molecular oscillators are connected both upstream and downstream is a central topic in circadian research today. That is, it is both important to find out how the local clocks are entrained by the SCN, but also how molecular oscillators relay their output functions in specific organs. Recent experimental developments have allowed genome-wide screens of rhythmic mRNAs, which has led to the finding that in higher eukaryotes about 10 percent of genes have rhythmic cytosolic mRNA accumulation, irrespective of organism or tissue type. At the same time imaging using fluorescent or bioluminescence reporters has allowed to observe self-sustained oscillators in individual cells. This has shown elegantly that oscillations are common in individual cells, in fact they occur by default.[12,13] In addition individual oscillators are somewhat noisy, such that their period is not exactly constant but fluctuates from one cycle to the next.[14] In the absence of intercellular interactions, this leads to desynchronization of the cells at the population level, i.e., the phase diffuse such that they cancel each other and the population appears globally arrhythmic. At the same time, strong enough coupling among oscillators counteracts the disorder and can leads to a synchrony in a cell population.

Chemical Kinetics Models

After the pioneering work by Winfree before the molecular era of circadian biology,[15] there has been a regain of interest in models for the circadian clock with the identification of genes involved in the molecular oscillator. An early paper developed a rate equation model to describe the negative feedback of the Period protein, including mRNA transcription, translation and phosphorylation of the protein, as well as nuclear translocation.[16] Subsequent models for gene circuits were developed that can be split somewhat artificially in two groups: those proposing simplified (low dimensional toy models) to focus on the role of common topological structure such as negative feedback loops,[17-19] and secondly more explicit and higher dimensional models that study detailed biochemical processes that were mapped experimentally.[20,21]

Phase Oscillators

Phase oscillators provide a coarser class of oscillator models, in which it is assumed that the microscopic processes lead to oscillatory behavior, and that one can focus on the phase dynamics to study important effects such as oscillator entrainment (forcing) and resetting, or oscillator coupling in cell populations which can lead to collective synchronization or phase locking.[15,22-24]

The focus of this chapter will be on the theory and applications of noisy phase models in which the individual oscillator frequencies fluctuate in time while cells are coupled, as in the Kuramoto model. Anaysis of bioluminescence recordings from populations of mouse fibroblasts will be considered as an example.

Mathematics of Phase Models

The Model

The chemical equations describing the core clock system possess a stable limit-cycle which we can re-parametrize using phase (φ) and frequency (f) variables.[22] The time-derivative of the phase is given by the instantaneous frequency, which is modeled by a Gaussian random process. We make the particular choice of an Ornstein-Uhlenbeck process, which has the properties of being stationary (the frequency distribution is time-independent) and markovian (frequency increments are independent of the past). Experimental support that frequencies drift was reported in zebrafish luciferase recordings (ref. 14). The frequency dynamics can thus be abstracted by a stochastic process $f(t)$ with the following three parameters: the mean $\mu = 1/24$

hours sets the circadian periodicity, the rate γ of decay of perturbations (or equivalently, the correlation decay time of the frequency fluctuations) and the variance σ of these fluctuations.

The phase dynamics is then also a Gaussian process with mean μt and time-dependent covariance.

$$\sigma_\varphi^2(t) = E\Big[\big(\varphi(t) - \mu t\big)\big(\varphi(t) - \mu t\big)\Big]$$

$$= \frac{2\sigma^2}{\gamma^2}\big(\gamma t + e^{-\gamma t} - 1\big).$$

Such a simple phase model already contains all the main ingredients of a circadian clock: the limit-cycle with period 24 hours and stability rate γ, the frequency fluctuations with variance σ which are caused by the finite size stochasticity combined with other noise effects from outside the core clock. In a large volume, near equilibrium situation, all additional degrees of freedom which one may want to integrate into a clock model are assumed to be slaved to the above phase dynamics.

Statistical Properties of Ensembles of Uncoupled Oscillators

Taking N independent cells, each of them described by its phase-frequency dynamics, we model the population signal as the average cosine of their phases. Remark that if the actual limit-cycle is somewhat non-circular as in Figure 1, we should in principle replace the cosine by another periodic function, which would in many cases only have a weak effect on the

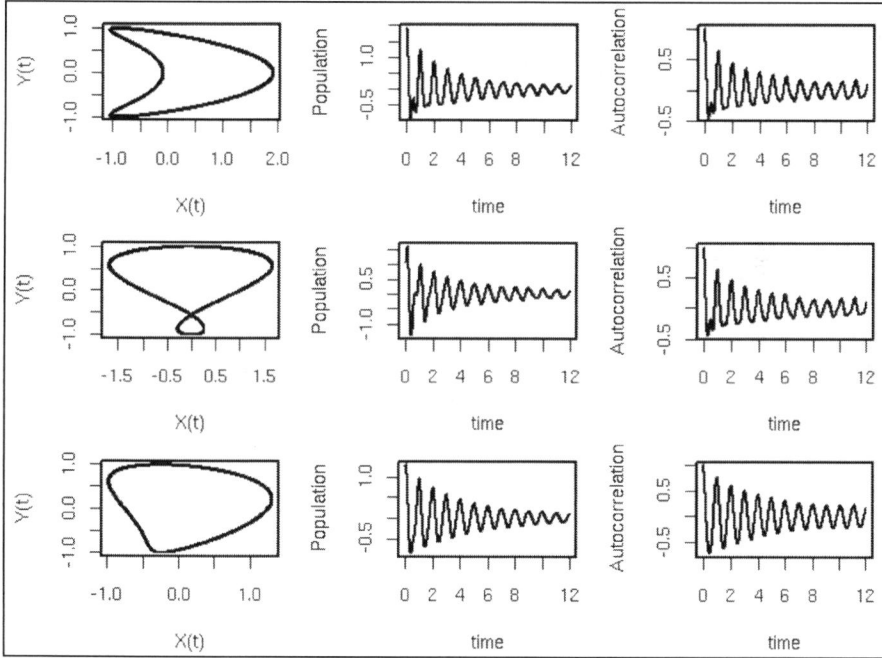

Figure 1. Non-circular limit-cycle with their population averages and autocorrelations. Curves were generated with $Y(t) = \sin(2pj(t))$ and $X(t) = \cos(2pj(t)) + b(2\,pi\,phi(t))$ where $b(x) = \cos(2x)/1.1$ (top), $b(x) = \sin(2x)/1.1$ (middle) or $b(x) = (\sin(2x) + \cos(2x))/4$ (bottom) and $j(t) = t + $(white noise). The population averages consists of 1000 independent replicates and the autocorrelations are averages of 3 independent replicates, both were applied to the $X(t)$ coordinate.

shape of the population average as the higher harmonics have a much larger decay rate in the population average:

$$Z(t) = \lim_{N \to \infty} \frac{1}{N} \sum_{i=1}^{N}$$

$$\left(\cos\left(2\pi\varphi_i(t)\right) + \sum_{k=2}^{\infty} a_k \cos\left(2\pi k\varphi_i(t)\right) + b_k \sin\left(2\pi k\varphi_i(t)\right) \right)$$

$$= \cos\left(2\pi\mu\tau\right) e^{-\frac{1}{2}\left(2\pi\sigma_\varphi(t)\right)^2}$$

$$+ \sum_{k=2}^{\infty} \left(a_k \cos\left(2\pi k\mu t\right) + b_k \sin\left(2\pi k\mu t\right) \right) e^{-\frac{k^2}{2}\left(2\pi\sigma_\varphi(t)\right)^2}$$

Considering only the first term of this series, we observe two limiting regimes: at short times the population's behavior resembles a pure static frequency dispersion (quadratic time dependence in the exponent) while in the long time limit we approach a phase diffusion (linear time dependence):

$$e^{-\frac{1}{2}\left(2\pi\sigma_\varphi(t)\right)^2} \approx \begin{cases} e^{-\left(2\pi\sigma\right)^2 t^2 / 2} & \text{for } t \to 0, \\ e^{-\left(2\pi\sigma/\gamma\right)^2 (\gamma t - 1)} & \text{for } t \to \infty. \end{cases}$$

The dephasing dynamics connecting these two asymptotic formulae provides a way to estimate the relevant parameters from experimental data.

Interacting Oscillators

We next introduce coupling inside the cell population, via an interaction term in the phase equations which is a simple sine function of the phase difference between coupled cells. This introduces a new parameter K to measure coupling strength (model 1).

$$\begin{cases} \dfrac{\partial \varphi_i(t)}{\partial t} = f_i(t) + \dfrac{K}{|N_i|} \sum_{j \in N_i} \sin\left(2\pi\left(\varphi_j(t) - \varphi_i(t)\right)\right), \\ \dfrac{\partial f_i(t)}{\partial t} = -\gamma\left(f_i(t) - u\right) + \sqrt{2\gamma}\,\sigma\eta_i(t). \end{cases}$$

Cell number i is coupled uniformly to either the N_i cells closest to it in a random tiling arrangement or to every other cell in the population ($N_i = N$). While the model cannot be explicitly solved anymore, we could however show[23] the existence of transition from a desynchronized state at low K to a synchronized population for K above a certain threshold K_c in the mean-field coupling.

The property of synchronization for stochastic phase evolutions is defined as the clustering of the phases and quantified by the norm of the average phase vector:

$$R(t) = \left| \frac{1}{N} \sum_{j=1}^{N} e^{2i\pi\varphi_j(t)} \right|$$

The time average of $R(t)$ will be asymptotically vanishing (tend to zero for large N) in the unsynchronized region and positive in the synchronized state. For local ($N_i < N$) coupling, numerical simulations show that a coupling extending to a few cell shells already results in a synchronization behavior close to the mean-field situation.

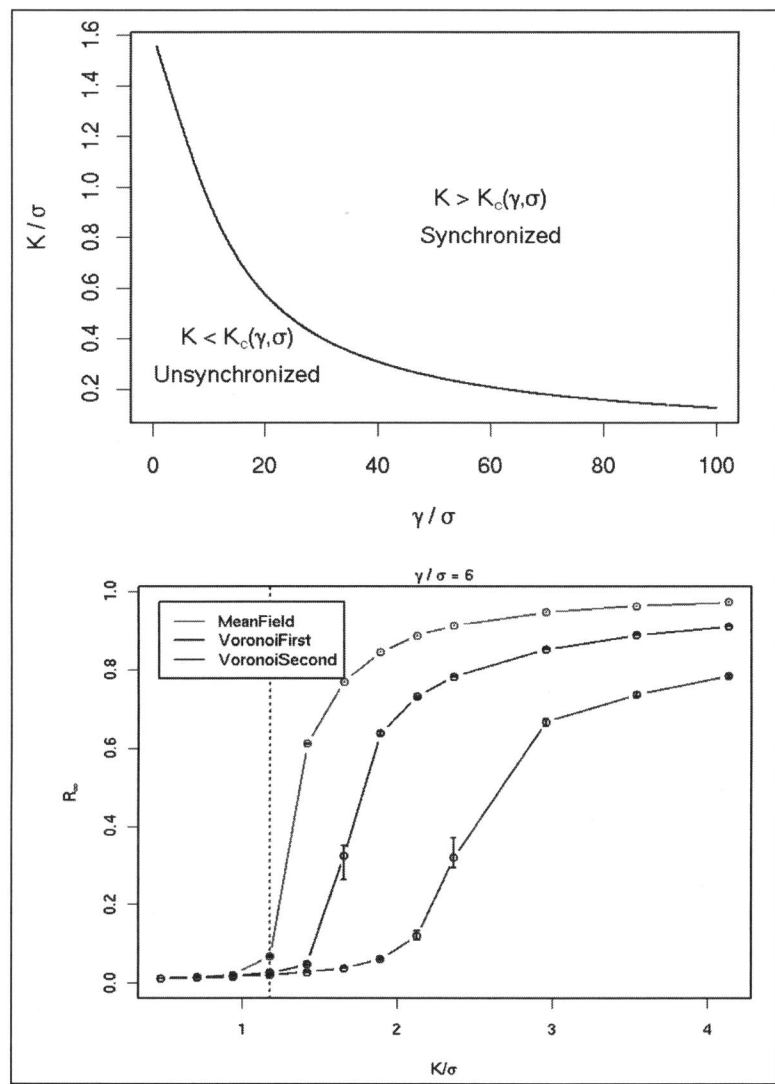

Figure 2. Synchronyzation thresholds in the coupled phase model. Top) the critical coupling above which the population starts to synchronize in the mean field model is shown in function of the damping rate γ. Bottom) Simulation using 10000 cells placed randomly on a plane. Neighbors are determined using a Voronoi tesselation. Error bars represent different variability from different samples of cells. Figures are adapted from reference 22 (top) and reference 25 (bottom).

Theory vs. Data

Bioluminescence Recordings

Bioluminescence reporters based on luciferase fusion genes were recently developed to address whether SCN oscillations were qualitatively different from those in peripheral tissues, even though the underlying molecular clocks seem to utilize the same genetic components. Recordings in immortalized[12] and primary[13] mouse fibroblasts showed that single cells generate cell-autonomous rhythms which could be resynchronized by a serum shock. Some of these conclusion could be reached by a mathematical analysis of long (19 days) bioluminescence recordings. These showed such good signal to noise ratios that it was possible to infer that dephasing rather than amplitude death was the dominant cause for amplitude reduction based on the decay properties of the oscillatory signal obtained from the whole population.

Envelope Analysis Using Phase Models

A 19 days bioluminescence recording from NIH3T3 fibroblasts stably transfected with a luceriferase reporter inserted in the Bmal1 locus (cf. Fig. 3B in ref. 12) was analysed using the phase model. This data are reproduced here in Figure 3A. The detrended signal $Z(t)$ was fit to the form predicted for the population average (Fig. 3B). All parameters could be estimated reliably and the error bars indicated in Figure 3C show that the model does not overfit the data. The frequency dispersion was found to be 0.1 days^{-1} which is close to values measured in single cells.[12] Furthermore, the estimated $\gamma=0.64 \pm 0.17$, reflecting a frequency damping time of 1.56 days implies that frequency disturbances take longer than a period length to decay. The model could also estimate inter-cell coupling which indicated that coupling in cell culture may be positive. However the values estimated were clearly below the synchronization threshold (Fig. 3C). This analysis is detailed in reference 25.

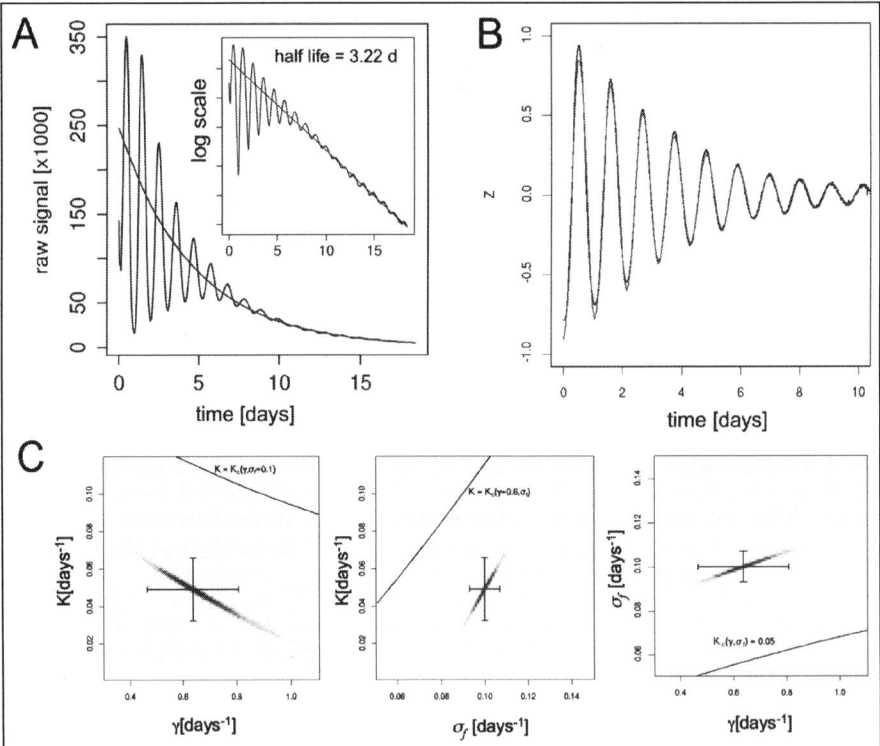

Figure 3. Analysis of population bioluminescence data. A) Raw bioluminescence counts for a recording of three week. The inset emphasizes exponential trend with half life of 3.2 days (shown in blue). B) detrended signal (black) ad the model best fit (red.) C) Parameter estimates, color coding shows the posterior probabilities and the black line indicates the lines of critical coupling. Reproduced from: Rougemont J, Naef F. Mol Syst Biol 2007; 3:93;[25] with permission from Nature Publishing Group. A color version of this figure is available at www.eurekah.com.

Co-Culture Experiment

In Nagoshi et al[12] a co-culture experiment was performed to study the question of inter-cellular coupling directly. Short-period (20 hours) mutant feeder cells were co-cultured with wild-type reporter cells, with a 20-fold relative excess of nonluminescent feeders. Bioluminescence recordings showed no significance phase shifts over approximately 3 days. To emphasize that intercellular coupling in itself does not imply population synchronization, we plotted the expected phase shift over time for several values of the coupling constant K. This is computed as follows:

$$\delta\varphi(t) = \varphi_{reporter}(t) - \frac{t}{24}$$

$$= K\int_0^t \sin\left(2\pi\left(\varphi_{feeder}(s) - \varphi_{reporter}(s)\right)\right)ds$$

$$= K\int_0^t \sin\left(s(1/20 - 1/24) - \delta\varphi(s)\right)ds$$

In the subcritical region, the coupling induces only a slow dephasing which can remain unmeasurable for several days. In particcular, a value of $K = 0.05$ as estimated from population recordings would only shift phases forward by 2.4 hours after 3 days. Remark that even a critical coupling of $K = 0.1183$ would still require of the order of 10 days to reverse the phase relative to a free-running wild-type cell.

It was noted in that tissue explants and dissociated cell cultures show similar decay rates of population bioluminescence signals, suggesting that coupling is of comparable intensity in the two situations. The presence of a positive, sub-critical coupling may play a role in peripheral organs, as this would facilitate resynchronization by systemic cues.

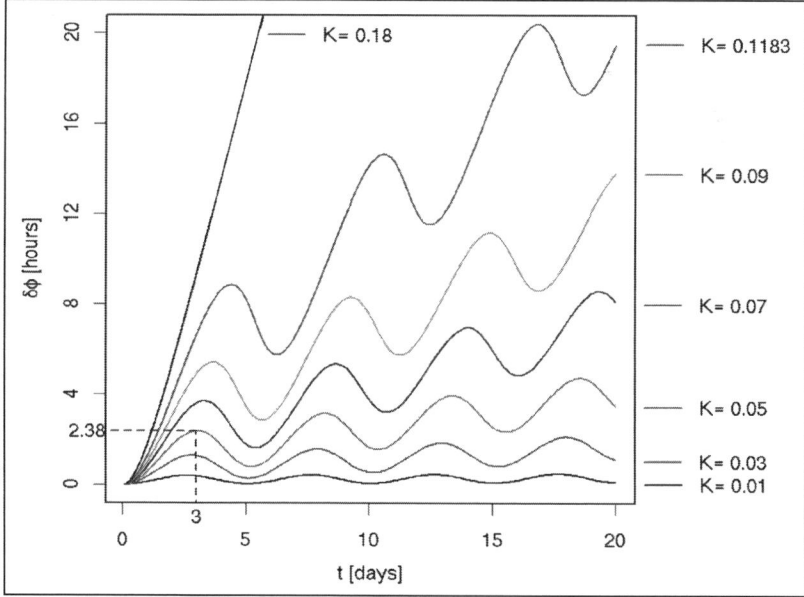

Figure 4. Simulation of the dephasing dynamics in a co-culture experiment. The value of δφ was computed numerically over 20 days for several values of K. The critical value of K for synchronisation is K=0.1183. Our estimation from population bioluminescence recordings was K=0.05, which leads to a phase-shift of 2.38 hours 3 days after the serum shock.

Conclusion

This chapter discussed how noisy phase models can be useful for circadian biology. Their main attractiveness is that they contain few parameters and can thus be relevant for analyzing effectively low dimensional signals, which is not uncommon in biology. Thus, their parameters can be determined accurately, but the downside is that the link between microscopic properties of biochemical networks such as rate constants and the more phenomenological parameters in the phase models is not immediately clear. In some case one can nevertheless use methods from dynamical systems to connect microscopic parameters with more macroscopic ones, such as the period dispersion or the decay rate of frequency fluctuations. For example, the computation of Floquet multipliers in ODE models for the mammalian circadian clock were used to identify which microscopic parameters most affect limit-cycle stability, which can be related to the rates of frequency fluctuations. Such approaches can have predictive values, e.g., it was found in the latter study that the parameters that are most potent to protect the mammalian circadian oscillator against noise are the transcription and phosphorylation rates of the Period mRNA and protein.[25] Most importantly, several interesting models systems exhibit molecular oscillation, e.g., the respiratory cycle in yeast or the segmentation clock in vertebrates, for which powerful molecular reporter techniques are being developed as in the circadian system. It is thus relevant to have a theoretical framework that allows not only to extract the most pertinent information from data, but also to bridge between the often unknown or too complex microscopic description, and a phenomenological lower dimensional description in terms of few highly informative parameters. Phase models definitely qualify for this purpose.

References

1. Konopka RJ, Benzer S. Clock mutants of Drosophila melanogaster. Proc Natl Acad Sci USA 1971; 68:2112-2116.
2. Young MW, Kay SA. Time zones: A comparative genetics of circadian clocks. Nat Rev Genet 2001; 2:702-715.
3. Locke JC, Kozma-Bognar L, Gould PD et al. Experimental validation of a predicted feedback loop in the multi-oscillator clock of Arabidopsis thaliana. Mol Syst Biol 2006; 2:59.
4. Zeilinger MN, Farre EM, Taylor SR et al. A novel computational model of the circadian clock in Arabidopsis that incorporates PRR7 and PRR9. Mol Syst Biol 2006; 2:58.
5. Wagner A. Circuit topology and the evolution of robustness in two-gene circadian oscillators. Proc Natl Acad Sci USA 2005; 102:11775 11780.
6. Nakajima M, Imai K, Ito H et al. Reconstitution of circadian oscillation of cyanobacterial KaiC phosphorylation in vitro. Science 2005; 308:414-415.
7. Tomita J, Nakajima M, Kondo T et al. No transcription-translation feedback in circadian rhythm of KaiC phosphorylation. Science 2005; 307:251-254.
8. Naef F. Circadian clocks go in vitro: Purely post-translational oscillators in cyanobacteria. Mol Syst Biol 2005; 1:2005-0019.
9. Merrow M, Mazzotta G, Chen Z et al. The right place at the right time: Regulation of daily timing by phosphorylation. Genes Dev 2006; 20:2629-2623.
10. Yoo SH, Yamazaki S, Lowrey PL et al. Period 2:Luciferase real-time reporting of circadian dynamics reveals persistent circadian oscillations in mouse peripheral tissues. Proc Natl Acad Sci USA 2004; 101:5339-5346.
11. Damiola F, Le Minh N, Preitner N et al. Restricted feeding uncouples circadian oscillators in peripheral tissues from the central pacemaker in the suprachiasmatic nucleus. Genes Dev 2000; 14:2950-2961.
12. Nagoshi E, Saini C, Bauer C et al. Circadian gene expression in individual fibroblasts: Cell-autonomous and self-sustained oscillators pass time to daughter cells. Cell 2004; 119:693-705.
13. Welsh DK, Yoo SH, Liu AC et al. Bioluminescence imaging of individual fibroblasts reveals persistent, independently phased circadian rhythms of clock gene expression. Curr Biol 2004; 14:2289-2295.
14. Carr AJ, Whitmore D. Imaging of single light-responsive clock cells reveals fluctuating free-running periods. Nat Cell Biol 2005; 7:319-321.
15. Winfree AT. Biological rhythms and the behavior of populations of coupled oscillators. J Theor Biol 1967; 16:15-42.

16. Goldbeter A. A model for circadian oscillations in the Drosophila period protein (PER). Proc Biol Sci 1995; 261:319-324.
17. Barkai N, Leibler S. Circadian clocks limited by noise. Nature 2000; 403:267-268.
18. Gonze D, Goldbeter A. Circadian rhythms and molecular noise. Chaos 2006; 16:026110.
19. Vilar JM, Kueh HY, Barkai N et al. Mechanisms of noise-resistance in genetic oscillators. Proc Natl Acad Sci USA 2002; 99:5988-5992.
20. Forger DB, Peskin CS. A detailed predictive model of the mammalian circadian clock. Proc Natl Acad Sci USA 2003; 100:14806-14811.
21. Leloup JC, Goldbeter A. Toward a detailed computational model for the mammalian circadian clock. Proc Natl Acad Sci USA 2003; 100:7051-7056.
22. Kuramoto Y. Chemical Oscillations, Waves, and Turbulence. Berlin: Springer, 1984.
23. Rougemont J, Naef F. Collective synchronization in populations of globally coupled phase oscillators with drifting frequencies. Phys Rev E Stat Nonlin Soft Matter Phys 2006; 73:011104.
24. Strogatz S. Nonlinear Dynamics and Chaos, with Applications to Physics, Biology, Chemistry and Engineering. Cambridge: Perseus Books, 2000.
25. Rougemont J, Naef F. Dynamical signatures of cellular fluctuations and oscillator stability in peripheral circadian clocks. Mol Syst Biol 2007; 3:93.

Index

U

V

Z